Biosignal and Biomedical Image Processing

Signal Processing and Communications

Additional Volumes in Preparation

To Lawrence Stark, M.D., who has shown me the many possibilities . . .

Series Introduction

Over the past 50 years, digital signal processing has evolved as a major engineering discipline. The fields of signal processing have grown from the origin of fast Fourier transform and digital filter design to statistical spectral analysis and array processing, image, audio, and multimedia processing, and shaped developments in high-performance VLSI signal processor design. Indeed, there are few fields that enjoy so many applications—signal processing is everywhere in our lives.

When one uses a cellular phone, the voice is compressed, coded, and modulated using signal processing techniques. As a cruise missile winds along hillsides searching for the target, the signal processor is busy processing the images taken along the way. When we are watching a movie in HDTV, millions of audio and video data are being sent to our homes and received with unbelievable fidelity. When scientists compare DNA samples, fast pattern recognition techniques are being used. On and on, one can see the impact of signal processing in almost every engineering and scientific discipline.

Because of the immense importance of signal processing and the fast-growing demands of business and industry, this series on signal processing serves to report up-to-date developments and advances in the field. The topics of interest include but are not limited to the following:

- Signal theory and analysis
- Statistical signal processing
- Speech and audio processing

- Image and video processing
- Multimedia signal processing and technology
- Signal processing for communications
- Signal processing architectures and VLSI design

We hope this series will provide the interested audience with high-quality, state-of-the-art signal processing literature through research monographs, edited books, and rigorously written textbooks by experts in their fields.

Preface

Signal processing can be broadly defined as the application of analog or digital techniques to improve the utility of a data stream. In biomedical engineering applications, improved utility usually means the data provide better diagnostic information. Analog techniques are applied to a data stream embodied as a time-varying electrical signal while in the digital domain the data are represented as an array of numbers. This array could be the digital representation of a time-varying signal, or an image. This text deals exclusively with signal processing of digital data, although Chapter 1 briefly describes analog processes commonly found in medical devices.

This text should be of interest to a broad spectrum of engineers, but it is written specifically for biomedical engineers (also known as bioengineers). Although the applications are different, the signal processing methodology used by biomedical engineers is identical to that used by other engineers such electrical and communications engineers. The major difference for biomedical engineers is in the level of understanding required for appropriate use of this technology. An electrical engineer may be required to expand or modify signal processing tools, while for biomedical engineers, signal processing techniques are tools to be used. For the biomedical engineer, a detailed understanding of the underlying theory, while always of value, may not be essential. Moreover, considering the broad range of knowledge required to be effective in this field, encompassing both medical and engineering domains, an in-depth understanding of all of the useful technology is not realistic. It is important is to know what tools are available, have a good understanding of what they do (if not how they do it), be aware of the most likely pitfalls and misapplications, and know how to implement these tools given available software packages. The basic concept of this text is that, just as the cardiologist can benefit from an oscilloscope-type display of the ECG without a deep understanding of electronics, so a biomedical engineer can benefit from advanced signal processing tools without always understanding the details of the underlying mathematics.

As a reflection of this philosophy, most of the concepts covered in this text are presented in two sections. The first part provides a broad, general understanding of the approach sufficient to allow intelligent application of the concepts. The second part describes how these tools can be implemented and relies primarily on the MATLAB® software package and several of its toolboxes.

This text is written for a single-semester course combining signal and image processing. Classroom experience using notes from this text indicates that this ambitious objective is possible for most graduate formats, although eliminating a few topics may be desirable. For example, some of the introductory or basic material covered in Chapters 1 and 2 could be skipped or treated lightly for students with the appropriate prerequisites. In addition, topics such as advanced spectral methods (Chapter 5), time-frequency analysis (Chapter 6), wavelets (Chapter 7), advanced filters (Chapter 8), and multivariate analysis (Chapter 9) are pedagogically independent and can be covered as desired without affecting the other material.

Although much of the material covered here will be new to most students, the book is not intended as an "introductory" text since the goal is to provide a working knowledge of the topics presented without the need for additional course work. The challenge of covering a broad range of topics at a useful, working depth is motivated by current trends in biomedical engineering education, particularly at the graduate level where a comprehensive education must be attained with a minimum number of courses. This has led to the development of "core" courses to be taken by all students. This text was written for just such a core course in the Graduate Program of Biomedical Engineering at Rutgers University. It is also quite suitable for an upper-level undergraduate course and would be of value for students in other disciplines who would benefit from a working knowledge of signal and image processing.

It would not be possible to cover such a broad spectrum of material to a depth that enables productive application without heavy reliance on MATLAB-based examples and problems. In this regard, the text assumes the student has some knowledge of MATLAB programming and has available the basic MATLAB software package including the Signal Processing and Image Processing Toolboxes. (MATLAB also produces a Wavelet Toolbox, but the section on wavelets is written so as not to require this toolbox, primarily to keep the number of required toolboxes to a minimum.) The problems are an essential part of this text and often provide a discovery-like experience regarding the associated topic. A few peripheral topics are introduced only though the problems. The code used for all examples is provided in the CD accompanying this text. Since many of the problems are extensions or modifications of examples given in the chapter, some of the coding time can be reduced by starting with the code of a related example. The CD also includes support routines and data files used in the examples and problems. Finally, the CD contains the code used to generate many of the figures. For instructors, there is a CD available that contains the problem solutions and Powerpoint® presentations from each of the chapters. These presentations include figures, equations, and text slides related to chapter. Presentations can be modified by the instructor as desired.

In addition to heavy reliance on MATLAB problems and examples, this text makes extensive use of simulated data. Except for the section on image processing, examples involving biological signals are rarely used. In my view, examples using biological signals provide motivation, but they are not generally very instructive. Given the wide range of material to be presented at a working depth, emphasis is placed on learning the tools of signal processing; motivation is left to the reader (or the instructor).

Organization of the text is straightforward. Chapters 1 through 4 are fairly basic. Chapter 1 covers topics related to analog signal processing and data acquisition while Chapter 2 includes topics that are basic to all aspects of signal and image processing. Chapters 3 and 4 cover classical spectral analysis and basic digital filtering, topics fundamental to any signal processing course. Advanced spectral methods, covered in Chapter 5, are important due to their widespread use in biomedical engineering. Chapter 6 and the first part of Chapter 7 cover topics related to spectral analysis when the signal's spectrum is varying in time, a condition often found in biological signals. Chapter 7 also covers both continuous and discrete wavelets, another popular technique used in the analysis of biomedical signals. Chapters 8 and 9 feature advanced topics. In Chapter 8, optimal and adaptive filters are covered, the latter's inclusion is also motivated by the time-varying nature of many biological signals. Chapter 9 introduces multivariate techniques, specifically principal component analysis and independent component analysis, two analysis approaches that are experiencing rapid growth with regard to biomedical applications. The last four chapters cover image processing, with the first of these, Chapter 10, covering the conventions used by MATLAB's Imaging Processing Toolbox. Image processing is a vast area and the material covered here is limited primarily to areas associated with medical imaging: image acquisition (Chapter 13); image filtering, enhancement, and transformation (Chapter 11); and segmentation, and registration (Chapter 12).

Many of the chapters cover topics that can be adequately covered only in a book dedicated solely to these topics. In this sense, every chapter represents a serious compromise with respect to comprehensive coverage of the associated topics. My only excuse for any omissions is that classroom experience with this approach seems to work: students end up with a working knowledge of a vast array of signal and image processing tools. A few of the classic or major books on these topics are cited in an Annotated bibliography at the end of the book. No effort has been made to construct an extensive bibliography or reference list since more current lists would be readily available on the Web.

TEXTBOOK PROTOCOLS

In most early examples that feature MATLAB code, the code is presented in full, while in the later examples some of the routine code (such as for plotting, display, and labeling operation) is omitted. Nevertheless, I recommend that students carefully label (and scale when appropriate) all graphs done in the problems. Some effort has been made to use consistent notation as described in Table 1. In general, lower-case letters n and k are used as data subscripts, and capital letters, N and K are used to indicate the length (or maximum subscript value) of a data set. In two-dimensional data sets, lower-case letters m and n are used to indicate the row and column subscripts of an array, while capital letters M and N are used to indicate vertical and horizontal dimensions, respectively. The letter m is also used as the index of a variable produced by a transformation, or as an index indicating a particular member of a family of related functions.* While it is common to use brackets to enclose subscripts of discrete variables (i.e., x[n]), ordinary parentheses are used here. Brackets are reserved to indicate vectors (i.e., $[x_1, x_2, x_3, \ldots]$) following MATLAB convention. Other notation follows standard conventions.

Italics (") are used to introduce important new terms that should be incorporated into the reader's vocabulary. If the meaning of these terms is not obvious from their use, they are explained where they are introduced. All MATLAB commands, routines, variables, and code are shown in the `Courier typeface`. Single quotes are used to highlight MATLAB filenames or string variables. Textbook protocols are summarized in Table 1.

I wish to thank Susanne Oldham who managed to edit this book, and provided strong, continuing encouragement and support. I would also like to acknowledge the patience and support of Peggy Christ and Lynn Hutchings. Professor Shankar Muthu Krishnan of Singapore provided a very thoughtful critique of the manuscript which led to significant improvements. Finally, I thank my students who provided suggestions and whose enthusiasm for the material provided much needed motivation.

---

*For example, m would be used to indicate the harmonic number of a family of harmonically related sine functions; i.e., $f_m(t) = \sin(2\pi m t)$.

TABLE 1 Textbook Conventions

Symbol	Description/General usage
$x(t)$, $y(t)$	General functions of time, usually a waveform or signal
k, n	Data indices, particularly for digitized time data
K, N	Maximum index or size of a data set
$x(n)$, $y(n)$	Waveform variable, usually digitized time variables (i.e., a discreet variable)
m	Index of variable produced by transformation, or the index of specifying the member number of a family of functions (i.e., $f_m(t)$)
$X(f)$, $Y(f)$	Frequency representation (complex) of a time function
$X(m)$, $Y(m)$	Frequency representation (complex) of a discreet variable
$h(t)$	Impulse response of a linear system
$h(n)$	Discrete impulse response of a linear system
$b(n)$	Digital filter coefficients representing the numerator of the discreet Transfer Function; hence the same as the impulse response
$a(n)$	Digital filter coefficients representing the denominator of the discreet Transfer Function
`Courier font`	MATLAB command, variable, routine, or program.
`Courier font`	MATLAB filename or string variable

John L. Semmlow

Contents

1

Introduction

TYPICAL MEASUREMENT SYSTEMS

A schematic representation of a typical biomedical measurement system is shown in Figure 1.1. Here we use the term measurement in the most general sense to include image acquisition or the acquisition of other forms of diagnostic information. The physiological process of interest is converted into an electric

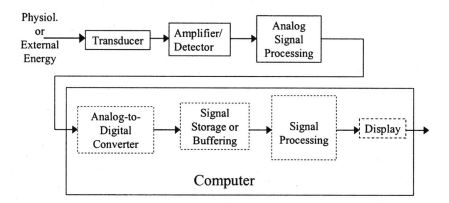

FIGURE 1.1 Schematic representation of typical bioengineering measurement system.

signal via the transducer (Figure 1.1). Some analog signal processing is usually required, often including amplification and lowpass (or bandpass) filtering. Since most signal processing is easier to implement using digital methods, the analog signal is converted to digital format using an analog-to-digital converter. Once converted, the signal is often stored, or *buffered*, in memory to facilitate subsequent signal processing. Alternatively, in some *real-time** applications, the incoming data must be processed as quickly as possible with minimal buffering, and may not need to be permanently stored. Digital signal processing algorithms can then be applied to the digitized signal. These signal processing techniques can take a wide variety of forms and various levels of sophistication, and they make up the major topic area of this book. Some sort of output is necessary in any useful system. This usually takes the form of a display, as in imaging systems, but may be some type of an effector mechanism such as in an automated drug delivery system.

With the exception of this chapter, this book is limited to digital signal and image processing concerns. To the extent possible, each topic is introduced with the minimum amount of information required to use and understand the approach, and enough information to apply the methodology in an intelligent manner. Understanding of strengths and weaknesses of the various methods is also covered, particularly through discovery in the problems at the end of the chapter. Hence, the problems at the end of each chapter, most of which utilize the MATLAB™ software package (Waltham, MA), constitute an integral part of the book: a few topics are introduced only in the problems.

A fundamental assumption of this text is that an in-depth mathematical treatment of signal processing methodology is not essential for effective and appropriate application of these tools. Thus, this text is designed to develop skills in the application of signal and image processing technology, but may not provide the skills necessary to develop new techniques and algorithms. References are provided for those who need to move beyond application of signal and image processing tools to the design and development of new methodology. In subsequent chapters, each major section is followed by a section on implementation using the MATLAB software package. Fluency with the MATLAB language is assumed and is essential for the use of this text. Where appropriate, a topic area may also include a more in-depth treatment including some of the underlying mathematics.

---

*Learning the vocabulary is an important part of mastering a discipline. In this text we highlight, using italics, terms commonly used in signal and image processing. Sometimes the highlighted term is described when it is introduced, but occasionally determination of its definition is left to responsibility of the reader. Real-time processing and buffering are described in the section on analog-to-digital conversion.

TRANSDUCERS

A *transducer* is a device that converts energy from one form to another. By this definition, a light bulb or a motor is a transducer. In signal processing applications, the purpose of energy conversion is to transfer information, not to transform energy as with a light bulb or a motor. In measurement systems, all transducers are so-called input transducers, they convert non-electrical energy into an electronic signal. An exception to this is the electrode, a transducer that converts electrical energy from ionic to electronic form. Usually, the output of a biomedical transducer is a voltage (or current) whose amplitude is proportional to the measured energy.

The energy that is converted by the input transducer may be generated by the physiological process itself, indirectly related to the physiological process, or produced by an external source. In the last case, the externally generated energy interacts with, and is modified by, the physiological process, and it is this alteration that produces the measurement. For example, when externally produced x-rays are transmitted through the body, they are absorbed by the intervening tissue, and a measurement of this absorption is used to construct an image. Many diagnostically useful imaging systems are based on this external energy approach.

In addition to passing external energy through the body, some images are generated using the energy of radioactive emissions of radioisotopes injected into the body. These techniques make use of the fact that selected, or *tagged*, molecules will collect in specific tissue. The areas where these radioisotopes collect can be mapped using a gamma camera, or with certain short-lived isotopes, better localized using positron emission tomography (PET).

Many physiological processes produce energy that can be detected directly. For example, cardiac internal pressures are usually measured using a pressure transducer placed on the tip of catheter introduced into the appropriate chamber of the heart. The measurement of electrical activity in the heart, muscles, or brain provides other examples of the direct measurement of physiological energy. For these measurements, the energy is already electrical and only needs to be converted from ionic to electronic current using an *electrode*. These sources are usually given the term ExG, where the 'x' represents the physiological process that produces the electrical energy: ECG–electrocardiogram, EEG–electroencephalogram; EMG–electromyogram; EOG–electrooculargram, ERG–electroretiniogram; and EGG–electrogastrogram. An exception to this terminology is the electrical activity generated by this skin which is termed the galvanic skin response, GSR. Typical physiological energies and the applications that use these energy forms are shown in Table 1.1

The *biotransducer* is often the most critical element in the system since it constitutes the interface between the subject or life process and the rest of the

TABLE 1.1   Energy Forms and Related Direct Measurements

Energy	Measurement
Mechanical	
length, position, and velocity	muscle movement, cardiovascular pressures, muscle contractility
force and pressure	valve and other cardiac sounds
Heat	body temperature, thermography
Electrical	EEG, ECG, EMG, EOG, ERG, EGG, GSR
Chemical	ion concentrations

system. The transducer establishes the risk, or *noninvasiveness*, of the overall system. For example, an imaging system based on differential absorption of x-rays, such as a CT (computed tomography) scanner is considered more *invasive* than an imagining system based on ultrasonic reflection since CT uses ionizing radiation that may have an associated risk. (The actual risk of ionizing radiation is still an open question and imaging systems based on x-ray absorption are considered *minimally invasive*.) Both ultrasound and x-ray imaging would be considered less invasive than, for example, monitoring internal cardiac pressures through cardiac catherization in which a small catheter is treaded into the heart chambers. Indeed many of the outstanding problems in biomedical measurement, such as noninvasive measurement of internal cardiac pressures, or the noninvasive measurement of intracranial pressure, await an appropriate (and undoubtedly clever) transducer mechanism.

Further Study: The Transducer

The transducer often establishes the major performance criterion of the system. In a later section, we list and define a number of criteria that apply to measurement systems; however, in practice, measurement resolution, and to a lesser extent bandwidth, are generally the two most important and troublesome measurement criteria. In fact, it is usually possible to trade-off between these two criteria. Both of these criteria are usually established by the transducer. Hence, although it is not the topic of this text, good system design usually calls for care in the choice or design of the transducer element(s). An efficient, low-noise transducer design can often reduce the need for extensive subsequent signal processing and still produce a better measurement.

Input transducers use one of two different fundamental approaches: the input energy causes the transducer element to generate a voltage or current, or the input energy creates a change in the electrical properties (i.e., the resistance, inductance, or capacitance) of the transducer element. Most optical transducers use the first approach. Photons strike a photo sensitive material producing free electrons (or holes) that can then be detected as an external current flow. Piezo-electric devices used in ultrasound also generate a charge when under mechanical stress. Many examples can be found of the use of the second category, a change in some electrical property. For example, metals (and semiconductors) undergo a consistent change in resistance with changes in temperature, and most temperature transducers utilize this feature. Other examples include the strain gage, which measures mechanical deformation using the small change in resistance that occurs when the sensing material is stretched.

Many critical problems in medical diagnosis await the development of new approaches and new transducers. For example, coronary artery disease is a major cause of death in developed countries, and its treatment would greatly benefit from early detection. To facilitate early detection, a biomedical instrumentation system is required that is inexpensive and easy to operate so that it could be used for general screening. In coronary artery disease, blood flow to the arteries of the heart (i.e., coronaries) is reduced due to partial or complete blockage (i.e., stenoses). One conceptually simple and inexpensive approach is to detect the sounds generated by turbulent blood flow through partially included coronary arteries (called *bruits* when detected in other arteries such as the carotids). This approach requires a highly sensitive transducer(s), in this case a cardiac microphone, as well as advanced signal processing methods. Results of efforts based on this approach are ongoing, and the problem of noninvasive detection of coronary artery disease is not yet fully solved.

Other holy grails of diagnostic cardiology include noninvasive measurement of cardiac output (i.e., volume of blood flow pumped by the heart per unit time) and noninvasive measurement of internal cardiac pressures. The former has been approached using Doppler ultrasound, but this technique has not yet been accepted as reliable. Financial gain and modest fame awaits the biomedical engineer who develops instrumentation that adequately addresses any of these three outstanding measurement problems.

ANALOG SIGNAL PROCESSING

While the most extensive signal processing is usually performed on digitized data using algorithms implemented in software, some analog signal processing is usually necessary. The first analog stage depends on the basic transducer operation. If the transducer is based on a variation in electrical property, the first stage must convert that variation in electrical property into a variation in voltage. If the transducer element is single ended, i.e., only one element changes, then a constant current source can be used and the detector equation follows ohm's law:

$$V_{out} = I(Z + \Delta Z) \qquad \text{where } \Delta Z = f(\text{input energy}). \qquad (1)$$

Figure 1.2 shows an example of a single transducer element used in operational amplifier circuit that provides constant current operation. The transducer element in this case is a thermistor, an element that changes its resistance with temperature. Using circuit analysis, it is easy to show that the thermistor is driven by a constant current of V_S/R amps. The output, V_{out}, is $[(R_T + \Delta R_T)/R]V_S$. Alternatively, an approximate constant current source can be generated using a voltage source and a large series resistor, R_S, where $R_S \gg \Delta R$.

If the transducer can be configured differentially so that one element increases with increasing input energy while the other element decreases, the bridge circuit is commonly used as a detector. Figure 1.3 shows a device made to measure intestinal motility using strain gages. A bridge circuit detector is used in conjunction with a pair of differentially configured strain gages: when the intestine contracts, the end of the cantilever beam moves downward and the upper strain gage (visible) is stretched and increases in resistance while the lower strain gage (not visible) compresses and decreases in resistance. The output of the bridge circuit can be found from simple circuit analysis to be: $V_{out} = V_S\Delta R/2$, where V_S is the value of the source voltage. If the transducer operates based on a change in inductance or capacitance, the above techniques are still useful except a sinusoidal voltage source must be used.

If the transducer element is a voltage generator, the first stage is usually an amplifier. If the transducer produces a current output, as is the case in many electromagnetic detectors, then a current-to-voltage amplifier (also termed a transconductance amplifier) is used to produce a voltage output.

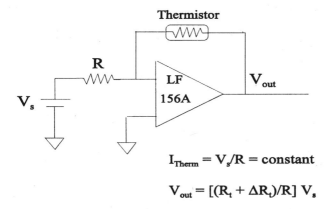

FIGURE 1.2 A thermistor (a semiconductor that changes resistance as a function of temperature) used in a constant current configuration.

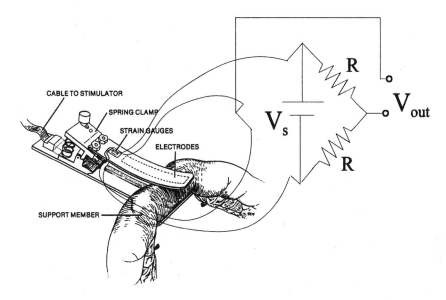

FIGURE 1.3 A strain gage probe used to measure motility of the intestine. The bridge circuit is used to convert differential change in resistance from a pair of strain gages into a change in voltage.

Figure 1.4 shows a photodiode transducer used with a *transconductance* amplifier. The output voltage is proportional to the current through the photodiode: $V_{out} = R_f I_{diode}$. Bandwidth can be increased at the expense of added noise by reverse biasing the photodiode with a small voltage.* More sophisticated detection systems such as phase sensitive detectors (PSD) can be employed in some cases to improve noise rejection. A software implementation of PSD is described in Chapter 8. In a few circumstances, additional amplification beyond the first stage may be required.

SOURCES OF VARIABILITY: NOISE

In this text, *noise* is a very general and somewhat relative term: noise is what you do not want and signal is what you do want. Noise is inherent in most measurement systems and often the limiting factor in the performance of a medical instrument. Indeed, many signal processing techniques are motivated by the

---

*A bias voltage improves movement of charge through the diode decreasing the response time. From −10 to −50 volts are used, except in the case of avalanche photodiodes where a higher voltage is required.

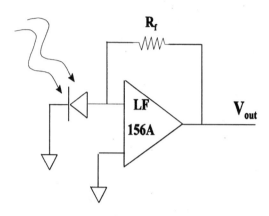

FIGURE 1.4 Photodiode used in a transconductance amplifier.

desire to minimize the variability in the measurement. In biomedical measurements, variability has four different origins: (1) physiological variability; (2) environmental noise or interference; (3) transducer artifact; and (4) electronic noise. Physiological variability is due to the fact that the information you desire is based on a measurement subject to biological influences other than those of interest. For example, assessment of respiratory function based on the measurement of blood pO_2 could be confounded by other physiological mechanisms that alter blood pO_2. Physiological variability can be a very difficult problem to solve, sometimes requiring a totally different approach.

Environmental noise can come from sources external or internal to the body. A classic example is the measurement of fetal ECG where the desired signal is corrupted by the mother's ECG. Since it is not possible to describe the specific characteristics of environmental noise, typical noise reduction techniques such as filtering are not usually successful. Sometimes environmental noise can be reduced using adaptive techniques such as those described in Chapter 8 since these techniques do not require prior knowledge of noise characteristics. Indeed, one of the approaches described in Chapter 8, *adaptive noise cancellation*, was initially developed to reduce the interference from the mother in the measurement of fetal ECG.

Transducer artifact is produced when the transducer responds to energy modalities other than that desired. For example, recordings of electrical potentials using electrodes placed on the skin are sensitive to *motion artifact*, where the electrodes respond to mechanical movement as well as the desired electrical signal. Transducer artifacts can sometimes be successfully addressed by modifications in transducer design. Aerospace research has led to the development of electrodes that are quite insensitive to motion artifact.

Unlike the other sources of variability, electronic noise has well-known sources and characteristics. Electronic noise falls into two broad classes: *thermal* or *Johnson noise*, and *shot noise*. The former is produced primarily in resistor or resistance materials while the latter is related to voltage barriers associated with semiconductors. Both sources produce noise with a broad range of frequencies often extending from DC to 10^{12}–10^{13} Hz. Such a broad spectrum noise is referred to as white noise since it contains energy at all frequencies (or at least all the frequencies of interest to biomedical engineers). Figure 1.5 shows a plot of power density versus frequency for white noise calculated from a noise waveform (actually an array of random numbers) using the spectra analysis methods described in Chapter 3. Note that its energy is fairly constant across the spectral range.

The various sources of noise or variability along with their causes and possible remedies are presented in Table 1.2 below. Note that in three out of four instances, appropriate transducer design was useful in the reduction of the

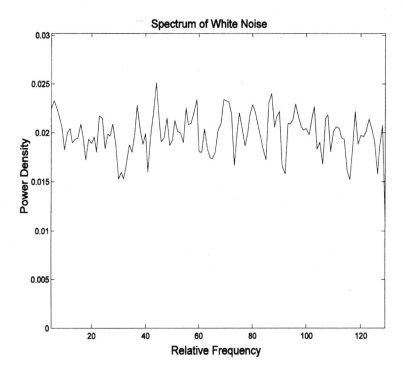

FIGURE 1.5 Power density (power spectrum) of digitizied white noise showing a fairly constant value over frequency.

TABLE 1.2   Sources of Variability

Source	Cause	Potential Remedy
Physiological variability	Measurement only indirectly related to variable of interest	Modify overall approach
Environmental (internal or external)	Other sources of similar energy form	Noise cancellation Transducer design
Artifact	Transducer responds to other energy sources	Transducer design
Electronic	Thermal or shot noise	Transducer or electronic design

variability or noise. This demonstrates the important role of the transducer in the overall performance of the instrumentation system.

Electronic Noise

Johnson or thermal noise is produced by resistance sources, and the amount of noise generated is related to the resistance and to the temperature:

$$V_J = \sqrt{4kT\,R\,B} \text{ volts} \tag{2}$$

where R is the resistance in ohms, T the temperature in degrees Kelvin, and k is Boltzman's constant ($k = 1.38 \times 10^{-23}$ J/°K).* B is the *bandwidth*, or range of frequencies, that is allowed to pass through the measurement system. The system bandwidth is determined by the filter characteristics in the system, usually the analog filtering in the system (see the next section).

If noise current is of interest, the equation for Johnson noise current can be obtained from Eq. (2) in conjunction with Ohm's law:

$$I_J = \sqrt{4kT\,B/R} \text{ amps} \tag{3}$$

Since Johnson noise is spread evenly over all frequencies (at least in theory), it is not possible to calculate a noise voltage or current without specifying B, the frequency range. Since the bandwidth is not always known in advance, it is common to describe a relative noise; specifically, the noise that would occur if the bandwidth were 1.0 Hz. Such relative noise specification can be identified by the unusual units required: volts/$\sqrt{\text{Hz}}$ or amps/$\sqrt{\text{Hz}}$.

---

*A temperature of 310 °K is often used as room temperature, in which case $4kT = 1.7 \times 10^{-20}$ J.

Shot noise is defined as a current noise and is proportional to the baseline current through a semiconductor junction:

$$I_s = \sqrt{2q\ I_d\ B} \text{ amps} \tag{4}$$

where q is the charge on an electron (1.662×10^{-19} coulomb), and I_d is the baseline semiconductor current. In photodetectors, the baseline current that generates shot noise is termed the *dark current*, hence, the symbol I_d in Eq. (4). Again, since the noise is spread across all frequencies, the bandwidth, BW, must be specified to obtain a specific value, or a relative noise can be specified in amps/$\sqrt{\text{Hz}}$.

When multiple noise sources are present, as is often the case, their voltage or current contributions to the total noise add as the square root of the sum of the squares, assuming that the individual noise sources are independent. For voltages:

$$V_T = (V_1^2 + V_2^2 + V_3^2 + \cdots + V_N^2)^{1/2} \tag{5}$$

A similar equation applies to current. Noise properties are discussed further in Chapter 2.

Signal-to-Noise Ratio

Most waveforms consist of signal plus noise mixed together. As noted previously, signal and noise are relative terms, relative to the task at hand: the signal is that portion of the waveform of interest while the noise is everything else. Often the goal of signal processing is to separate out signal from noise, to identify the presence of a signal buried in noise, or to detect features of a signal buried in noise.

The relative amount of signal and noise present in a waveform is usually quantified by the signal-to-noise ratio, *SNR*. As the name implies, this is simply the ratio of signal to noise, both measured in RMS (root-mean-squared) amplitude. The SNR is often expressed in "db" (short for decibels) where:

$$SNR = 20 \log \left(\frac{\text{Signal}}{\text{Noise}}\right) \tag{6}$$

To convert from db scale to a linear scale:

$$SNR_{\text{linear}} = 10^{\text{db}/20} \tag{7}$$

For example, a ratio of 20 db means that the RMS value of the signal was 10 times the RMS value of the noise ($10^{20/20} = 10$), +3 db indicates a ratio of 1.414 ($10^{3/20} = 1.414$), 0 db means the signal and noise are equal in RMS value,

−3 db means that the ratio is 1/1.414, and −20 db means the signal is 1/10 of the noise in RMS units. Figure 1.6 shows a sinusoidal signal with various amounts of white noise. Note that is it is difficult to detect presence of the signal visually when the SNR is −3 db, and impossible when the SNR is −10 db. The ability to detect signals with low SNR is the goal and motivation for many of the signal processing tools described in this text.

ANALOG FILTERS: FILTER BASICS

The analog signal processing circuitry shown in Figure 1.1 will usually contain some filtering, both to remove noise and appropriately condition the signal for

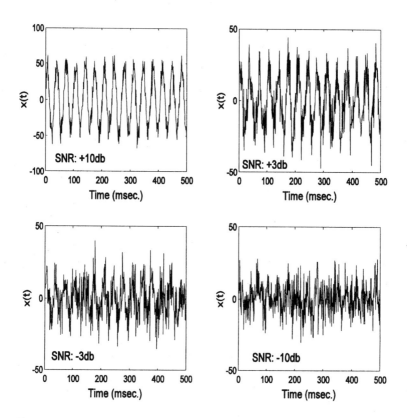

FIGURE 1.6   A 30 Hz sine wave with varying amounts of added noise. The sine wave is barely discernable when the SNR is −3db and not visible when the SNR is −10 db.

analog-to-digital conversion (ADC). It is this filtering that usually establishes the bandwidth of the system for noise calculations [the bandwidth used in Eqs. (2)–(4)]. As shown later, accurate conversion of the analog signal to digital format requires that the signal contain frequencies no greater than ½ the sampling frequency. This rule applies to the analog waveform as a whole, not just the signal of interest. Since all transducers and electronics produce some noise and since this noise contains a wide range of frequencies, analog lowpass filtering is usually essential to limit the bandwidth of the waveform to be converted. Waveform bandwidth and its impact on ADC will be discussed further in Chapter 2. Filters are defined by several properties: filter type, bandwidth, and attenuation characteristics. The last can be divided into initial and final characteristics. Each of these properties is described and discussed in the next section.

Filter Types

Analog *filters* are electronic devices that remove selected frequencies. Filters are usually termed according to the range of frequencies they do not suppress. Thus, *lowpass* filters allow low frequencies to pass with minimum attenuation while higher frequencies are attenuated. Conversely, *highpass* filters pass high frequencies, but attenuate low frequencies. *Bandpass* filters reject frequencies above and below a *passband* region. An exception to this terminology is the *bandstop* filter, which passes frequencies on either side of a range of attenuated frequencies.

Within each class, filters are also defined by the frequency ranges that they pass, termed the filter *bandwidth*, and the sharpness with which they increase (or decrease) attenuation as frequency varies. Spectral sharpness is specified in two ways: as an initial sharpness in the region where attenuation first begins and as a *slope* further along the attenuation curve. These various filter properties are best described graphically in the form of a frequency plot (sometimes referred to as a *Bode* plot), a plot of filter gain against frequency. Filter gain is simply the ratio of the output voltage divided by the input voltage, V_{out}/V_{in}, often taken in db. Technically this ratio should be defined for all frequencies for which it is nonzero, but practically it is usually stated only for the frequency range of interest. To simplify the shape of the resultant curves, frequency plots sometimes plot gain in db against the log of frequency.* When the output/input ratio is given analytically as a function of frequency, it is termed the *transfer function*. Hence, the frequency plot of a filter's output/input relationship can be

---

*When gain is plotted in db, it is in logarithmic form, since the db operation involves taking the log [Eq. (6)]. Plotting gain in db against log frequency puts the two variables in similar metrics and results in straighter line plots.

viewed as a graphical representation of the transfer function. Frequency plots for several different filter types are shown in Figure 1.7.

Filter Bandwidth

The bandwidth of a filter is defined by the range of frequencies that are not attenuated. These unattenuated frequencies are also referred to as *passband* frequencies. Figure 1.7A shows that the frequency plot of an ideal filter, a filter that has a perfectly flat passband region and an infinite attenuation slope. Real filters may indeed be quite flat in the passband region, but will attenuate with a

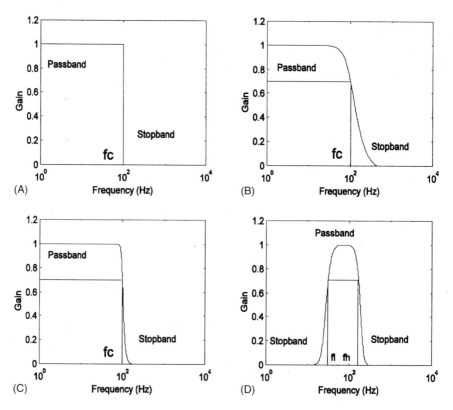

FIGURE 1.7 Frequency plots of ideal and realistic filters. The frequency plots shown here have a linear vertical axis, but often the vertical axis is plotted in db. The horizontal axis is in log frequency. (A) Ideal lowpass filter. (B) Realistic lowpass filter with a gentle attenuation characteristic. (C) Realistic lowpass filter with a sharp attenuation characteristic. (D) Bandpass filter.

more gentle slope, as shown in Figure 1.7B. In the case of the ideal filter, Figure 1.7A, the bandwidth or region of unattenuated frequencies is easy to determine; specifically, it is between 0.0 and the sharp attenuation at f_c Hz. When the attenuation begins gradually, as in Figure 1.7B, defining the passband region is problematic. To specify the bandwidth in this filter we must identify a frequency that defines the boundary between the attenuated and non-attenuated portion of the frequency characteristic. This boundary has been somewhat arbitrarily defined as the frequency when the attenuation is 3 db.* In Figure 1.7B, the filter would have a bandwidth of 0.0 to f_c Hz, or simply f_c Hz. The filter in Figure 1.7C has a sharper attenuation characteristic, but still has the same bandwidth (f_c Hz). The bandpass filter of Figure 1.7D has a bandwidth of $f_h - f_l$ Hz.

Filter Order

The slope of a filter's attenuation curve is related to the complexity of the filter: more complex filters have a steeper slope better approaching the ideal. In analog filters, complexity is proportional to the number of energy storage elements in the circuit (which could be either inductors or capacitors, but are generally capacitors for practical reasons). Using standard circuit analysis, it can be shown that each energy storage device leads to an additional order in the polynomial of the denominator of the transfer function that describes the filter. (The denominator of the transfer function is also referred to as the *characteristic equation*.) As with any polynomial equation, the number of roots of this equation will depend on the order of the equation; hence, filter complexity (i.e., the number of energy storage devices) is equivalent to the number of roots in the denominator of the Transfer Function. In electrical engineering, it has long been common to call the roots of the denominator equation *poles*. Thus, the complexity of the filter is also equivalent to the number of poles in the transfer function. For example, a second-order or two-pole filter has a transfer function with a second-order polynomial in the denominator and would contain two independent energy storage elements (very likely two capacitors).

Applying asymptote analysis to the transfer function, is not difficult to show that the slope of a second-order lowpass filter (the slope for frequencies much greater than the cutoff frequency, f_c) is 40 db/decade specified in log-log terms. (The unusual units, db/decade are a result of the log-log nature of the typical frequency plot.) That is, the attenuation of this filter increases linearly on a log-log scale by 40 db (a factor of 100 on a linear scale) for every order of magnitude increase in frequency. Generalizing, for each filter pole (or order)

---

*This defining point is not entirely arbitrary because when the signal is attenuated 3 db, its amplitude is 0.707 ($10^{-3/20}$) of what it was in the passband region and it has half the power of the unattenuated signal (since $0.707^2 = 1/2$). Accordingly this point is also known as the *half-power point*.

the downward slope (sometimes referred to as the *rolloff*) is increased by 20 db/decade. Figure 1.8 shows the frequency plot of a second-order (two-pole with a slope of 40 db/decade) and a 12th-order lowpass filter, both having the same cutoff frequency, f_c, and hence, the same bandwidth. The steeper slope or rolloff of the 12-pole filter is apparent. In principle, a 12-pole lowpass filter would have a slope of 240 db/decade (12×20 db/decade). In fact, this frequency characteristic is theoretical because in real analog filters parasitic components and inaccuracies in the circuit elements limit the actual attenuation that can be obtained. The same rationale applies to highpass filters except that the frequency plot decreases with decreasing frequency at a rate of 20 db/decade for each highpass filter pole.

Filter Initial Sharpness

As shown in Figure 1.8, both the slope and the initial sharpness increase with filter order (number of poles), but increasing filter order also increases the com-

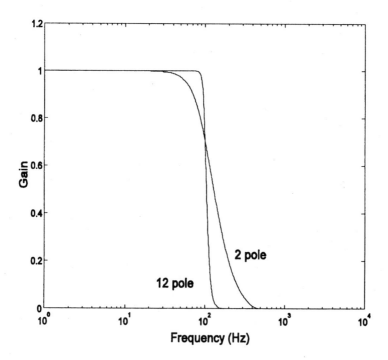

FIGURE 1.8 Frequency plot of a second-order (2-pole) and a 12th-order lowpass filter with the same cutoff frequency. The higher order filter more closely approaches the sharpness of an ideal filter.

plexity, hence the cost, of the filter. It is possible to increase the initial sharpness of the filter's attenuation characteristics without increasing the order of the filter, if you are willing to except some unevenness, or *ripple*, in the passband. Figure 1.9 shows two lowpass, 4th-order filters, differing in the initial sharpness of the attenuation. The one marked Butterworth has a smooth passband, but the initial attenuation is not as sharp as the one marked Chebychev; which has a passband that contains ripples. This property of analog filters is also seen in digital filters and will be discussed in detail in Chapter 4.

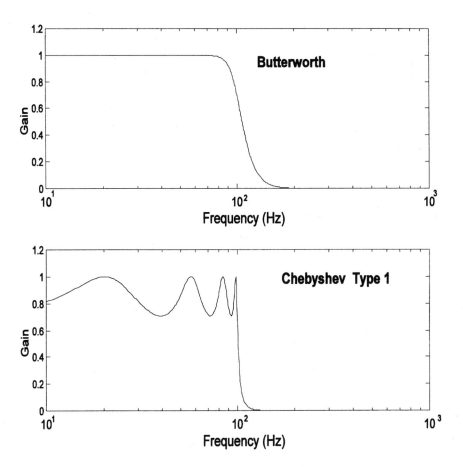

FIGURE 1.9 Two filters having the same order (4-pole) and cutoff frequency, but differing in the sharpness of the initial slope. The filter marked Chebychev has a steeper initial slope or rolloff, but contains ripples in the passband.

ANALOG-TO-DIGITAL CONVERSION: BASIC CONCEPTS

The last analog element in a typical measurement system is the analog-to-digital converter (ADC), Figure 1.1. As the name implies, this electronic component converts an analog voltage to an equivalent digital number. In the process of analog-to-digital conversion an analog or continuous waveform, $x(t)$, is converted into a discrete waveform, $x(n)$, a function of real numbers that are defined only at discrete integers, n. To convert a continuous waveform to digital format requires slicing the signal in two ways: slicing in time and slicing in amplitude (Figure 1.10).

Slicing the signal into discrete points in time is termed *time sampling* or simply *sampling*. Time slicing *samples* the continuous waveform, $x(t)$, at discrete prints in time, nT_s, where T_s is the sample interval. The consequences of time slicing are discussed in the next chapter. The same concept can be applied to images wherein a continuous image such as a photograph that has intensities that vary continuously across spatial distance is sampled at distances of S mm. In this case, the digital representation of the image is a two-dimensional array. The consequences of spatial sampling are discussed in Chapter 11.

Since the binary output of the ADC is a discrete integer while the analog signal has a continuous range of values, analog-to-digital conversion also requires the analog signal to be sliced into discrete levels, a process termed *quantization*, Figure 1.10. The equivalent number can only approximate the level of

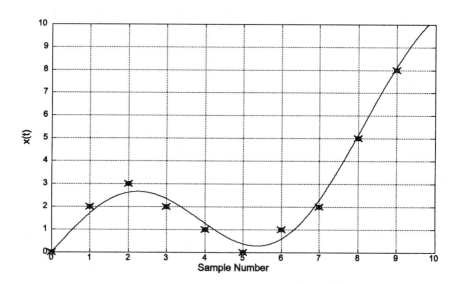

FIGURE 1.10 Converting a continuous signal (solid line) to discrete format requires slicing the signal in time and amplitude. The result is a series of discrete points (X's) that approximate the original signal.

the analog signal, and the degree of approximation will depend on the range of binary numbers and the amplitude of the analog signal. For example, if the output of the ADC is an 8-bit binary number capable of 2^8 or 256 discrete states, and the input amplitude range is 0.0–5.0 volts, then the quantization interval will be 5/256 or 0.0195 volts. If, as is usually the case, the analog signal is time varying in a continuous manner, it must be approximated by a series of binary numbers representing the approximate analog signal level at discrete points in time (Figure 1.10). The errors associated with amplitude slicing, or quantization, are described in the next section, and the potential error due to sampling is covered in Chapter 2. The remainder of this section briefly describes the hardware used to achieve this approximate conversion.

Analog-to-Digital Conversion Techniques

Various conversion rules have been used, but the most common is to convert the voltage into a proportional binary number. Different approaches can be used to implement the conversion electronically; the most common is the successive approximation technique described at the end of this section. ADC's differ in conversion range, speed of conversion, and resolution. The range of analog voltages that can be converted is frequently software selectable, and may, or may not, include negative voltages. Typical ranges are from 0.0–10.0 volts or less, or if negative values are possible ± 5.0 volts or less. The speed of conversion is specified in terms of samples per second, or conversion time. For example, an ADC with a conversion time of 10 µsec should, logically, be able to operate at up to 100,000 samples per second (or simply 100 kHz). Typical conversion rates run up to 500 kHz for moderate cost converters, but *off-the-shelf* converters can be obtained with rates up to 10–20 MHz. Except for image processing systems, lower conversion rates are usually acceptable for biological signals. Even image processing systems may use *downsampling* techniques to reduce the required ADC conversion rate and, hence, the cost.

A typical ADC system involves several components in addition to the actual ADC element, as shown in Figure 1.11. The first element is an N-to-1 analog switch that allows multiple input channels to be converted. Typical ADC systems provide up to 8 to 16 channels, and the switching is usually software-selectable. Since a single ADC is doing the conversion for all channels, the conversion rate for any given channel is reduced in proportion to the number of channels being converted. Hence, an ADC system with converter element that had a conversion rate of 50 kHz would be able to sample each of eight channels at a theoretical maximum rate of 50/8 = 6.25 kHz.

The Sample and Hold is a high-speed switch that momentarily records the input signal, and retains that signal value at its output. The time the switch is closed is termed the *aperture time*. Typical values range around 150 ns, and, except for very fast signals, can be considered basically instantaneous. This

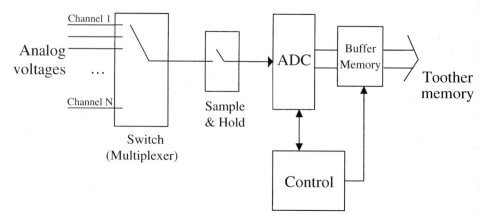

FIGURE 1.11   Block diagram of a typical analog-to-digital conversion system.

instantaneously sampled voltage value is held (as a charge on a capacitor) while the ADC element determines the equivalent binary number. Again, it is the ADC element that determines the overall speed of the conversion process.

Quantization Error

Resolution is given in terms of the number of bits in the binary output with the assumption that the least significant bit (LSB) in the output is accurate (which may not always be true). Typical converters feature 8-, 12-, and 16-bit output with 12 bits presenting a good compromise between conversion resolution and cost. In fact, most signals do not have a sufficient signal-to-noise ratio to justify a higher resolution; you are simply obtaining a more accurate conversion of the noise. For example, assuming that converter resolution is equivalent to the LSB, then the minimum voltage that can be resolved is the same as the quantization voltage described above: the voltage range divided by 2^N, where N is the number of bits in the binary output. The resolution of a 5-volt, 12-bit ADC is $5.0/2^{12} = 5/4096 = 0.0012$ volts. The dynamic range of a 12-bit ADC, the range from the smallest to the largest voltage it can convert, is from 0.0012 to 5 volts: in db this is $20 * \log|10^{12}| = 167$ db. Since typical signals, especially those of biological origin, have dynamic ranges rarely exceeding 60 to 80 db, a 12-bit converter with the dynamic range of 167 db may appear to be overkill. However, having this extra resolution means that not all of the range need be used, and since 12-bit ADC's are only marginally more expensive than 8-bit ADC's they are often used even when an 8-bit ADC (with dynamic range of over 100 DB, would be adequate). A 12-bit output does require two bytes to store and will double the memory requirements over an 8-bit ADC.

The number of bits used for conversion sets a lower limit on the resolution, and also determines the quantization error (Figure 1.12). This error can be thought of as a noise process added to the signal. If a sufficient number of quantization levels exist (say $N > 64$), the distortion produced by quantization error may be modeled as additive independent white noise with zero mean with the variance determined by the quantization step size, $\delta = V_{MAX}/2^N$. Assuming that the error is uniformly distributed between $-\delta/2$ $+\delta/2$, the variance, σ, is:

$$\sigma = \int_{-\delta/2}^{\delta/2} \eta^2/\delta \, d\eta = V_{Max}^2 \, (2^{-2N})/12 \qquad (8)$$

Assuming a uniform distribution, the RMS value of the noise would be just twice the standard deviation, σ.

Further Study: Successive Approximation

The most popular analog-to-digital converters use a rather roundabout strategy to find the binary number most equivalent to the input analog voltage—a *digital-to-analog converter* (DAC) is placed in a feedback loop. As shown Figure 1.13, an initial binary number stored in the buffer is fed to a DAC to produce a

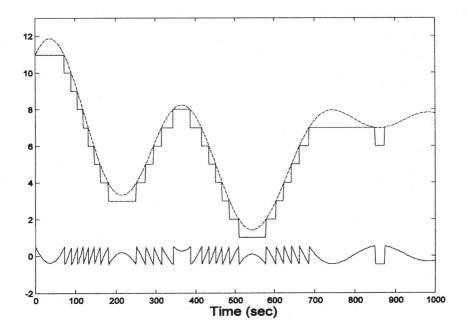

FIGURE 1.12 Quantization (amplitude slicing) of a continuous waveform. The lower trace shows the error between the quantized signal and the input.

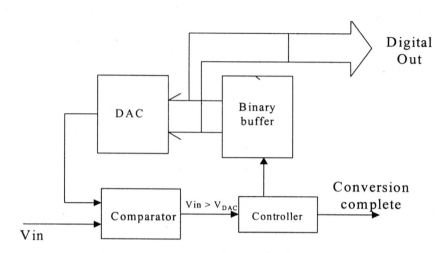

FIGURE 1.13 Block diagram of an analog-to-digital converter. The input analog voltage is compared with the output of a digital-to-analog converter. When the two voltages match, the number held in the *binary buffer* is equivalent to the input voltage with the resolution of the converter. Different strategies can be used to adjust the contents of the binary buffer to attain a match.

proportional voltage, V_{DAC}. This DAC voltage, V_{DAC}, is then compared to the input voltage, and the binary number in the buffer is adjusted until the desired level of match between V_{DAC} and V_{in} is obtained. This approach begs the question "How are DAC's constructed?" In fact, DAC's are relatively easy to construct using a simple *ladder* network and the principal of current superposition.

The controller adjusts the binary number based on whether or not the comparator finds the voltage out of the DAC, V_{DAC}, to be greater or less than the input voltage, V_{in}. One simple adjustment strategy is to increase the binary number by one each cycle if $V_{DAC} < V_{in}$, or decrease it otherwise. This so-called *tracking* ADC is very fast when V_{in} changes slowly, but can take many cycles when V_{in} changes abruptly (Figure 1.14). Not only can the conversion time be quite long, but it is variable since it depends on the dynamics of the input signal. This strategy would not easily allow for sampling an analog signal at a fixed rate due to the variability in conversion time.

An alternative strategy termed *successive approximation* allows the conversion to be done at a fixed rate and is well-suited to digital technology. The successive approximation strategy always takes the same number of cycles irrespective of the input voltage. In the first cycle, the controller sets the most significant bit (MSB) of the buffer to 1; all others are cleared. This binary number is half the maximum possible value (which occurs when all the bits are

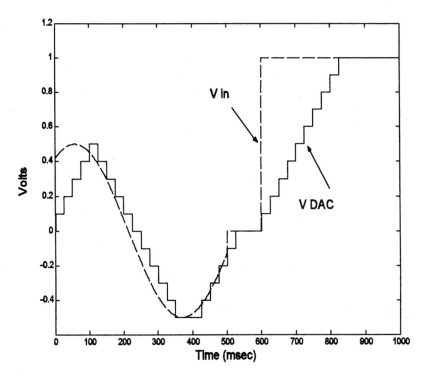

FIGURE 1.14 Voltage waveform of an ADC that uses a tracking strategy. The ADC voltage (solid line) follows the input voltage (dashed line) fairly closely when the input voltage varies slowly, but takes many cycles to "catch up" to an abrupt change in input voltage.

1), so the DAC should output a voltage that is half its maximum voltage—that is, a voltage in the middle of its range. If the comparator tells the controller that $V_{in} > V_{DAC}$, then the input voltage, V_{in}, must be greater than half the maximum range, and the MSB is left set. If $V_{in} < V_{DAC}$, then that the input voltage is in the lower half of the range and the MSB is cleared (Figure 1.15). In the next cycle, the next most significant bit is set, and the same comparison is made and the same bit adjustment takes place based on the results of the comparison (Figure 1.15).

After N cycles, where N is the number of bits in the digital output, the voltage from the DAC, V_{DAC}, converges to the best possible fit to the input voltage, V_{in}. Since $V_{in} \approx V_{DAC}$, the number in the buffer, which is proportional to V_{DAC}, is the best representation of the analog input voltage within the resolution of the converter. To signal the end of the conversion process, the ADC puts

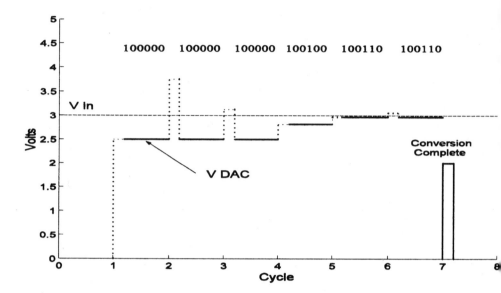

FIGURE 1.15 V_{in} and V_{DAC} in a 6-bit ADC using the successive approximation strategy. In the first cycle, the MSB is set (solid line) since $V_{in} > V_{DAC}$. In the next two cycles, the bit being tested is cleared because $V_{in} < V_{DAC}$ when this bit was set. For the fourth and fifth cycles the bit being tested remained set and for the last cycle it was cleared. At the end of the sixth cycle a *conversion complete* flag is set to signify the end of the conversion process.

out a digital signal or *flag* indicating that the conversion is complete (Figure 1.15).

TIME SAMPLING: BASICS

Time sampling transforms a continuous analog signal into a discrete time signal, a sequence of numbers denoted as $x(n) = [x_1, x_2, x_3, \ldots x_N]$,* Figure 1.16 (lower trace). Such a representation can be thought of as an array in computer memory. (It can also be viewed as a vector as shown in the next chapter.) Note that the array position indicates a relative position in time, but to relate this number sequence back to an absolute time both the sampling interval and sampling onset time must be known. However, if only the time relative to conversion onset is important, as is frequently the case, then only the sampling interval needs to be

---

*In many textbooks brackets, [ ], are used to denote digitized variables; i.e., $x[n]$. Throughout this text we reserve brackets to indicate a series of numbers, or vector, following the MATLAB format.

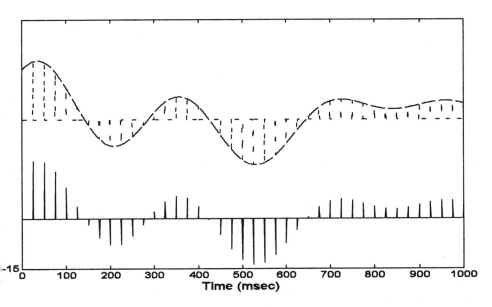

FIGURE 1.16 A continuous signal (upper trace) is sampled at discrete points in time and stored in memory as an array of proportional numbers (lower trace).

known. Converting back to relative time is then achieved by multiplying the sequence number, n, by the sampling interval, T_s: $x(t) = x(nT_s)$.

Sampling theory is discussed in the next chapter and states that a sinusoid can be uniquely reconstructed providing it has been sampled by at least two equally spaced points over a cycle. Since Fourier series analysis implies that any signal can be represented is a series of sin waves (see Chapter 3), then by extension, a signal can be uniquely reconstructed providing the sampling frequency is twice that of the highest frequency in the signal. Note that this highest frequency component may come from a noise source and could be well above the frequencies of interest. The inverse of this rule is that any signal that contains frequency components greater than twice the sampling frequency cannot be reconstructed, and, hence, its digital representation is in error. Since this error is introduced by undersampling, it is inherent in the digital representation and no amount of digital signal processing can correct this error. The specific nature of this *under*-sampling error is termed *aliasing* and is described in a discussion of the consequences of sampling in Chapter 2.

From a practical standpoint, aliasing must be avoided either by the use of very high sampling rates—rates that are well above the bandwidth of the analog system—or by filtering the analog signal before analog-to-digital conversion. Since extensive sampling rates have an associated cost, both in terms of the

ADC required and memory costs, the latter approach is generally preferable. Also note that the sampling frequency must be twice the highest frequency present in the input signal, not to be confused with the bandwidth of the analog signal. All frequencies in the sampled waveform greater than one half the sampling frequency (one-half the sampling frequency is sometimes referred to as the *Nyquist* frequency) must be essentially zero, not merely attenuated. Recall that the bandwidth is defined as the frequency for which the amplitude is reduced by only 3 db from the nominal value of the signal, while the sampling criterion requires that the value be reduced to zero. Practically, it is sufficient to reduce the signal to be less than quantization noise level or other acceptable noise level. The relationship between the sampling frequency, the order of the anti-aliasing filter, and the system bandwidth is explored in a problem at the end of this chapter.

Example 1.1. An ECG signal of 1 volt peak-to-peak has a bandwidth of 0.01 to 100 Hz. (Note this frequency range has been established by an official standard and is meant to be conservative.) Assume that broadband noise may be present in the signal at about 0.1 volts (i.e., −20 db below the nominal signal level). This signal is filtered using a four-pole lowpass filter. What sampling frequency is required to insure that the error due to aliasing is less than −60 db (0.001 volts)?

Solution. The noise at the sampling frequency must be reduced another 40 db (20 * log (0.1/0.001)) by the four-pole filter. A four-pole filter with a cutoff of 100 Hz (required to meet the fidelity requirements of the ECG signal) would attenuate the waveform at a rate of 80 db per decade. For a four-pole filter the asymptotic attenuation is given as:

Attenuation = $80 \log(f_2/f_c)$ db

To achieve the required additional 40 db of attenuation required by the problem from a four-pole filter:

$80 \log(f_2/f_c) = 40$ $\log(f_2/f_c) = 40/80 = 0.5$
$f_2/f_c = 10.5 =;$ $f_2 = 3.16 \times 100 = 316$ Hz

Thus to meet the sampling criterion, the sampling frequency must be at least 632 Hz, twice the frequency at which the noise is adequately attenuated. The solution is approximate and ignores the fact that the initial attenuation of the filter will be gradual. Figure 1.17 shows the frequency response characteristics of an actual 4-pole analog filter with a cutoff frequency of 100 Hz. This figure shows that the attenuation is 40 db at approximately 320 Hz. Note the high sampling frequency that is required for what is basically a relatively low frequency signal (the ECG). In practice, a filter with a sharper cutoff, perhaps

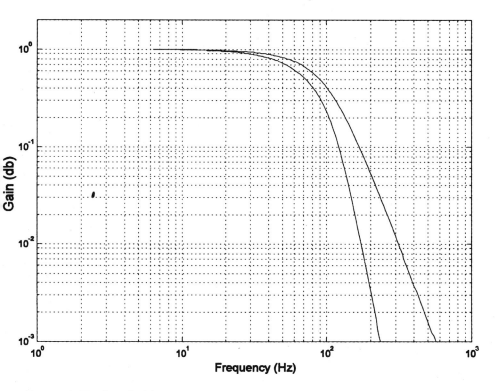

FIGURE 1.17   Detailed frequency plot (on a log-log scale) of a 4-pole and 8-pole filter, both having a cutoff frequency of 100 Hz.

an 8-pole filter, would be a better choice in this situation. Figure 1.17 shows that the frequency response of an 8-pole filter with the same 100 Hz frequency provides the necessary attenuation at less than 200 Hz. Using this filter, the sampling frequency could be lowered to under 400 Hz.

FURTHER STUDY: BUFFERING AND REAL-TIME DATA PROCESSING

Real-time data processing simply means that the data is processed and results obtained in sufficient time to influence some ongoing process. This influence may come directly from the computer or through human intervention. The processing time constraints naturally depend on the dynamics of the process of interest. Several minutes might be acceptable for an automated drug delivery system, while information on the electrical activity the heart needs to be immediately available.

The term *buffer*, when applied digital technology, usually describes a set of memory locations used to temporarily store incoming data until enough data is acquired for efficient processing. When data is being acquired continuously, a technique called *double buffering* can be used. Incoming data is alternatively sent to one of two memory arrays, and the one that is not being filled is processed (which may involve simply transfer to disk storage). Most ADC software packages provide a means for determining which element in an array has most recently been filled to facilitate buffering, and frequently the ability to determine which of two arrays (or which half of a single array) is being filled to facilitate double buffering.

DATA BANKS

With the advent of the World Wide Web it is not always necessary to go through the analog-to-digital conversion process to obtain digitized data of physiological signals. A number of data banks exist that provide physiological signals such as ECG, EEG, gait, and other common biosignals in digital form. Given the volatility and growth of the Web and the ease with which searches can be made, no attempt will be made to provide a comprehensive list of appropriate Websites. However, a good source of several common biosignals, particularly the ECG, is the Physio Net Data Bank maintained by MIT—http://www.physionet.org. Some data banks are specific to a given set of biosignals or a given signal processing approach. An example of the latter is the ICALAB Data Bank in Japan—http://www.bsp.brain.riken.go.jp/ICALAB/—which includes data that can be used to evaluate independent component analysis (see Chapter 9) algorithms.

Numerous other data banks containing biosignals and/or images can be found through a quick search of the Web, and many more are likely to come online in the coming years. This is also true for some of the signal processing algorithms as will be described in more detail later. For example, the ICALAB Website mentioned above also has algorithms for independent component analysis in MATLAB m-file format. A quick Web search can provide both signal processing algorithms and data that can be used to evaluate a signal processing system under development. The Web is becoming an evermore useful tool in signal and image processing, and a brief search of the Web can save considerable time in the development process, particularly if the signal processing system involves advanced approaches.

PROBLEMS

1.   A single sinusoidal signal is contained in noise. The RMS value of the noise is 0.5 volts and the SNR is 10 db. What is the peak-to-peak amplitude of the sinusoid?

2. A resistor produces 10 μV noise when the room temperature is 310°K and the bandwidth is 1 kHz. What current noise would be produced by this resistor?

3. The noise voltage out of a 1 MΩ resistor was measured using a digital volt meter as 1.5 μV at a room temperature of 310 °K. What is the effective bandwidth of the voltmeter?

4. The photodetector shown in Figure 1.4 has a sensitivity of 0.3μA/μW (at a wavelength of 700 nm). In this circuit, there are three sources of noise. The photodetector has a dark current of 0.3 nA, the resistor is 10 MΩ, and the amplifier has an input current noise of 0.01 pA/√Hz. Assume a bandwidth of 10 kHz. (a) Find the total noise current input to the amplifier. (b) Find the minimum light flux signal that can be detected with an SNR = 5.

5. A lowpass filter is desired with the cutoff frequency of 10 Hz. This filter should attenuate a 100 Hz signal by a factor of 85. What should be the order of this filter?

6. You are given a box that is said to contain a highpass filter. You input a series of sine waves into the box and record the following output:

Frequency (Hz):	2	10	20	60	100	125	150	200	300	400
V_{out} volts rms:	$.15 \times 10^{-7}$	0.1×10^{-3}	0.002	0.2	1.5	3.28	4.47	4.97	4.99	5.0

What is the cutoff frequency and order of this filter?

7. An 8-bit ADC converter that has an input range of ± 5 volts is used to convert a signal that varies between ± 2 volts. What is the SNR of the input if the input noise equals the quantization noise of the converter?

8. As elaborated in Chapter 2, time sampling requires that the maximum frequency present in the input be less than $f_s/2$ for proper representation in digital format. Assume that the signal must be attenuated by a factor of 1000 to be considered "not present." If the sampling frequency is 10 kHz and a 4th-order lowpass anti-aliasing filter is used prior to analog-to-digital conversion, what should be the bandwidth of the sampled signal? That is, what must the cutoff frequency be of the anti-aliasing lowpass filter?

2

Basic Concepts

NOISE

In Chapter 1 we observed that noise is an inherent component of most measurements. In addition to physiological and environmental noise, electronic noise arises from the transducer and associated electronics and is intermixed with the signal being measured. Noise is usually represented as a random variable, $x(n)$. Since the variable is random, describing it as a function of time is not very useful. It is more common to discuss other properties of noise such as its probability distribution, range of variability, or frequency characteristics. While noise can take on a variety of different probability distributions, the Central Limit Theorem implies that most noise will have a *Gaussian* or *normal* distribution*. The Central Limit Theorem states that when noise is generated by a large number of independent sources it will have a Gaussian probability distribution regardless of the probability distribution characteristics of the individual sources. Figure 2.1A shows the distribution of 20,000 uniformly distributed random numbers between −1 and +1. The distribution is approximately flat between the limits of ±1 as expected. When the data set consists of 20,000 numbers, each of which is the average of two uniformly distributed random numbers, the distribution is much closer to Gaussian (Figure 2.1B, upper right). The distribution

---

*Both terms are used and reader should be familiar with both. We favor the term "Gaussian" to avoid the value judgement implied by the word "normal."

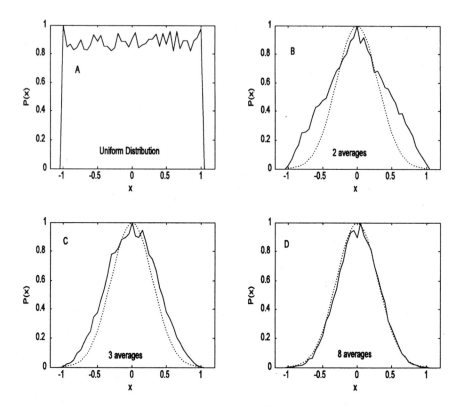

FIGURE 2.1   (A) The distribution of 20,000 uniformly distributed random numbers. (B) The distribution of 20,000 numbers, each of which is the average of two uniformly distributed random numbers. (C) and (D) The distribution obtained when 3 and 8 random numbers, still uniformly distributed, are averaged together. Although the underlying distribution is uniform, the averages of these uniformly distributed numbers tend toward a Gaussian distribution (dotted line). This is an example of the Central Limit Theorem at work.

constructed from 20,000 numbers that are averages of only 8 random numbers appears close to Gaussian, Figure 2.1D, even though the numbers being averaged have a uniform distribution.

The probability of a Gaussianly distributed variable, x, is specified in the well-known normal or Gaussian distribution equation:

$$p(x) = \frac{1}{\sigma\sqrt{2\pi}}\, e^{-x^2/2\sigma^2} \tag{1}$$

Two important properties of a random variable are its *mean*, or average value, and its *variance*, the term σ^2 in Eq. (1). The arithmetic quantities of mean and variance are frequently used in signal processing algorithms, and their computation is well-suited to discrete data.

The mean value of a discrete array of N samples is evaluated as:

$$\bar{x} = \frac{1}{N} \sum_{k=1}^{N} x_k \tag{2}$$

Note that the summation in Eq. (2) is made between 1 and N as opposed to 0 and $N - 1$. This protocol will commonly be used throughout the text to be compatible with MATLAB notation where the first element in an array has an index of 1, not 0.

Frequently, the mean will be subtracted from the data sample to provide data with zero mean value. This operation is particularly easy in MATLAB as described in the next section. The sample variance, σ^2, is calculated as shown in Eq. (3) below, and the standard deviation, σ, is just the square root of the variance.

$$\sigma^2 = \frac{1}{N - 1} \sum_{k=1}^{N} (x_k - \bar{x})^2 \tag{3}$$

Normalizing the standard deviation or variance by $1/N - 1$ as in Eq. (3) produces the best estimate of the variance, if x is a sample from a Gaussian distribution. Alternatively, normalizing the variance by $1/N$ produces the second moment of the data around x. Note that this is the equivalent of the RMS value of the data if the data have zero as the mean.

When multiple measurements are made, multiple random variables can be generated. If these variables are combined or added together, the means add so that the resultant random variable is simply the mean, or average, of the individual means. The same is true for the variance—the variances add and the average variance is the mean of the individual variances:

$$\bar{\sigma}^2 = \frac{1}{N} \sum_{k=1}^{N} \sigma_k^2 \tag{4}$$

However, the standard deviation is the square root of the variance and the standard deviations add as the $\sqrt{N}$ times the average standard deviation [Eq. (5)]. Accordingly, the mean standard deviation is the average of the individual standard deviations divided by $\sqrt{N}$ [Eq. (6)].

From Eq. (4):

$$\sum_{k=1}^{N} \sigma_k^2, \quad \text{hence:} \quad \sum_{k=1}^{N} \sigma_k = \sqrt{N \bar{\sigma}^2} = \sqrt{N} \, \bar{\sigma} \tag{5}$$

$$\text{Mean Standard Deviation} = \frac{1}{N} \sum_{k=1}^{N} \sigma_k = \frac{1}{N} \sqrt{N} \, \overline{\sigma} = \frac{\overline{\sigma}}{\sqrt{N}} \tag{6}$$

In other words, averaging noise from different sensors, or multiple observations from the same source, will reduce the standard deviation of the noise by the square root of the number of averages.

In addition to a mean and standard deviation, noise also has a spectral characteristic—that is, its energy distribution may vary with frequency. As shown below, the frequency characteristics of the noise are related to how well one instantaneous value of noise correlates with the adjacent instantaneous values: for digitized data how much one data point is correlated with its neighbors. If the noise has so much randomness that each point is independent of its neighbors, then it has a flat spectral characteristic and vice versa. Such noise is called *white noise* since it, like white light, contains equal energy at all frequencies (see Figure 1.5). The section on Noise Sources in Chapter 1 mentioned that most electronic sources produce noise that is essentially white up to many megahertz. When white noise is filtered, it becomes bandlimited and is referred to as *colored* noise since, like colored light, it only contains energy at certain frequencies. Colored noise shows some correlation between adjacent points, and this correlation becomes stronger as the bandwidth decreases and the noise becomes more *monochromatic*. The relationship between bandwidth and correlation of adjacent points is explored in the section on autocorrelation.

ENSEMBLE AVERAGING

Eq. (6) indicates that averaging can be a simple, yet powerful signal processing technique for reducing noise when multiple observations of the signal are possible. Such multiple observations could come from multiple sensors, but in many biomedical applications, the multiple observations come from repeated responses to the same stimulus. In *ensemble averaging*, a group, or ensemble, of time responses are averaged together on a point-by-point basis; that is, an average signal is constructed by taking the average, for each point in time, over all signals in the ensemble (Figure 2.2). A classic biomedical engineering example of the application of ensemble averaging is the visual evoked response (VER) in which a visual stimulus produces a small neural signal embedded in the EEG. Usually this signal cannot be detected in the EEG signal, but by averaging hundreds of observations of the EEG, time-locked to the visual stimulus, the visually evoked signal emerges.

There are two essential requirements for the application of ensemble averaging for noise reduction: the ability to obtain multiple observations, and a reference signal closely time-linked to the response. The reference signal shows how the multiple observations are to be aligned for averaging. Usually a time

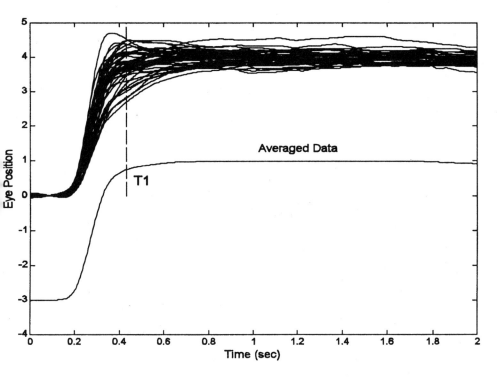

FIGURE 2.2 Upper traces: An ensemble of individual (vergence) eye movement responses to a step change in stimulus. Lower trace: The ensemble average, displaced downward for clarity. The ensemble average is constructed by averaging the individual responses at each point in time. Hence, the value of the average response at time T1 (vertical line) is the average of the individual responses at that time.

signal linked to the stimulus is used. An example of ensemble averaging is shown in Figure 2.2, and the code used to produce this figure is presented in the following MATLAB implementation section.

MATLAB IMPLEMENTATION

In MATLAB the mean, variance, and standard deviations are implemented as shown in the three code lines below.

```
xm = mean(x);        % Evaluate mean of x
xvar = var(x)        % Evaluate the variance of x normalizing by
                     %   N-1
```

```
xnorm = var(x,1);       % Evaluate the variance of x
xstd = std(x);          % Evaluate the standard deviation of x,
```

If **x** is an array (also termed a vector for reasons given later) the output of these function calls is a scalar representing the mean, variance, or standard deviation. If **x** is a matrix then the output is a row vector resulting from applying the appropriate calculation (mean, variance, or standard deviation) to each column of the matrix.

Example 2.1 below shows the implementation of ensemble averaging that produced the data in Figure 2.2. The program first loads the eye movement data (**load verg1**), then plots the ensemble. The ensemble average is determined using the MATLAB **mean** routine. Note that the data matrix, **data_out,** must be in the correct orientation (the responses must be in rows) for routine **mean**. If that were not the case (as in Problem 1 at the end of this chapter), the matrix transposition operation should be performed*. The ensemble average, **avg**, is then plotted displaced by 3 degrees to provide a clear view. Otherwise it would overlay the data.

Example 2.1 Compute and display the Ensemble average of an ensemble of vergence eye movement responses to a step change in stimulus. These responses are stored in MATLAB file **verg1.mat**.

```
% Example 2.1 and Figure 2.2 Load eye movement data, plot
%     the data then generate and plot the ensemble average.
%
close all; clear all;
load verg1;                       % Get eye movement data;
Ts = .005;                        % Sample interval = 5 msec
[nu,N] = size(data_out);          % Get data length (N)
t = (1:N)*Ts;                     % Generate time vector
%
% Plot ensemble data superimposed
plot(t,data_out,'k');
hold on;
%
% Construct and plot the ensemble average
avg = mean(data_out);             % Calculate ensemble average
plot(t,avg-3,'k');                %   and plot, separated from
                                  %   the other data
xlabel('Time (sec)');             % Label axes
ylabel('Eye Position');
```

---

*In MATLAB, matrix or vector transposition is indicated by an apostrophe following the variable. For example if *x* is a row vector, *x′* is a column vector and visa versa. If *X* is a matrix, *X′* is that matrix with rows and columns switched.

```
plot([.43 .43],[0 5],'-k');    % Plot horizontal line
text(1,1.2,'Averaged Data');   % Label data average
```

DATA FUNCTIONS AND TRANSFORMS

To mathematicians, the term *function* can take on a wide range of meanings. In signal processing, most functions fall into two categories: waveforms, images, or other data; and entities that operate on waveforms, images, or other data (Hubbard, 1998). The latter group can be further divided into functions that modify the data, and functions used to analyze or probe the data. For example, the basic filters described in Chapter 4 use functions (the filter coefficients) that modify the spectral content of a waveform while the Fourier Transform detailed in Chapter 3 uses functions (harmonically related sinusoids) to analyze the spectral content of a waveform. Functions that modify data are also termed *operations* or *transformations*.

Since most signal processing operations are implemented using digital electronics, functions are represented in discrete form as a sequence of numbers:

$$x(n) = [x(1),x(2),x(3), \ldots ,x(N)] \tag{5}$$

Discrete data functions (waveforms or images) are usually obtained through analog-to-digital conversion or other data input, while analysis or modifying functions are generated within the computer or are part of the computer program. (The consequences of converting a continuous time function into a discrete representation are described in the section below on sampling theory.)

In some applications, it is advantageous to think of a function (of whatever type) not just as a sequence, or array, of numbers, but as a *vector*. In this conceptualization, $x(n)$ is a single vector defined by a single point, the endpoint of the vector, in N-dimensional space, Figure 2.3. This somewhat curious and highly mathematical concept has the advantage of unifying some signal processing operations and fits well with matrix methods. It is difficult for most people to imagine higher-dimensional spaces and even harder to present them graphically, so operations and functions in higher-dimensional space are usually described in 2 or 3 dimensions, and the extension to higher dimensional space is left to the imagination of the reader. (This task can sometimes be difficult for non-mathematicians: try and imagine a data sequence of even a 32-point array represented as a single vector in 32-dimensional space!)

A *transform* can be thought of as a re-mapping of the original data into a function that provides more information than the original.* The Fourier Transform described in Chapter 3 is a classic example as it converts the original time

---

*Some definitions would be more restrictive and require that a transform be bilateral; that is, it must be possible to recover the original signal from the transformed data. We will use the looser definition and reserve the term *bilateral transform* to describe reversible transformations.

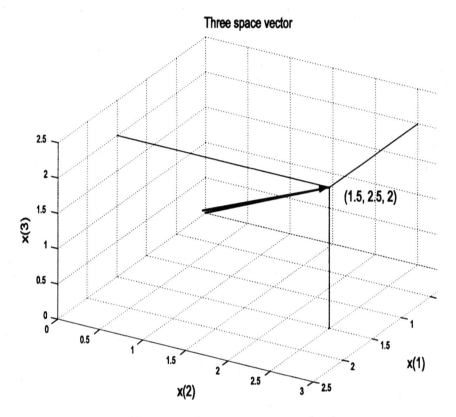

FIGURE 2.3 The data sequence $x(n) = [1.5,2.5,2]$ represented as a vector in three-dimensional space.

data into frequency information which often provides greater insight into the nature and/or origin of the signal. Many of the transforms described in this text are achieved by comparing the signal of interest with some sort of probing function. This comparison takes the form of a correlation (produced by multiplication) that is averaged (or integrated) over the duration of the waveform, or some portion of the waveform:

$$X(m) = \int_{-\infty}^{\infty} x(t)\ f_m(t)\ dt \tag{7}$$

where $x(t)$ is the waveform being analyzed, $f_m(t)$ is the probing function and m is some variable of the probing function, often specifying a particular member in a family of similar functions. For example, in the Fourier Transform $f_m(t)$ is a family of harmonically related sinusoids and m specifies the frequency of an individual sinusoid in that family (e.g., sin(*mft*)). A family of probing functions is also termed a *basis*. For discrete functions, a probing function consists of a sequence of values, or vector, and the integral becomes summation over a finite range:

$$X(m) = \sum_{n=1}^{N} x(n) f_m(n) \qquad (8)$$

where $x(n)$ is the discrete waveform and $f_m(n)$ is a discrete version of the family of probing functions. This equation assumes the probe and waveform functions are the same length. Other possibilities are explored below.

When either $x(t)$ or $f_m(t)$ are of infinite length, they must be truncated in some fashion to fit within the confines of limited memory storage. In addition, if the length of the probing function, $f_m(n)$, is shorter than the waveform, $x(n)$, then $x(n)$ must be shortened in some way. The length of either function can be shortened by simple truncation or by multiplying the function by yet another function that has zero value beyond the desired length. A function used to shorten another function is termed a window function, and its action is shown in Figure 2.4. Note that simple truncation can be viewed as multiplying the function by a *rectangular window*, a function whose value is one for the portion of the function that is retained, and zero elsewhere. The consequences of this artificial shortening will depend on the specific window function used. Consequences of *data windowing* are discussed in Chapter 3 under the heading Window Functions. If a window function is used, Eq. (8) becomes:

$$X(m) = \sum_{n=1}^{N} x(n) \; f_m(n) \; W(n) \qquad (9)$$

where $W(n)$ is the window function. In the Fourier Transform, the length of $W(n)$ is usually set to be the same as the available length of the waveform, $x(n)$, but in other applications it can be shorter than the waveform. If $W(n)$ is a rectangular function, then $W(n) = 1$ over the length of the summation ($1 \leq n \leq N$), and it is usually omitted from the equation. The rectangular window is implemented implicitly by the summation limits.

If the probing function is of finite length (in mathematical terms such a function is said to have *finite support*) and this length is shorter than the waveform, then it might be appropriate to translate or slide it over the signal and perform the comparison (correlation, or multiplication) at various relative positions between the waveform and probing function. In the example shown in Figure 2.5, a single probing function is shown (representing a single family member), and a single output function is produced. In general, the output would be a family of functions, or a two-variable function, where one variable corresponds to the relative position between the two functions and the other to the

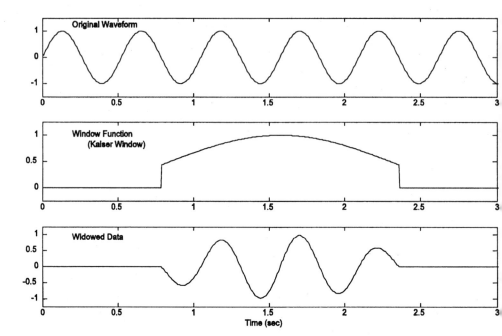

FIGURE 2.4 A waveform (upper plot) is multiplied by a window function (middle plot) to create a truncated version (lower plot) of the original waveform. The window function is shown in the middle plot. This particular window function is called the *Kaiser Window*, one of many popular window functions.

specific family member. This sliding comparison is similar to convolution described in the next section, and is given in discrete form by the equation:

$$X(m,k) = \sum_{n=1}^{N} x(n) \, f_m(n - k) \tag{10}$$

where the variable k indicates the relative position between the two functions and m is the family member as in the above equations. This approach will be used in the filters described in Chapter 4 and in the Continuous Wavelet Transform described in Chapter 7. A variation of this approach can be used for long—or even infinite—probing functions, provided the probing function itself is shortened by windowing to a length that is less than the waveform. Then the shortened probing function can be translated across the waveform in the same manner as a probing function that is naturally short. The equation for this condition becomes:

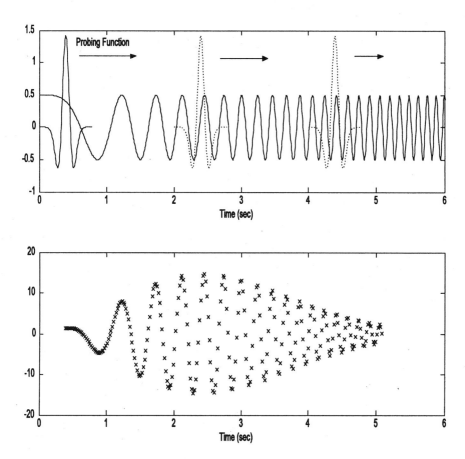

FIGURE 2.5 The probing function slides over the waveform of interest (upper panel) and at each position generates the summed, or averaged, product of the two functions (lower panel), as in Eq. (10). In this example, the probing function is one member of the "Mexican Hat" family (see Chapter 7) and the waveform is a sinusoid that increases its frequency linearly over time (known as a *chirp*.) The summed product (lower panel), also known as the *scalar product*, shows the relative correlation between the waveform and the probing function as it slides across the waveform. Note that this relative correlation varies sinusoidally as the phase between the two functions varies, but reaches a maximum around 2.5 sec, the time when the waveform is most like the probing function.

$$X(m,k) = \sum_{n=1}^{N} x(n)\,[W(n-k)\,f_m(n)] \tag{11}$$

where $f_m(n)$ is a longer function that is shortened by the sliding window function, $(W(n-k)$, and the variables m and k have the same meaning as in Eq. (10). This is the approach taken in the Short-Term Fourier Transform described in Chapter 6.

All of the discrete equations above, Eqs. (7) to (11), have one thing in common: they all feature the multiplication of two (or sometimes three) functions and the summation of the product over some finite interval. Returning to the vector conceptualization for data sequences mentioned above (see Figure 2.3), this multiplication and summation is the same as *scalar product* of the two vectors.*

The scalar product is defined as:

$$\text{Scalar product of a \& b} \equiv \langle a,b \rangle = \begin{bmatrix} a_1 \\ a_2 \\ \vdots \\ a_n \end{bmatrix} \begin{bmatrix} b_1 \\ b_2 \\ \vdots \\ b_n \end{bmatrix}$$

$$= a_1b_1 + a_2b_2 + \cdots + a_nb_n \tag{12}$$

Note that the scalar product results in a single number (i.e., a scalar), not a vector. The scalar product can also be defined in terms of the magnitude of the two vectors and the angle between them:

$$\text{Scalar product of a and b} \equiv \langle a,b \rangle = |a|\,|b|\,\cos\theta \tag{13}$$

where θ is the angle between the two vectors. If the two vectors are perpendicular to one another, i.e., they are *orthogonal*, then $\theta = 90°$, and their salar product will be zero. Eq. (13) demonstrates that the scalar product between waveform and probe function is mathematically the same as a projection of the waveform vector onto the probing function vector (after normalizing by probe vector length). When the probing function consists of a family of functions, then the scalar product operations in Eqs. (7)–(11) can be thought of as projecting the waveform vector onto vectors representing the various family members. In this vector-based conceptualization, the probing function family, or *basis*, can be thought of as the axes of a coordinate system. This is the motivation behind the development of probing functions that have family members that are orthogonal,

---

*The scalar product is also termed the *inner product*, the *standard inner product*, or the *dot product*.

or *orthonormal*:† the scalar product computations (or projections) can be done on each axes (i.e., on each family member) independently of the others.

CONVOLUTION, CORRELATION, AND COVARIANCE

Convolution, correlation, and covariance are similar-sounding terms and are similar in the way they are calculated. This similarity is somewhat misleading—at least in the case of convolution—since the areas of application and underlying concepts are not the same.

Convolution and the Impulse Response

Convolution is an important concept in linear systems theory, solving the need for a time domain operation equivalent to the Transfer Function. Recall that the Transfer Function is a frequency domain concept that is used to calculate the output of a linear system to any input. Convolution can be used to define a general input–output relationship in the time domain analogous to the Transfer Function in the frequency domain. Figure 2.6 demonstrates this application of convolution. The input, $x(t)$, the output, $y(t)$, and the function linking the two through convolution, $h(t)$, are all functions of time; hence, convolution is a time domain operation. (Ironically, convolution algorithms are often implemented in the frequency domain to improve the speed of the calculation.)

The basic concept behind convolution is superposition. The first step is to determine a time function, $h(t)$, that tells how the system responds to an infinitely short segment of the input waveform. If superposition holds, then the output can be determined by summing (integrating) all the response contributions calculated from the short segments. The way in which a linear system responds to an infinitely short segment of data can be determined simply by noting the system's response to an infinitely short input, an infinitely short pulse. An infinitely short pulse (or one that is at least short compared to the dynamics of the system) is termed an impulse or *delta* function (commonly denoted $\delta(t)$), and the response it produces is termed the *impulse response*, $h(t)$.

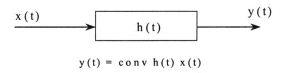

$$y(t) = conv\ h(t)\ x(t)$$

FIGURE 2.6 Convolution as a linear process.

---

†Orthonormal vectors are orthogonal, but also have unit length.

Given that the impulse response describes the response of the system to an infinitely short segment of data, and any input can be viewed as an infinite string of such infinitesimal segments, the impulse response can be used to determine the output of the system to any input. The response produced by an infinitely small data segment is simply this impulse response scaled by the magnitude of that data segment. The contribution of each infinitely small segment can be summed, or integrated, to find the response created by all the segments.

The convolution process is shown schematically in Figure 2.7. The left graph shows the input, $x(n)$ (dashed curve), to a linear system having an impulse response of $h(n)$ (solid line). The right graph of Figure 2.7 shows three partial responses (solid curves) produced by three different infinitely small data segments at $N1$, $N2$, and $N3$. Each partial response is an impulse response scaled by the associated input segment and shifted to the position of that segment. The output of the linear process (right graph, dashed line) is the summation of the individual

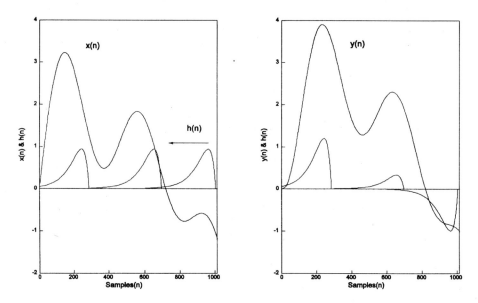

FIGURE 2.7   (A) The input, $x(n)$, to a linear system (dashed line) and the impulse response of that system, $h(n)$ (solid line). Three points on the input data sequence are shown: N1, N2, and N3. (B) The partial contributions from the three input data points to the output are impulse responses scaled by the value of the associated input data point (solid line). The overall response of the system, $y(n)$ (dashed line, scaled to fit on the graph), is obtained by summing the contributions from all the input points.

impulse responses produced by each of the input data segments. (The output is scaled down to produce a readable plot).

Stated mathematically, the output $y(t)$, to any input, $x(t)$ is given by:

$$y(t) = \int_{-\infty}^{+\infty} h(\tau)\, x(t - \tau)\, d\tau = \int_{-\infty}^{+\infty} h(t - \tau)\, x(\tau)\, d\tau \qquad (14)$$

To determine the impulse of each infinitely small data segment, the impulse response is shifted a time τ with respect to the input, then scaled (i.e., multiplied) by the magnitude of the input at that point in time. It does not matter which function, the input or the impulse response, is shifted.* Shifting and multiplication is sometimes referred to as the *lag product*. For most systems, $h(\tau)$ is finite, so the limit of integration is finite. Moreover, a real system can only respond to past inputs, so $h(\tau)$ must be 0 for $\tau < 0$ (negative τ implies future times in Eq. (14), although for computer-based operations, where future data may be available in memory, τ can be negative.

For discrete signals, the integration becomes a summation and the convolution equation becomes:

$$y(n) = \sum_{k=1}^{N} h(n - k)\, x(k) \qquad \text{or....}$$

$$y(n) = \sum_{k=1}^{N} h(n)\, x(k - n) \equiv h(n) * x(n) \qquad (15)$$

Again either $h(n)$ or $x(n)$ can be shifted. Also for discrete data, both $h(n)$ and $x(n)$ must be finite (since they are stored in finite memory), so the summation is also finite (where N is the length of the shorter function, usually $h(n)$).

In signal processing, convolution can be used to implement some of the basic filters described in Chapter 4. Like their analog counterparts, digital filters are just linear processes that modify the input spectra in some desired way (such as reducing noise). As with all linear processes, the filter's impulse response, $h(n)$, completely describes the filter. The process of sampling used in analog-to-digital conversion can also be viewed in terms of convolution: the sampled output $x(n)$ is just the convolution of the analog signal, $x(t)$, with a very short pulse (i.e., an impulse function) that is periodic with the sampling frequency. Convolution has signal processing implications that extend beyond the determination of input-output relationships. We will show later that convolution in the time domain is equivalent to multiplication in the frequency domain, and vice versa. The former has particular significance to sampling theory as described latter in this chapter.

---

*Of course, shifting both would be redundant.

Covariance and Correlation

The word correlation connotes similarity: how one thing is like another. Mathematically, correlations are obtained by multiplying and normalizing. Both *covariance* and *correlation* use multiplication to compare the linear relationship between two variables, but in correlation the coefficients are normalized to fall between zero and one. This makes the correlation coefficients insensitive to variations in the gain of the data acquisition process or the scaling of the variables. However, in many signal processing applications, the variable scales are similar, and covariance is appropriate. The operations of correlation and covariance can be applied to two or more waveforms, to multiple observations of the same source, or to multiple segments of the same waveform. These comparisons between data sequences can also result in a correlation or covariance matrix as described below.

Correlation/covariance operations can not only be used to compare different waveforms at specific points in time, they can also make comparisons over a range of times by shifting one signal with respect the other. The *crosscorrelation function* is an example of this process. The correlation function is the lagged product of two waveforms, and the defining equation, given here in both continuous and discrete form, is quite similar to the convolution equation above (Eqs. (14) and (15):

$$r_{xx}(t) = \int_0^T y(t) \ x(t + \tau) d\tau \tag{16a}$$

$$r_{xx}(n) = \sum_{k=1}^M y(k + n) \ x(k) \tag{16b}$$

Eqs. (16a) and (16b) show that the only difference in the computation of the crosscorrelation versus convolution is the direction of the shift. In convolution the waveforms are shifted in opposite directions. This produces a *causal* output: the output function is the creation of past values of the input function (the output is caused by the input). This form of shifting is reflected in the negative sign in Eq. (15). Crosscorrelation shows the similarity between two waveforms at all possible relative positions of one waveform with respect to the other, and it is useful in identifying segments of similarity. The output of Eq. (16) is sometimes termed the *raw correlation* since there is no normalization involved. Various scalings can be used (such as dividing by N, the number of in the sum), and these are described in the section on MATLAB implementation.

A special case of the correlation function occurs when the comparison is between two waveforms that are one in the same; that is, a function is correlated with different shifts of itself. This is termed the *autocorrelation function* and it provides a description of how similar a waveform is to itself at various time shifts, or *time lags*. The autocorrelation function will naturally be maximum for zero lag ($n = 0$) because at zero lag the comparison is between identical waveforms. Usually the autocorrelation is scaled so that the correlation at zero lag is 1. The function must be symmetric about $n = 0$, since shifting one version of the same waveform in the negative direction is the same as shifting the other version in the positive direction.

The autocorrelation function is related to the bandwidth of the waveform. The sharper the peak of the autocorrelation function the broader the bandwidth. For example, in white noise, which has infinite bandwidth, adjacent points are uncorrelated, and the autocorrelation function will be nonzero only for zero lag (see Problem 2). Figure 2.8 shows the autocorrelation functions of noise that has been filtered to have two different bandwidths. In statistics, the crosscorrelation and autocorrelation sequences are derived from the *expectation* operation applied to infinite data. In signal processing, data lengths are finite, so the *expec-*

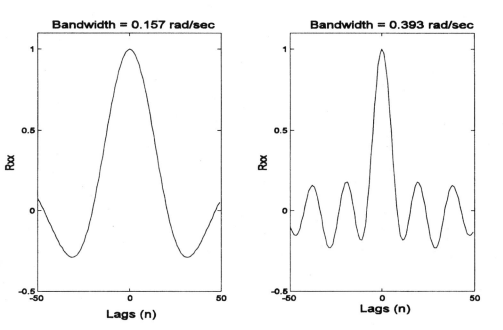

FIGURE 2.8 Autocorrelation functions of a random time series with a narrow bandwidth (left) and broader bandwidth (right). Note the inverse relationship between the autocorrelation function and the spectrum: the broader the bandwidth the narrower the first peak. These figures were generated using the code in Example 2.2 below.

tation operation becomes summation (with or without normalization), and the crosscorrelation and autocorrelation functions are necessarily estimations.

The crosscovariance function is the same as crosscorrelation function except that the means have been removed from the data before calculation. Accordingly, the equation is a slight modification of Eq. (16b), as shown below:

$$\text{Cov}(n) = \sum_{k=1}^{M} [y(k+n) - \bar{y}] [x(k) - \bar{x}] \tag{17}$$

The terms correlation and covariance, when used alone (i.e., without the term function), imply operations similar to those described in Eqs. (16) and (17), but without the lag operation. The result will be a single number. For example, the covariance between two functions is given by:

$$\text{Cov} = \sigma_{x,y} = \sum_{k=1}^{M} [y(k) - \bar{y}] [x(k) - \bar{x}] \tag{18}$$

Of particular interest is the covariance and correlation matrices. These analysis tools can be applied to *multivariate* data where multiple responses, or observations, are obtained from a single process. A representative example in biosignals is the EEG where the signal consists of a number of related waveforms taken from different positions on the head. The covariance and correlation matrices assume that the multivariate data are arranged in a matrix where the columns are different variables and the rows are different *observations* of those variables. In signal processing, the rows are the waveform time samples, and the columns are the different signal channels or observations of the signal. The covariance matrix gives the variance of the columns of the data matrix in the diagonals while the covariance between columns is given by the off-diagonals:

$$S = \begin{bmatrix} \sigma_{1,1} & \sigma_{1,2} & \cdots & \sigma_{1,N} \\ \sigma_{2,1} & \sigma_{2,2} & \cdots & \sigma_{2,N} \\ \vdots & \vdots & \ddots & \vdots \\ \sigma_{N,1} & \sigma_{N,2} & \cdots & \sigma_{N,N} \end{bmatrix} \tag{19}$$

An example of the use of the covariance matrix to compare signals is given in the section on MATLAB implementation.

In its usual signal processing definition, the correlation matrix is a normalized version of the covariance matrix. Specifically, the correlation matrix is related to the covariance matrix by the equation:

$$C(i,j) = \frac{C(i,j)}{\sqrt{C(i,i)\,C(j,j)}} \tag{20}$$

The correlation matrix is a set of correlation coefficients between waveform observations or channels and has a similar positional relationship as in the covariance matrix:

$$
R_{xx} = \begin{bmatrix} r_{xx}(0) & r_{xx}(1) & \cdots & r_{xx}(L) \\ r_{xx}(1) & r_{xx}(0) & \cdots & r_{xx}(L-1) \\ \vdots & \vdots & \ddots & \vdots \\ r_{xx}(L) & r_{xx}(L-1) & \cdots & r_{xx}(0) \end{bmatrix} \tag{21}
$$

Since the diagonals in the correlation matrix give the correlation of a given variable or waveform with itself, they will all equal 1 ($r_{xx}(0) = 1$), and the off-diagonals will vary between ± 1.

MATLAB Implementation

MATLAB has specific functions for performing convolution, crosscorrelation/autocorrelation, crossvariance/autocovariance, and construction of the correlation and covariance matrices. To implement convolution in MATLAB, the code is straightforward using the `conv` function:

```
y = conv(x,h)
```

where `x` and `h` are vectors containing the waveforms to be convolved and `y` is the output waveform. The length of the output waveform is equal to the length of `x` plus the length of `h` minus 1. This will produce additional data points, and methods for dealing with these extra points are presented at the end of this chapter, along with other problems associated with finite data. Frequently, the additional data points can simply be discarded. An example of the use of this routine is given in Example 2.2. Although the algorithm performs the process defined in equation in Eq. (15), it actually operates in the frequency domain to improve the speed of the operation.

The crosscorrelation and autocorrelation operations are both performed with the same MATLAB routine, with autocorrelation being treated as a special case:

```
[c,lags] = xcorr(x,y,maxlags,'options')
```

Only the first input argument, `x`, is required. If no `y` variable is specified, autocorrelation is performed. The optional argument `maxlags` specifies the shifting range. The shifted waveform is shifted between $\pm$ `maxlags`, or the default value which is $-N + 1$ to $N - 1$ where N is length of the input vector, `x`. If a `y` vector is specified then crosscorrelation is performed, and the same shifting range applies. If one of the waveforms the shorter than the other (as is usually the case), it is *zero padded* (defined and described at the end of this chapter) to be the same length as the longer segment; hence, N would be the length of longer waveform. A number of scaling operations can be specified by the argument `options`. If `options` equals `biased`, the output is divided by $1/N$ which gives a biased estimate of the crosscorrelation/autocorrelation function. If `options` equals `unbiased`, the output is scaled by $1/|N - M|$ where M is the length of the data output as defined below. Setting `options` to `coeff` is used in autocorrelation and scales the autocorrelation function so that the zero lag autocorrelation has a value equal to one. Finally `options` equals `none` indicates no scaling, which is the default.

The `xcorr` function produces an output argument, `c`, that is a vector of length 2 `maxlags` + 1 if `maxlags` is specified or $2N - 1$ if the default range is used. The optional output argument, `lags`, is simply a vector containing the lag values (i.e., a vector of integers ranging between $\pm$`maxlags` and is useful in plotting.

Autocovariance or crosscovariance is obtained using the `xcov` function:

```
[c,lags] = xcov(x,y,maxlags,'options')
```

The arguments are identical to those described above for the `xcorr` function.

Correlation or covariance matrices are calculated using the `corrcoef` or `cov` functions respectively. Again, the calls are similar for both functions:

```
Rxx = corrcoef(x)
S = cov(x), or S = cov(x,1);
```

Without the additional `1` in the calling argument, `cov` normalizes by $N - 1$, which provides the best unbiased estimate of the covariance matrix if the observations are from a Gaussian distribution. When the second argument is present, `cov` normalizes by N which produces the second moment of the observations about their mean.

Example 2.2 shows the use of both the convolution and autocorrelation functions. The program produces autocorrelation functions of noise bandlimited at two different frequencies. To generate the bandlimited (i.e., colored) noise used for the autocorrelation, an impulse response function is generated in the form of $\sin(x)/x$ (i.e., the sinc function). We will see in Chapter 4 that this is the impulse response of one type of lowpass filter. Convolution of this impulse response with a white noise sequence is used to generate bandlimited noise. A vector containing Gaussian white noise is produced using the `randn` routine and the lowpass filter is implemented by convolving the noise with the filter's impulse response. The result is noise bandlimited by the cutoff frequency of the filter. The output of the filter is then processed by the autocorrelation routine to produce the autocorrelation curves shown in Figure 2.8 above. The two figures were obtained for bandlimited noise having bandwidths of $\pi/20$ rad/sec and $\pi/8$ rad/sec. The variable wc specifies the cutoff frequency of the lowpass filter in the code below. The theory and implementation of a lowpass filter such as used below are presented in Chapter 4.

Example 2.2 Generate bandlimited noise and compute and plot the auto-correlation function for two different bandwidths.

```
% Example 2.2 and Figure 2.8
% Generate colored noise having two different bandwidths
%    and evaluate using autocorrelation.
%
close all; clear all;
N = 1024;               % Size of arrays
L = 100;                % FIR filter length
w = pi/20;              % Lowpass filter cutoff frequency
noise = randn(N,1);     % Generate noise
%
% Compute the impulse response of a lowpass filter
% This type of filter is covered in Chapter 4
%
wn = pi*[1/20 1/8];     % Use cutoff frequencies of π/20 and
                        %   π/8
for k = 1:2             % Repeat for two different cutoff
                        %   frequencies
 wc = wn(k);            % Assigning filter cutoff frequency
 for i = 1:L+1          % Generate sin(x)/x function
  n = i-L/2;            %   and make symmetrical
  if n = = 0
    hn(i) = wc/pi;
  else
    hn(i) = (sin(wc*(n)))/(pi*n); % Filter impulse response
  end
 end
 out = conv(hn,noise);              % Filter
 [cor, lags] = xcorr(out,'coeff'); % Calculate autocorrela-
                                    %   tion, normalized
 % Plot the autocorrelation functions
 subplot (1,2,k);
 plot(lags(1,:),cor(:,1),'k');     % Plot using 'lags' vector
 axis([-50 50 -.5 1.1]);           % Define axes scale
```

```
    ylabel('Rxx');                    % Labels
    xlabel('Lags(n)');
    title(['Bandwidth =
    'num2str(wc)]);
end
```

Example 2.3 evaluates the covariance and correlation of sinusoids that are, and are not, orthogonal. Specifically, this example demonstrates the lack of correlation and covariance between sinusoids that are orthogonal such as a sine and cosine at the same frequency and harmonically related sinusoids (i.e., those having multiple frequencies of one another). It also shows correlation and covariance for sinusoids that are not orthogonal such as sines that are not at harmonically related frequencies.

Example 2.3 Generate a data matrix where the columns consist of orthogonal and non-orthogonal sinusoids. Specifically, the data matrix should consist of a 1 Hz sine and a cosine, a 2 Hz sine and cosine, and a 1.5 Hz sine and cosine. The six sinusoids should all be at different amplitudes. The first four sinusoids are orthogonal and should show negligible correlation while the two 1.5 Hz sinusoids should show some correlation with the other sinusoids.

```
% Example 2.3
% Application of the correlation and covariance matrices to
% sinusoids that are orthogonal and non-orthogonal
%
clear all; close all;
N = 256;                           % Number of data points in
                                   %   each waveform
fs = 256;                          % Sample frequency
n = (1:N)/fs;                      % Generate 1 sec of data
%
% Generate the sinusoids as columns of the matrix
x(:,1) = sin(2*pi*n)';             % Generate a 1 Hz sin
x(:,2) = 2*cos(2*pi*n);            % Generate a 1 Hx cos
x(:,3) = 1.5*sin(4*pi*n)';         % Generate a 2 Hz sin
x(:,4) = 3*cos(4*pi*n)';           % Generate a 2 Hx cos
x(:,5) = 2.5*sin(3*pi*n)';         % Generate a 1.5 Hx sin
x(:,6) = 1.75*cos(3*pi*n)';        % Generate a 1.5 Hz cos
%
S = cov(x)                         % Print covariance matrix
C = corrcoef(x)                    %   and correlation matrix
```

The output from this program is a covariance and correlation matrix. The covariance matrix is:

```
S =
    0.5020    0.0000    0.0000    0.0000    0.0000   -0.4474
    0.0000    2.0078   -0.0000   -0.0000    1.9172   -0.0137
    0.0000   -0.0000    1.1294    0.0000   -0.0000    0.9586
    0.0000   -0.0000    0.0000    4.5176   -2.0545   -0.0206
    0.0000    1.9172   -0.0000   -2.0545    2.8548    0.0036
   -0.4474   -0.0137    0.9586   -0.0206    0.0036    1.5372
```

In the covariance matrix, the diagonals which give the variance of the six signals vary since the amplitudes of the signals are different. The covariance between the first four signals is zero, demonstrating the orthogonality of these signals. The correlation between the 5th and 6th signals and the other sinusoids can be best observed from the correlation matrix:

```
Rxx =
    1.0000    0.0000    0.0000    0.0000    0.0000   -0.5093
    0.0000    1.0000   -0.0000   -0.0000    0.8008   -0.0078
    0.0000   -0.0000    1.0000    0.0000   -0.0000    0.7275
    0.0000   -0.0000    0.0000    1.0000   -0.5721   -0.0078
    0.0000    0.8008   -0.0000   -0.5721    1.0000    0.0017
   -0.5093   -0.0078    0.7275   -0.0078    0.0017    1.0000
```

In the correlation matrix, the correlation of each signal with itself is, of course, 1.0. The 1.5 Hz sine (the 5th column of the data matrix) shows good correlation with the 1.0 and 2.0 Hz cosine (2nd and 4th rows) but not the other sinewaves, while the 1.5 Hz cosine (the 6th column) shows the opposite. Hence, sinusoids that are not harmonically related are not orthogonal and do show some correlation.

SAMPLING THEORY AND FINITE DATA CONSIDERATIONS

To convert an analog waveform into a digitized version residing in memory requires two operations: sampling the waveform at discrete points in time,* and, if the waveform is longer than the computer memory, isolating a segment of the analog waveform for the conversion. The waveform segmentation operation is *windowing* as mentioned previously, and the consequences of this operation are discussed in the next chapter. If the purpose of sampling is to produce a digitized copy of the original waveform, then the critical issue is how well does this copy represent the original? Stated another way, can the original be reconstructed from the digitized copy? If so, then the copy is clearly adequate. The

---

*As described in Chapter 1, this operation involves both time slicing, termed *sampling*, and amplitude slicing, termed *quantization*.

answer to this question depends on the frequency at which the analog waveform is sampled relative to the frequencies that it contains.

The question of what sampling frequency should be used can be best addressed assuming a simple waveform, a single sinusoid.* All finite, continuous waveforms can be represented by a series of sinusoids (possibly an infinite series), so if we can determine the appropriate sampling frequency for a single sinusoid, we have also solved the more general problem. The "Shannon Sampling Theorem" states that any sinusoidal waveform can be uniquely reconstructed provided it is sampled at least twice in one period. (Equally spaced samples are assumed). That is, the sampling frequency, f_s, must be $\geq 2f_{\text{sinusoid}}$. In other words, only two equally spaced samples are required to uniquely specify a sinusoid, and these can be taken anywhere over the cycle. Extending this to a general analog waveform, Shannon's Sampling Theorem states that a continuous waveform can be reconstructed without loss of information provided the sampling frequency is greater than twice the highest frequency in the analog waveform:

$$f_s > 2f_{\text{max}} \tag{22}$$

As mentioned in Chapter 1, in practical situations, f_{max} is usually taken as the highest frequency in the analog waveform for which less than a negligible amount of energy exists.

The sampling process is equivalent to multiplying the analog waveform by a repeating series of short pulses. This repeating series of short pulses is sometimes referred to as the sampling function. Recall that the ideal short pulse is called the impulse function, $\delta(t)$. In theory, the impulse function is infinitely short, but is also infinitely tall, so that its total area equals 1. (This must be justified using limits, but any pulse that is very short compared to the dynamics of the sampled waveform will due. Recall the sampling pulse produced in most modern analog-to-digital converters, termed the *aperture time*, is typically less than 100 nsec.) The sampling function can be stated mathematically using the impulse response.

$$S_{\text{amp}}(n) = \sum_{k=-\infty}^{\infty} \delta(n - kT_s) \tag{23}$$

where T_s is the sample interval and equals $1/f_s$.

For an analog waveform, $x(t)$, the sampled version, $x(n)$, is given by multiplying $x(t)$ by the sampling function in Eq. (22):

---

*A sinusoid has a straightforward frequency domain representation: only a single complex point at the frequency of the sinusoid. Classical methods of frequency analysis described in the next chapter make use of this fact.

$$x(n) = \sum_{k=-\infty}^{\infty} x(nT_s) \, \delta \, (n - kT_s) \tag{24}$$

The frequency spectrum of the sampling process represented by Eq. (23) can be determined by taking advantage of fact that multiplication in the time domain is equivalent to convolution in frequency domain (and vice versa). Hence, the frequency characteristic of a sampled waveform is just the convolution of the analog waveform spectrum with the sampling function spectrum. Figure 2.9A shows the spectrum of a sampling function having a repetition rate of T_s, and Figure 2.9B shows the spectrum of a hypothetical signal that has a well-defined maximum frequency, f_{max}. Figure 2.9C shows the spectrum of the sampled waveform assuming $f_s = 1/T_s \geq 2f_{max}$. Note that the frequency characteristic of the sampled waveform is the same as the original for the lower frequencies, but the sampled spectrum now has a repetition of the original spectrum reflected on either side of f_s and at multiples of f_s. Nonetheless, it would be possible to recover the original spectrum simply by filtering the sampled data by an ideal lowpass filter with a bandwidth $> f_{max}$ as shown in Figure 2.9E. Figure 2.9D shows the spectrum that results if the digitized data were sampled at $f_s < 2f_{max}$, in this case $f_s = 1.5f_{max}$. Note that the reflected portion of the spectrum has become intermixed with the original spectrum, and no filter can un-mix them.* When $f_s < 2f_{max}$, the sampled data suffers from spectral overlap, better known as *aliasing*. The sampled data no longer provides a unique representation of the analog waveform, and recovery is not possible.

When correctly sampled, the original spectrum can by recovered by applying an ideal lowpass filter (digital filter) to the digitized data. In Chapter 4, we show that an ideal lowpass filter has an impulse response given by:

$$h(n) = \frac{\sin(2\pi f_c T_s n)}{\pi n} \tag{25}$$

where T_s is the sample interval and f_c is the filter's cutoff frequency.

Unfortunately, in order for this impulse function to produce an ideal filter, it must be infinitely long. As demonstrated in Chapter 4, truncating $h(n)$ results in a filter that is less than ideal. However if $f_s \gg f_{max}$, as is often the case, then any reasonable lowpass filter would suffice to recover the original waveform, Figure 2.9F. In fact, using sampling frequencies much greater than required is the norm, and often the lowpass filter is provided only by the response characteristics of the output, or display device which is sufficient to reconstruct an adequate looking signal.

---

*You might argue that you could recover the original spectrum if you knew exactly the spectrum of the original analog waveform, but with this much information, why bother to sample the waveform in the first place!

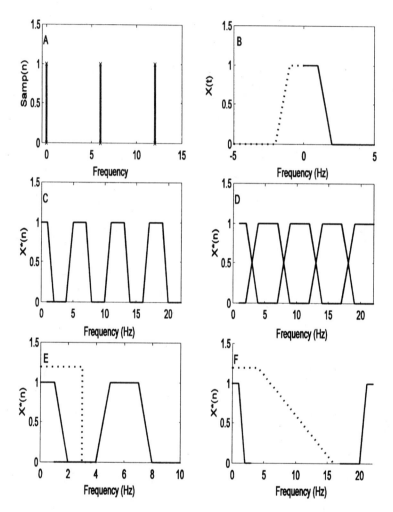

FIGURE 2.9 Consequences of sampling expressed in the frequency domain. (A) Frequency spectrum of a repetitive impulse function sampling at 6 Hz. (B) Frequency spectrum of a hypothetical time signal that has a maximum frequency, f_{max}, around 2 Hz. (Note negative frequencies occur with complex representation). (C) Frequency spectrum of sampled waveform when the sampling frequency was greater that twice the highest frequency component in the sampled waveform. (D) Frequency spectrum of sampled waveform when the sampling frequency was less that twice the highest frequency component in the sampled waveform. Note the overlap. (E) Recovery of correctly sampled waveform using an ideal lowpass filter (dotted line). (F) Recovery of a waveform when the sampling frequency is much much greater that twice the highest frequency in the sampled waveform ($f_s = 10 f_{max}$). In this case, the lowpass filter (dotted line) need not have as sharp a cutoff.

Edge Effects

An advantage of dealing with infinite data is that one need not be concerned with the end points since there are no end points. However, finite data consist of numerical sequences having a fixed length with fixed end points at the beginning and end of the sequence. Some operations, such as convolution, may produce additional data points while some operations will require additional data points to complete their operation on the data set. The question then becomes how to add or eliminate data points, and there are a number of popular strategies for dealing with these edge effects.

There are three common strategies for extending a data set when additional points are needed: extending with zeros (or a constant), termed *zero padding*; extending using periodicity or *wraparound*; and extending by reflection, also known as *symmetric extension*. These options are illustrated in Figure 2.10. In the zero padding approach, zeros are added to the end or beginning of the data sequence (Figure 2.10A). This approach is frequently used in spectral analysis and is justified by the implicit assumption that the waveform is zero outside of the sample period anyway. A variant of zero padding is *constant padding*, where the data sequence is extended using a constant value, often the last (or first) value in the sequence. If the waveform can be reasonably thought of as one cycle of a periodic function, then the wraparound approach is clearly justified (Figure 2.10B). Here the data are extended by tacking on the initial data sequence to the end of the data set and visa versa. This is quite easy to implement numerically: simply make all operations involving the data sequence index modulo N, where N is the initial length of the data set. These two approaches will, in general, produce a discontinuity at the beginning or end of the data set, which can lead to artifact in certain situations. The symmetric reflection approach eliminates this discontinuity by tacking on the end points in reverse order (or beginning points if extending the beginning of the data sequence) (Figure 2.10C).*

To reduce the number of points in cases where an operation has generated additional data, two strategies are common: simply eliminate the additional points at the end of the data set, or eliminate data from both ends of the data set, usually symmetrically. The latter is used when the data are considered periodic and it is desired to retain the same period or when other similar concerns are involved. An example of this is *circular* or *periodic convolution*. In this case, the original data set is extended using the wraparound strategy, convolution is performed on the extended data set, then the additional points are removed

---

*When using this extension, there is a question as to whether or not to repeat the last point in the extension; either strategy will produce a smooth extension. The answer to this question will depend on the type of operation being performed and the number of data points involved, and determining the best approach may require empirical evaluation.

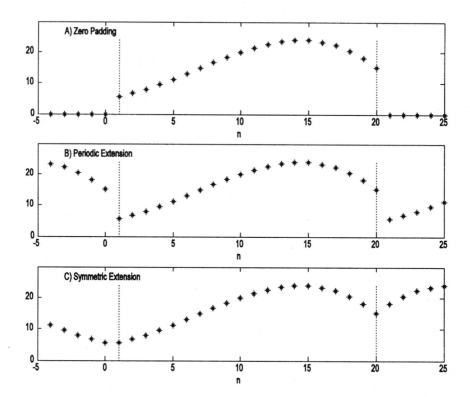

FIGURE 2.10 Three strategies for extending the length of a finite data set. (A) *Zero padding*: Zeros are added at the ends of the data set. (B) *Periodic* or *wrap-around*: The waveform is assumed periodic so the end points are added at the beginning, and beginning points are added at the end. (C) *Symmetric*: Points are added to the ends in reverse order. Using this strategy the edge points may be repeated as was done at the beginning of the data set, or not repeated as at the end of the set.

symmetrically. The goal is to preserve the relative phase between waveforms pre- and post-convolution. Periodic convolution is often used in wavelet analysis where a data set may be operated on sequentially a number of times, and examples are found in Chapter 7.

PROBLEMS

1. Load the data in `ensemble_data.mat` found in the CD. This file contains a data matrix labeled *data*. The data matrix contains 100 responses of a second-

order system buried in noise. In this matrix each row is a separate response. Plot several randomly selected samples of these responses. Is it possible to evaluate the second-order response from any single record? Construct and plot the ensemble average for this data. Also construct and plot the ensemble standard deviation.

2.   Use the MATLAB autocorrelation and random number routine to plot the autocorrelation sequence of white noise. Use arrays of 2048 and 256 points to show the affect of data length on this operation. Repeat for both uniform and Gaussian (normal) noise. (Use the MATLAB routines `rand` and `randn`, respectively.)

3.   Construct a 512-point noise arrray then filter by averaging the points three at a time. That is, construct a new array in which every point is the average of the preceding three points in the noise array: $y(n) = 1/3\ x(n) + 1/3\ x(n-1) + 1/3\ x(n-2)$. Note that the new array will be two points shorter than the original noise array. Construct and plot the autocorrelation of this filtered array. You may want to save the output, or the code that generates it, for use in a spectral analysis problem at the end of Chapter 3. (See Problem 2, Chapter 3.)

4.   Repeat the operation of Problem 3 to find the autocorrelation, but use convolution to implement the filter. That is, construct a filter function consisting of 3 equal coefficients of 1/3: (`h(n)` = `[1/3 1/3 1/3]`). Then convolve this weighting function with the random array using `conv`.

5.   Repeat the process in Problem 4 using a 10-weight averaging *filter*. (Note that it is much easier to implement such a *running average* filter with this many weights using convolution.)

6.   Construct an array containing the impulse response of a first-order process. The impulse of a first-order process is given by the equation: $y(t) = e^{-t/\tau}$ (scaled for unit amplitude). Assume a sampling frequency of 200 Hz and a time constant, τ, of 1 sec. Make sure the array is at least 5 time constants long. Plot this impulse response to verify its exponential shape. Convolve this impulse response with a 512-point noise array and construct and plot the autocorrelation function of this array. Repeat this analysis for an impulse response with a time constant of 0.2 sec. Save the outputs for use in a spectral analysis problem at the end of Chapter 3. (See Problems 4 and 5, Chapter 3.)

7.   Repeat Problem 5 above using the impulse response of a second-order underdamped process. The impulse response of a second-order underdamped system is given by:

$$y(t) = \frac{\delta}{\delta - 1}\ e^{-\delta 2\pi f_n t}\ \sin(2\pi f_n \sqrt{1 - \delta^2} t)$$

Use a sampling rate of 500 Hz and set the damping factor, δ, to 0.1 and the frequency, f_n (termed the undamped natural frequency), to 10 Hz. The array should be equivalent of at least 2.0 seconds of data. Plot the impulse response to check its shape. Again, convolve this impulse response with a 512-point noise array and construct and plot the autocorrelation function of this array. Save the outputs for use in a spectral analysis problem at the end of Chapter 3. (See Problem 6, Chapter 3.)

8. Construct 4 damped sinusoids similar to the signal, $y(t)$, in Problem 7. Use a damping factor of 0.04 and generate two seconds of data assuming a sampling frequency of 500 Hz. Two of the 4 signals should have an f_n of 10 Hz and the other two an f_n of 20 Hz. The two signals at the same frequency should be 90 degrees out of phase (replace the sin with a cos). Are any of these four signals orthogonal?

3

Spectral Analysis: Classical Methods

INTRODUCTION

Sometimes the frequency content of the waveform provides more useful information than the time domain representation. Many biological signals demonstrate interesting or diagnostically useful properties when viewed in the so-called *frequency domain*. Examples of such signals include heart rate, EMG, EEG, ECG, eye movements and other motor responses, acoustic heart sounds, and stomach and intestinal sounds. In fact, just about all biosignals have, at one time or another, been examined in the frequency domain. Figure 3.1 shows the time response of an EEG signal and an estimate of spectral content using the classical Fourier transform method described later. Several peaks in the frequency plot can be seen indicating significant energy in the EEG at these frequencies.

Determining the frequency content of a waveform is termed *spectral analysis*, and the development of useful approaches for this frequency decomposition has a long and rich history (Marple, 1987). Spectral analysis can be thought of as a *mathematical prism* (Hubbard, 1998), decomposing a waveform into its constituent frequencies just as a prism decomposes light into its constituent colors (i.e., specific frequencies of the electromagnetic spectrum).

A great variety of techniques exist to perform spectral analysis, each having different strengths and weaknesses. Basically, the methods can be divided into two broad categories: classical methods based on the Fourier transform and modern methods such as those based on the estimation of model parameters.

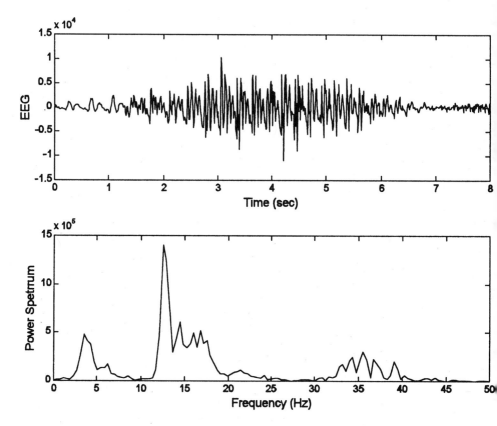

FIGURE 3.1   Upper plot: Segment of an EEG signal from the PhysioNet data bank (Golberger et al.), and the resultant power spectrum (lower plot).

The accurate determination of the waveform's spectrum requires that the signal be periodic, or of finite length, and noise-free. The problem is that in many biological applications the waveform of interest is either infinite or of sufficient length that only a portion of it is available for analysis. Moreover, biosignals are often corrupted by substantial amounts of noise or artifact. If only a portion of the actual signal can be analyzed, and/or if the waveform contains noise along with the signal, then all spectral analysis techniques must necessarily be approximate; they are estimates of the true spectrum. The various spectral analysis approaches attempt to improve the estimation accuracy of specific spectral features.

Intelligent application of spectral analysis techniques requires an understanding of what spectral features are likely to be of interest and which methods provide the most accurate determination of those features. Two spectral features of potential interest are the overall shape of the spectrum, termed the spectral estimate, and/or local features of the spectrum sometimes referred to as parametric estimates. For example, signal detection, finding a narrowband signal in broadband noise, would require a good estimate of local features. Unfortunately, techniques that provide good spectral estimation are poor local estimators and vice versa. Figure 3.2A shows the spectral estimate obtained by applying the traditional Fourier transform to a waveform consisting of a 100 Hz sine wave buried in white noise. The SNR is minus 14 db; that is, the signal amplitude is 1/5 of the noise. Note that the 100 Hz sin wave is readily identified as a peak in the spectrum at that frequency. Figure 3.2B shows the spectral estimate obtained by a smoothing process applied to the same signal (the Welch method, described later in this chapter). In this case, the waveform was divided into 32

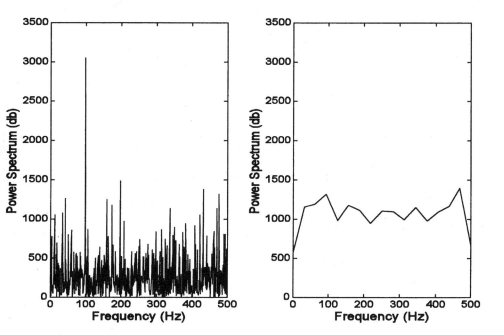

FIGURE 3.2 Spectra obtained from a waveform consisting of a 100 Hz sine wave and white noise using two different methods. The Fourier transform method was used to produce the left-hand spectrum and the spike at 100 Hz is clearly seen. An averaging technique was used to create the spectrum on the right side, and the 100 Hz component is no longer visible. Note, however, that the averaging technique produces a better estimate of the white noise spectrum. (The spectrum of white noise should be flat.)

segments, the Fourier transform was applied to each segment, then the 32 spectra were averaged. The resulting spectrum provides a more accurate representation of the overall spectral features (predominantly those of the white noise), but the 100 Hz signal is lost. Figure 3.2 shows that the smoothing approach is a good spectral estimator in the sense that it provides a better estimate of the dominant noise component, but it is not a good signal detector.

The classical procedures for spectral estimation are described in this chapter with particular regard to their strengths and weaknesses. These methods can be easily implemented in MATLAB as described in the following section. Modern methods for spectral estimation are covered in Chapter 5.

THE FOURIER TRANSFORM: FOURIER SERIES ANALYSIS

Periodic Functions

Of the many techniques currently in vogue for spectral estimation, the classical Fourier transform (FT) method is the most straightforward. The Fourier transform approach takes advantage of the fact that sinusoids contain energy at only one frequency. If a waveform can be broken down into a series of sines or cosines of different frequencies, the amplitude of these sinusoids must be proportional to the frequency component contained in the waveform at those frequencies.

From Fourier series analysis, we know that any periodic waveform can be represented by a series of sinusoids that are at the same frequency as, or multiples of, the waveform frequency. This family of sinusoids can be expressed either as sines and cosines, each of appropriate amplitude, or as a single sine wave of appropriate amplitude and phase angle. Consider the case where sines and cosines are used to represent the frequency components: to find the appropriate amplitude of these components it is only necessary to correlate (i.e., multiply) the waveform with the sine and cosine family, and average (i.e., integrate) over the complete waveform (or one period if the waveform is periodic). Expressed as an equation, this procedure becomes:

$$a(m) = \frac{1}{T} \int_0^T x(t) \cos(2\pi m f_T t) \, dt \tag{1}$$

$$b(m) = \frac{1}{T} \int_0^T x(t) \sin(2\pi m f_T t) \, dt \tag{2}$$

where T is the period or time length of the waveform, $f_T = 1/T$, and m is set of integers, possibly infinite: $m = 1, 2, 3, \ldots$, defining the family member. This gives rise to a family of sines and cosines having harmonically related frequencies, $m f_T$.

In terms of the general transform discussed in Chapter 2, the Fourier series analysis uses a probing function in which the family consists of harmonically related sinusoids. The sines and cosines in this family have valid frequencies only at values of m/T, which is either the same frequency as the waveform (when $m = 1$) or higher multiples (when $m > 1$) that are termed *harmonics*. Since this approach represents waveforms by harmonically related sinusoids, the approach is sometimes referred to as *harmonic decomposition*. For periodic functions, the Fourier transform and Fourier series constitute a bilateral transform: the Fourier transform can be applied to a waveform to get the sinusoidal components and the Fourier series sine and cosine components can be summed to reconstruct the original waveform:

$$x(t) = a(0)/2 + \sum_{m=0}^{\infty} a(k) \cos(2\pi m f_T t) + \sum_{m=0}^{\infty} b(k) \sin(2\pi m f_T t) \qquad (3)$$

Note that for most real waveforms, the number of sine and cosine components that have significant amplitudes is limited, so that a finite, sometimes fairly short, summation can be quite accurate. Figure 3.3 shows the construction

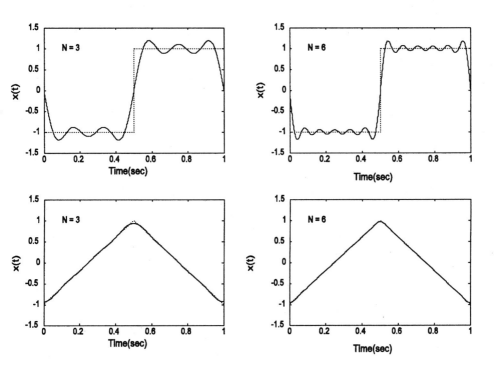

FIGURE 3.3 Two periodic functions and their approximations constructed from a limited series of sinusoids. Upper graphs: A square wave is approximated by a series of 3 and 6 sine waves. Lower graphs: A triangle wave is approximated by a series of 3 and 6 cosine waves.

of a square wave (upper graphs) and a triangle wave (lower graphs) using Eq. (3) and a series consisting of only 3 (left side) or 6 (right side) sine waves. The reconstructions are fairly accurate even when using only 3 sine waves, particularly for the triangular wave.

Spectral information is usually presented as a frequency plot, a plot of sine and cosine amplitude vs. component number, or the equivalent frequency. To convert from component number, m, to frequency, f, note that $f = m/T$, where T is the period of the fundamental. (In digitized signals, the sampling frequency can also be used to determine the spectral frequency). Rather than plot sine and cosine amplitudes, it is more intuitive to plot the amplitude and phase angle of a sinusoidal wave using the rectangular-to-polar transformation:

$$a \cos(x) + b \sin(x) = C \sin(x + \Theta) \tag{4}$$

where $C = (a^2 + b^2)^{1/2}$ and $\Theta = \tan^{-1}(b/a)$.

Figure 3.4 shows a periodic triangle wave (sometimes referred to as a *sawtooth*), and the resultant frequency plot of the magnitude of the first 10 components. Note that the magnitude of the sinusoidal component becomes quite small after the first 2 components. This explains why the triangle function can be so accurately represented by only 3 sine waves, as shown in Figure 3.3.

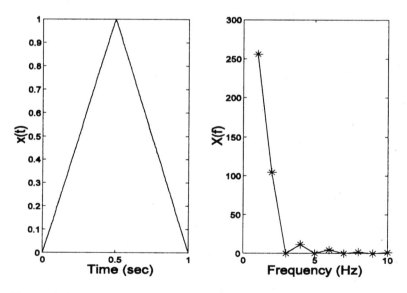

FIGURE 3.4 A triangle or sawtooth wave (left) and the first 10 terms of its Fourier series (right). Note that the terms become quite small after the second term.

Symmetry

Some waveforms are symmetrical or anti-symmetrical about $t = 0$, so that one or the other of the components, $a(k)$ or $b(k)$ in Eq. (3), will be zero. Specifically, if the waveform has mirror symmetry about $t = 0$, that is, $x(t) = x(-t)$, than multiplications by a sine functions will be zero irrespective of the frequency, and this will cause all $b(k)$ terms to be zeros. Such mirror symmetry functions are termed *even* functions. Similarly, if the function has anti-symmetry, $x(t) = -x(t)$, a so-called *odd* function, then all multiplications with cosines of any frequency will be zero, causing all $a(k)$ coefficients to be zero. Finally, functions that have *half-wave* symmetry will have no even coefficients, and both $a(k)$ and $b(k)$ will be zero for even m. These are functions where the second half of the period looks like the first half flipped left to right; i.e., $x(t) = x(T - t)$. Functions having half-wave symmetry can also be either odd or even functions. These symmetries are useful for reducing the complexity of solving for the coefficients when such computations are done manually. Even when the Fourier transform is done on a computer (which is usually the case), these properties can be used to check the correctness of a program's output. Table 3.1 summarizes these properties.

Discrete Time Fourier Analysis

The discrete-time Fourier series analysis is an extension of the continuous analysis procedure described above, but modified by two operations: sampling and windowing. The influence of sampling on the frequency spectra has been covered in Chapter 2. Briefly, the sampling process makes the spectra repetitive at frequencies mf_T ($m = 1,2,3, \ldots$), and symmetrically reflected about these frequencies (see Figure 2.9). Hence the discrete Fourier series of any waveform is theoretically infinite, but since it is periodic and symmetric about $f_s/2$, all of the information is contained in the frequency range of 0 to $f_s/2$ ($f_s/2$ is the *Nyquist* frequency). This follows from the sampling theorem and the fact that the original analog waveform must be bandlimited so that its highest frequency, f_{MAX}, is $<f_s/2$ if the digitized data is to be an accurate representation of the analog waveform.

TABLE 3.1 Function Symmetries

Function Name	Symmetry	Coefficient Values
Even	$x(t) = x(-t)$	$b(k) = 0$
Odd	$x(t) = -x(-t)$	$a(k) = 0$
Half-wave	$x(t) = x(T-t)$	$a(k) = b(k) = 0$; for m even

The digitized waveform must necessarily be truncated at least to the length of the memory storage array, a process described as *windowing*. The windowing process can be thought of as multiplying the data by some window shape (see Figure 2.4). If the waveform is simply truncated and no further shaping is performed on the resultant digitized waveform (as is often the case), then the window shape is rectangular by default. Other shapes can be imposed on the data by multiplying the digitized waveform by the desired shape. The influence of such windowing processes is described in a separate section below.

The equations for computing Fourier series analysis of digitized data are the same as for continuous data except the integration is replaced by summation. Usually these equations are presented using complex variables notation so that both the sine and cosine terms can be represented by a single exponential term using Euler's identity:

$$e^{jx} = \cos x + j \sin x \tag{5}$$

(Note mathematicians use i to represent $\sqrt{-1}$ while engineers use j; i is reserved for current.) Using complex notation, the equation for the discrete Fourier transform becomes:

$$X(m) = \sum_{n=0}^{N-1} x(n)e^{(-j2\pi mn/N)} \tag{6}$$

where N is the total number of points and m indicates the family member, i.e., the harmonic number. This number must now be allowed to be both positive and negative when used in complex notation: $m = -N/2, \ldots, N/2-1$. Note the similarity of Eq. (6) with Eq. (8) of Chapter 2, the general transform in discrete form. In Eq. (6), $f_m(n)$ is replaced by $e^{-j2\pi mn/N}$. The inverse Fourier transform can be calculated as:

$$x(n) = \frac{1}{N} \sum_{n=0}^{N-1} X(m) \, e^{-j2\pi n f_m T_s} \tag{7}$$

Applying the rectangular-to-polar transformation described in Eq. (4), it is also apparent $|X(m)|$ gives the magnitude for the sinusoidal representation of the Fourier series while the angle of $X(m)$ gives the phase angle for this representation, since $X(m)$ can also be written as:

$$X(m) = \sum_{n=0}^{N-1} x(n) \cos(2\pi mn/N) - j \sum_{n=0}^{N-1} x(n) \sin(2\pi mn/N) \tag{8}$$

As mentioned above, for computational reasons, $X(m)$ must be allowed to have both positive and negative values for m; negative values imply negative frequencies, but these are only a computational necessity and have no physical meaning. In some versions of the Fourier series equations shown above, Eq. (6)

is multiplied by T_s (the sampling time) while Eq. (7) is divided by T_s so that the sampling interval is incorporated explicitly into the Fourier series coefficients. Other methods of scaling these equations can be found in the literature.

The discrete Fourier transform produces a function of m. To convert this to frequency note that:

$$f_m = mf_1 = m/T_P = m/NT_s = mf_s/N \tag{9}$$

where $f_1 \equiv f_T$ is the fundamental frequency, T_s is the sample interval; f_s is the sample frequency; N is the number of points in the waveform; and $T_P = NTs$ is the period of the waveform. Substituting $m = f_m T_s$ into Eq. (6), the equation for the discrete Fourier transform (Eq. (6)) can also be written as:

$$X(f) = \sum_{n=0}^{N-1} x(n) \, e^{(-j2\pi n f_m T_s)} \tag{10}$$

which may be more useful in manual calculations.

If the waveform of interest is truly periodic, then the approach described above produces an accurate spectrum of the waveform. In this case, such analysis should properly be termed Fourier series analysis, but is usually termed Fourier transform analysis. This latter term more appropriately applies to aperiodic or truncated waveforms. The algorithms used in all cases are the same, so the term Fourier transform is commonly applied to all spectral analyses based on decomposing a waveform into sinusoids.

Originally, the Fourier transform or Fourier series analysis was implemented by direct application of the above equations, usually using the complex formulation. Currently, the Fourier transform is implemented by a more computationally efficient algorithm, the fast Fourier transform (FFT), that cuts the number of computations from N^2 to $2 \log N$, where N is the length of the digital data.

Aperiodic Functions

If the function is not periodic, it can still be accurately decomposed into sinusoids if it is aperiodic; that is, it exists only for a well-defined period of time, and that time period is fully represented by the digitized waveform. The only difference is that, theoretically, the sinusoidal components can exist at all frequencies, not just multiple frequencies or harmonics. The analysis procedure is the same as for a periodic function, except that the frequencies obtained are really only samples along a continuous frequency spectrum. Figure 3.5 shows the frequency spectrum of a periodic triangle wave for three different periods. Note that as the period gets longer, approaching an aperiodic function, the spectral shape does not change, but the points get closer together. This is reasonable

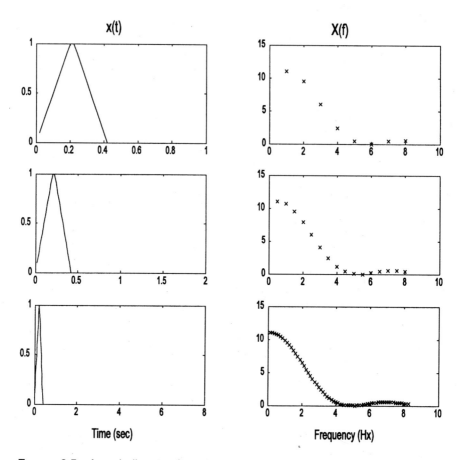

FIGURE 3.5 A periodic waveform having three different periods: 2, 2.5, and 8 sec. As the period gets longer, the shape of the frequency spectrum stays the same but the points get closer together.

since the space between the points is inversely related to the period (m/T).* In the limit, as the period becomes infinite and the function becomes truly aperiodic, the points become infinitely close and the curve becomes continuous. The analysis of waveforms that are not periodic and that cannot be completely represented by the digitized data is described below.

---

*The trick of adding zeros to a waveform to make it appear to a have a longer period (and, therefore, more points in the frequency spectrum) is another example of zero padding.

Frequency Resolution

From the discrete Fourier series equation above (Eq. (6)), the number of points produced by the operation is N, the number of points in the data set. However, since the spectrum produced is symmetrical about the midpoint, $N/2$ (or $f_s/2$ in frequency), only half the points contain unique information.* If the sampling time is T_s, then each point in the spectra represents a frequency increment of $1/(NT_s)$. As a rough approximation, the frequency resolution of the spectra will be the same as the frequency spacing, $1/(NT_s)$. In the next section we show that frequency resolution is also influenced by the type of windowing that is applied to the data.

As shown in Figure 3.5, frequency spacing of the spectrum produced by the Fourier transform can be decreased by increasing the length of the data, N. Increasing the sample interval, T_s, should also improve the frequency resolution, but since that means a decrease in f_s, the maximum frequency in the spectra, $f_s/2$ is reduced limiting the spectral range. One simple way of increasing N even after the waveform has been sampled is to use zero padding, as was done in Figure 3.5. Zero padding is legitimate because the undigitized portion of the waveform is always assumed to be zero (whether true or not). Under this assumption, zero padding simply adds more of the unsampled waveform. The zero-padded waveform appears to have improved resolution because the frequency interval is smaller. In fact, zero padding does not enhance the underlying resolution of the transform since the number of points that actually provide information remains the same; however, zero padding does provide an interpolated transform with a smoother appearance. In addition, it may remove ambiguities encountered in practice when a narrowband signal has a center frequency that lies between the $1/NT_s$ frequency evaluation points (compare the upper two spectra in Figure 3.5). Finally, zero padding, by providing interpolation, can make it easier to estimate the frequency of peaks in the spectra.

Truncated Fourier Analysis: Data Windowing

More often, a waveform is neither periodic or aperiodic, but a segment of a much longer—possibly infinite—time series. Biomedical engineering examples are found in EEG and ECG analysis where the waveforms being analyzed continue over the lifetime of the subject. Obviously, only a portion of such waveforms can be represented in the finite memory of the computer, and some attention must be paid to how the waveform is truncated. Often a segment is simply

---

*Recall that the Fourier transform contains magnitude and phase information. There are $N/2$ unique magnitude data points and $N/2$ unique phase data points, so the same number of actual data points is required to fully represent the data. Both magnitude and phase data are required to reconstruct the original time function, but we are often only interested in magnitude data for analysis.

cut out from the overall waveform; that is, a portion of the waveform is truncated and stored, without modification, in the computer. This is equivalent to the application of a rectangular *window* to the overall waveform, and the analysis is restricted to the *windowed* portion of the waveform. The window function for a rectangular window is simply 1.0 over the length of the window, and 0.0 elsewhere, (Figure 3.6, left side). Windowing has some similarities to the sampling process described previously and has well-defined consequences on the resultant frequency spectrum. Window shapes other than rectangular are possible simply by multiplying the waveform by the desired shape (sometimes these shapes are referred to as *tapering* functions). Again, points outside the window are assumed to be zero even if it is not true.

When a data set is windowed, which is essential if the data set is larger than the memory storage, then the frequency characteristics of the window become part of the spectral result. In this regard, all windows produce artifact. An idea of the artifact produced by a given window can be obtained by taking the Fourier transform of the window itself. Figure 3.6 shows a rectangular window on the left side and its spectrum on the right. Again, the absence of a window function is, by default, a rectangular window. The rectangular window, and in fact all windows, produces two types of artifact. The actual spectrum is widened by an artifact termed the *mainlobe*, and additional peaks are generated termed

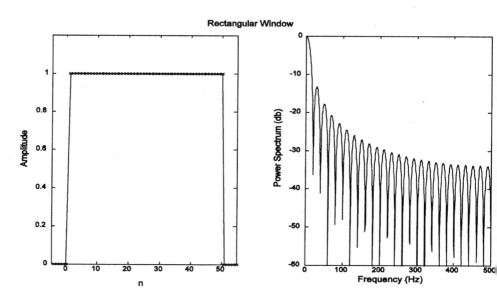

FIGURE 3.6 The time function of a rectangular window (left) and its frequency characteristics (right).

the *sidelobes*. Most alternatives to the rectangular window reduce the sidelobes (they decay away more quickly than those of Figure 3.6), but at the cost of wider mainlobes. Figures 3.7 and 3.8 show the shape and frequency spectra produced by two popular windows: the *triangular window* and the raised cosine or *Hamming window*. The algorithms for these windows are straightforward:

Triangular window:
for odd n:

$$w(k) = \begin{cases} 2k/(n - 1) & 1 \leq k \leq (n + 1)/2 \\ 2(n - k - 1)/(n + 1) & (n + 1)/2 \leq k \leq n \end{cases} \tag{11}$$

for even n:

$$w(k) = \begin{cases} (2k - 1)/n & 1 \leq k \leq n/2 \\ 2(n - k + 1)/n & (n/2) + 1 \leq k \leq n \end{cases} \tag{12}$$

Hamming window:

$$w(k + 1) = 0.54 - 0.46(2\pi k/(n - 1))k = 0, 1, \ldots, n - 1 \tag{13}$$

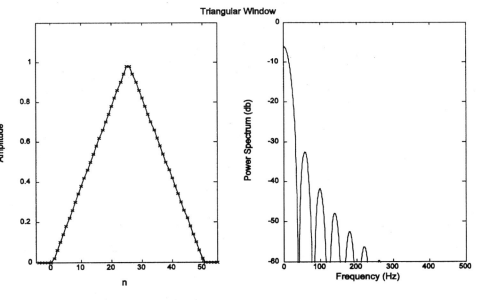

FIGURE 3.7 The triangular window in the time domain (left) and its spectral characteristic (right). The sidelobes diminish faster than those of the rectangular window (Figure 3.6), but the mainlobe is wider.

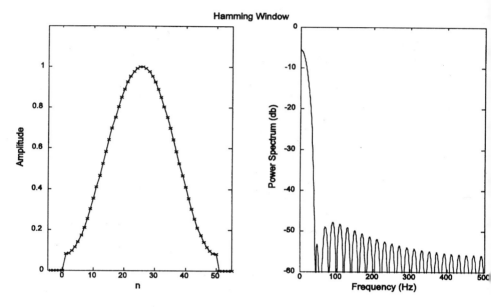

FIGURE 3.8 The Hamming window in the time domain (left) and its spectral characteristic (right).

These and several others are easily implemented in MATLAB, especially with the Signal Processing Toolbox as described in the next section. A MATLAB routine is also described to plot the spectral characteristics of these and other windows. Selecting the appropriate window, like so many other aspects of signal analysis, depends on what spectral features are of interest. If the task is to resolve two narrowband signals closely spaced in frequency, then a window with the narrowest mainlobe (the rectangular window) is preferred. If there is a strong and a weak signal spaced a moderate distance apart, then a window with rapidly decaying sidelobes is preferred to prevent the sidelobes of the strong signal from overpowering the weak signal. If there are two moderate strength signals, one close and the other more distant from a weak signal, then a compromise window with a moderately narrow mainlobe and a moderate decay in sidelobes could be the best choice. Often the most appropriate window is selected by trial and error.

Power Spectrum

The power spectrum is commonly defined as the Fourier transform of the autocorrelation function. In continuous and discrete notation, the power spectrum equation becomes:

$$PS(f) = \int_0^T r_{xx}(\tau) \, e^{-2\pi f_T \tau^\tau} \, d\tau$$

$$PS(f) = \sum_{n=0}^{N-1} r_{xx}(n) \, e^{-j2\pi n f_T T_s} \tag{14}$$

where $r_{xx}(n)$ is the autocorrelation function described in Chapter 2. Since the autocorrelation function has odd symmetry, the sine terms, b(k) will all be zero (see Table 3.1) and Eq. (14) can be simplified to include only real cosine terms.

$$PS(f) = \int_0^T r_{xx}(\tau) \, \cos(2\pi m f_T t) \, d\tau$$

$$PS(f) = \sum_{n=0}^{N-1} r_{xx}(n) \, \cos(2\pi n f_T T_s) \tag{15}$$

These equations in continuous and discrete form are sometimes referred to as the *cosine transform*. This approach to evaluating the power spectrum has lost favor to the so-called *direct approach*, given by Eq. (18) below, primarily because of the efficiency of the fast Fourier transform. However, a variation of this approach is used in certain time–frequency methods described in Chapter 6. One of the problems compares the power spectrum obtained using the direct approach of Eq. (18) with the traditional method represented by Eq. (14).

The direct approach is motivated by the fact that the energy contained in an analog signal, $x(t)$, is related to the magnitude of the signal squared, integrated over time:

$$E = \int_{-\infty}^{\infty} |x(t)|^2 \, dt \tag{16}$$

By an extension of Parseval's theorem it is easy to show that:

$$\int_{-\infty}^{\infty} |x(t)|^2 \, dt = \int_{-\infty}^{\infty} |X(f)|^2 \, df \tag{17}$$

Hence $|X(f)|^2$ equals the energy density function over frequency, also referred to as the energy spectral density, the *power spectral density*, or simply the *power spectrum*. In the direct approach, the power spectrum is calculated as the magnitude squared of the Fourier transform of the waveform of interest:

$$PS(f) = |X(f)|^2 \tag{18}$$

Power spectral analysis is commonly applied to truncated data, particularly when the data contains some noise, since phase information is less useful in such situations.

While the power spectrum can be evaluated by applying the FFT to the entire waveform, averaging is often used, particularly when the available waveform is only a sample of a longer signal. In such very common situations, power spectrum evaluation is necessarily an estimation process, and averaging improves the statistical properties of the result. When the power spectrum is based on a direct application of the Fourier transform followed by averaging, it is commonly referred to as an average *periodogram*. As with the Fourier transform, evaluation of power spectra involves necessary trade-offs to produce statistically reliable spectral estimates that also have high resolution. These trade-offs are implemented through the selection of the data window and the averaging strategy. In practice, the selection of data window and averaging strategy is usually based on experimentation with the actual data.

Considerations regarding data windowing have already been described and apply similarly to power spectral analysis. Averaging is usually achieved by dividing the waveform into a number of segments, possibly overlapping, and evaluating the Fourier transform on each of these segments (Figure 3.9). The final spectrum is taken from an average of the Fourier transforms obtained from the various segments. Segmentation necessarily reduces the number of data sam-

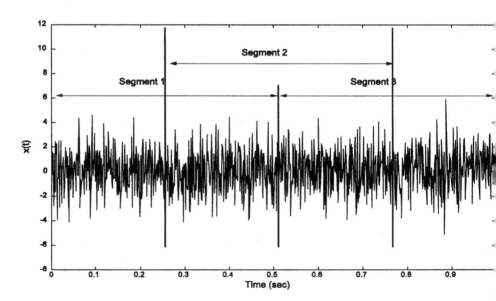

FIGURE 3.9 A waveform is divided into three segments with a 50% overlap between each segment. In the Welch method of spectral analysis, the Fourier transform of each segment would be computed separately, and an average of the three transforms would provide the output.

ples evaluated by the Fourier transform in each segment. As mentioned above, frequency resolution of a spectrum is approximately equal to $1/NT_s$, where N is now the number samples per segment. Choosing a short segment length (a small N) will provide more segments for averaging and improve the reliability of the spectral estimate, but it will also decrease frequency resolution. Figure 3.2 shows spectra obtained from a 1024-point data array consisting of a 100 Hz sinusoid and white noise. In Figure 3.2A, the periodogram is taken from the entire waveform, while in Figure 3.2B the waveform is divided into 32 non-overlapping segments; a Fourier transform is calculated from each segment, then averaged. The periodogram produced from the segmented and averaged data is much smoother, but the loss in frequency resolution is apparent as the 100 Hz sine wave is no longer visible.

One of the most popular procedures to evaluate the average periodogram is attributed to Welch and is a modification of the segmentation scheme origi-nally developed by Bartlett. In this approach, overlapping segments are used, and a window is applied to each segment. By overlapping segments, more seg-ments can be averaged for a given segment and data length. Averaged periodo-grams obtained from noisy data traditionally average spectra from half-overlap-ping segments; that is, segments that overlap by 50%. Higher amounts of overlap have been recommended in other applications, and, when computing time is not factor, maximum overlap has been recommended. Maximum overlap means shifting over by just a single sample to get the new segment. Examples of this approach are provided in the next section on implementation.

The use of data windowing for sidelobe control is not as important when the spectra are expected to be relatively flat. In fact, some studies claim that data windows give some data samples more importance than others and serve only to decrease frequency resolution without a significant reduction in estima-tion error. While these claims may be true for periodograms produced using all the data (i.e., no averaging), they are not true for the Welch periodograms be-cause overlapping segments serves to equalize data treatment and the increased number of segments decreases estimation errors. In addition, windows should be applied whenever the spectra are expected have large amplitude differences.

MATLAB IMPLEMENTATION

Direct FFT and Windowing

MATLAB provides a variety of methods for calculating spectra, particularly if the Signal Processing Toolbox is available. The basic Fourier transform routine is implemented as:

```
X = fft(x,n)
```

where **x** is the input waveform and **x** is a complex vector providing the sinusoidal coefficients. The argument **n** is optional and is used to modify the length of data analyzed: if **n** < **length(x)**, then the analysis is performed over the first **n** points; or, if **n** > **length(x)**, **x** is padded with trailing zeros to equal **n**. The **fft** routine implements Eq. (6) above and employs a high-speed algorithm. Calculation time is highly dependent on data length and is fastest if the data length is a power of two, or if the length has many prime factors. For example, on one machine a 4096-point FFT takes 2.1 seconds, but requires 7 seconds if the sequence is 4095 points long, and 58 seconds if the sequence is for 4097 points. If at all possible, it is best to stick with data lengths that are powers of two.

The magnitude of the frequency spectra can be easily obtained by applying the absolute value function, **abs**, to the complex output **X**:

```
Magnitude = abs(X)
```

This MATLAB function simply takes the square root of the sum of the real part of **x** squared and the imaginary part of **x** squared. The phase angle of the spectra can be obtained by application of the MATLAB **angle** function:

```
Phase = angle(X)
```

The **angle** function takes the arctangent of the imaginary part divided by the real part of **y**. The magnitude and phase of the spectrum can then be plotted using standard MATLAB plotting routines. An example applying the MATLAB **fft** to a array containing sinusoids and white noise is provided below and the resultant spectra is given in Figure 3.10. Other applications are explored in the problem set at the end of this chapter. This example uses a special routine, **sig_noise,** found on the disk. The routine generates data consisting of sinusoids and noise that are useful in evaluating spectral analysis algorithms. The calling structure for **sig_noise** is:

```
[x,t] = sig_noise([f],[SNR],N);
```

where **f** specifies the frequency of the sinusoid(s) in Hz, **SNR** specifies the desired noise associated with the sinusoid(s) in db, and **N** is the number of points. The routine assumes a sample frequency of 1 kHz. If **f** and **SNR** are vectors, multiple sinusoids are generated. The output waveform is in **x** and **t** is a time vector useful in plotting.

Example 3.1   Plot the power spectrum of a waveform consisting of a single sine wave and white noise with an SNR of −7 db.

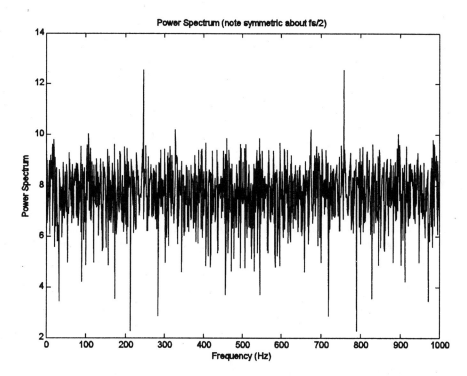

FIGURE 3.10 Plot produced by the MATLAB program above. The peak at 250 Hz is apparent. The sampling frequency of this data is 1 kHz, hence the spectrum is symmetric about the Nyquist frequency, $f_s/2$ (500 Hz). Normally only the first half of this spectrum would be plotted (SNR = −7 db; N = 1024).

```
% Example 3.1 and Figure 3.10 Determine the power spectrum
%   of a noisy waveform
% First generates a waveform consisting of a single sine in
%   noise, then calculates the power spectrum from the FFT
%   and plots
clear all; close all;
N = 1024;                        % Number of data points
% Generate data using sig_noise
%   250 Hz sin plus white noise; N data points ; SNR = -7 db
[x,t] = sig_noise (250,-7,N);
fs = 1000;                       % The sample frequency of data
                                 %   is 1 kHz.
Y = fft(x);                      % Calculate FFT
PS = abs(Y).^2;                  % Calculate PS as magnitude
                                 %   squared
```

```
freq = (1:N)/fs;                    % Frequency vector for plot-
                                      ting
plot(freq,20*log10(PS),'k');        % Plot PS in log scale
title('Power Spectrum (note symmetric about fs/2)');
xlabel('Frequency (Hz)');
ylabel('Power Spectrum (db)');
```

The Welch Method for Power Spectral Density Determination

As described above, the Welch method for evaluating the power spectrum divides the data in several segments, possibly overlapping, performs an FFT on each segment, computes the magnitude squared (i.e., power spectrum), then averages these spectra. Coding these in MATLAB is straightforward, but this is unnecessary as the Signal Processing Toolbox features a function that performs these operations. In its more general form, the pwelch* function is called as:

$$[PS,f] = pwelch(x,window,noverlap,nfft,fs)$$

Only the first input argument, the name of the data vector, is required as the other arguments have default values. By default, x is divided into eight sections with 50% overlap, each section is windowed with a Hamming window and eight periodograms are computed and averaged. If window is an integer, it specifies the segment length, and a Hamming window of that length is applied to each segment. If window is a vector, then it is assumed to contain the window function (easily implemented using the window routines described below). In this situation, the window size will be equal to the length of the vector, usually set to be the same as nfft. If the window length is specified to be less than nfft (greater is not allowed), then the window is zero padded to have a length equal to nfft. The argument noverlap specifies the overlap in samples. The sampling frequency is specified by the optional argument fs and is used to fill the frequency vector, f, in the output with appropriate values. This output variable can be used in plotting to obtain a correctly scaled frequency axis (see Example 3.2). As is always the case in MATLAB, any variable can be omitted, and the default selected by entering an empty vector, [ ].

If pwelch is called with no output arguments, the default is to plot the power spectral estimate in dB per unit frequency in the current figure window. If PS is specified, then it contains the power spectra. PS is only half the length of the data vector, x, specifically, either (nfft/2)+1 if nfft is even, or (nfft+1)/2 for nfft odd, since the additional points would be redundant. (An

---

*The calling structure for this function is different in MATLAB versions less than 6.1. Use the 'Help' command to determine the calling structure if you are using an older version of MATLAB.

exception is made if x is complex data in which case the length of PS is equal to nfft.) Other options are available and can be found in the help file for pwelch.

Example 3.2 Apply Welch's method to the sine plus noise data used in Example 3.1. Use 124-point data segments and a 50% overlap.

```
% Example 3.2 and Figure 3.11
% Apply Welch's method to sin plus noise data of Figure 3.10
clear all; close all;
N = 1024;                   % Number of data points
fs = 1000;                  % Sampling frequency (1 kHz)
```

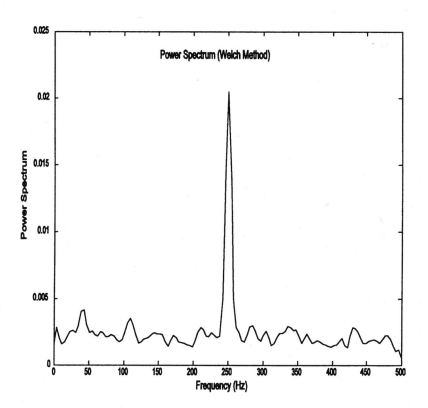

FIGURE 3.11 The application of the Welch power spectral method to data containing a single sine wave plus noise, the same as the one used to produce the spectrum of Figure 3.10. The segment length was 128 points and segments overlapped by 50%. A triangular window was applied. The improvement in the background spectra is obvious, although the 250 Hz peak is now broader.

```
% Generate data (250 Hz sin plus noise)
[x,t,] = sig_noise(250,-7,N);
%
% Estimate the Welch spectrum using 128 point segments,
%   a the triangular filter, and a 50% overlap.
%
[PS,f] = (x, triang(128),[ ],128,fs);
plot(f,PS,'k');            % Plot power spectrum
title('Power Spectrum (Welch Method)');
xlabel('Frequency (Hz)');
ylabel('Power Spectrum');
```

Comparing the spectra in Figure 3.11 with that of Figure 3.10 shows that the background noise is considerably smoother and reduced. The sine wave at 250 Hz is clearly seen, but the peak is now slightly broader indicating a loss in frequency resolution.

Window Functions

MATLAB has a number of data windows available including those described in Eqs. (11–13). The relevant MATLAB routine generates an n-point vector array containing the appropriate window shape. All have the same form:

```
w = window_name(N);      % Generate vector w of length N
                         %   containing the window function
                         %   of the associated name
```

where **N** is the number of points in the output vector and `window_name` is the name, or an abbreviation of the name, of the desired window. At this writing, thirteen different windows are available in addition to rectangular (`rectwin`) which is included for completeness. Using `help window` will provide a list of window names. A few of the more popular windows are: `bartlett`, `blackman`, `gausswin`, `hamming` (a common MATLAB default window), `hann`, `kaiser`, and `triang`. A few of the routines have additional optional arguments. In particular, `chebwin` (Chebyshev window), which features a nondecaying, constant level of sidelobes, has a second argument to specify the sidelobe amplitude. Of course, the smaller this level is set, the wider the mainlobe, and the poorer the frequency resolution. Details for any given window can be found through the `help` command. In addition to the individual functions, all of the window functions can be constructed with one call:

```
w = window(@name,N,opt) % Get N-point window 'name.'
```

where name is the name of the specific window function (preceded by ⓐ), **N** the number of points desired, and **opt** possible optional argument(s) required by some specific windows.

To apply a window to the Fourier series analysis such as in Example 2.1, simply point-by-point multiply the digitized waveform by the output of the MATLAB **window_name** routine before calling the FFT routine. For example:

```
w = triang (N);    % Get N-point triangular window curve
x = x .* w';       % Multiply (point-by-point) data by window
X = fft(x);        % Calculate FFT
```

Note that in the example above it was necessary to transpose the window function **w** so that it was in the same format as the data. The window function produces a row vector.

Figure 3.12 shows two spectra obtained from a data set consisting of two sine waves closely spaced in frequency (235 Hz and 250 Hz) with added white noise in a 256 point array sampled at 1 kHz. Both spectra used the Welch method with the same parameters except for the windowing. (The window func-

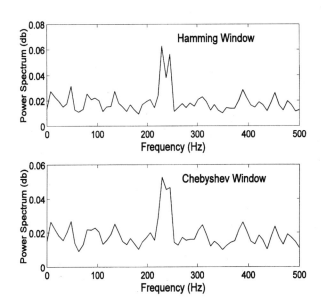

FIGURE 3.12 Two spectra computed for a waveform consisting of two closely spaced sine waves (235 and 250 Hz) in noise (SNR = –10 db). Welch's method was used for both methods with the same parameters (nfft = 128, overlap = 64) except for the window functions.

tion can be embedded in the `pwelch` calling structure.) The upper spectrum was obtained using a Hamming window (`hamming`) which has large sidelobes, but a fairly narrow mainlobe while the lower spectrum used a Chebyshev window (`chebwin`) which has small sidelobes but a larger mainlobe.

A small difference is seen in the ability to resolve the two peaks. The Hamming window with a smaller main lobe gives rise to a spectrum that shows two peaks while the presence of two peaks might be missed in the Chebyshev windowed spectrum.

PROBLEMS

1. (A) Construct two arrays of white noise: one 128 points in length and the other 1024 points in length. Take the FT of both. Does increasing the length improve the spectral estimate of white noise?

(B) Apply the Welch methods to the longer noise array using a Hanning window with an nfft of 128 with no overlap. Does this approach improve the spectral estimate? Now change the overlap to 64 and note any changes in the spectrum. Submit all frequency plots appropriately labeled.

2. Find the power spectrum of the filtered noise data from Problem 3 in Chapter 2 using the standard FFT. Show frequency plots appropriately labeled. Scale, or rescale, the frequency axis to adequately show the frequency response of this filter.

3. Find the power spectrum of the filtered noise data in Problem 2 above using the FFT, but zero pad the data so that $N = 2048$. Note the visual improvement in resolution.

4. Repeat Problem 2 above using the data from Problem 6 in Chapter 2. Applying the Hamming widow to the data before calculating the FFT.

5. Repeat problem 4 above using the Welch method with 256 and 65 segment lengths and the window of your choice.

6. Repeat Problem 4 above using the data from Problem 7, Chapter 2.

7. Use routine `sig_noise` noise to generate a 256-point array that contains two closely spaced sinusoids at 140 and 180 Hz both with an SNR of -10 db. (Calling structure: `data = sig_noise([140 180], [-10 -10], 256);`) `sig_noise` assumes a sampling rate of 1 kHz. Use the Welch method. Find the spectrum of the waveform for segment lengths of 256 (no overlap) and 64 points with 0%, 50% and 99% overlap.

8. Use `sig_noise` to generate a 512-point array that contains a single sinusoid at 200 Hz with an SNR of -12 db. Find the power spectrum first by taking the

FFT of the autocorrelation function. Compare this power spectrum with the one obtained using the direct method. Plot the two spectra side-by-side.

9. Using the data of Problem 7 above, find the power spectrum applying the Welch method with 64-point segments, and no overlap. Using the Chebyshev (`chebwin`), Kaiser (`kaiser`), and Gauss (`gausswin`) windows, find the best window in terms of frequency separation. Submit frequency plots obtained using the best and worse windows (in terms of separation). For the Chebyshev window use a ripple of 40 db, and for the Kaiser window use a beta of 0 (minimum mainlobe option).

10. Use routine `sig_noise` to generate a 512-point array containing one sinusoid at 150 Hz and white noise; SNR = −15db. Generate the power spectrum as the square of the magnitude obtained using the Fourier transform. Put the signal generator commands and spectral analysis commands in a loop and calculate the spectrum five times plotting the five spectra superimposed. Repeat using the Welch method and data segment length of 128 and a 90% overlap.

4

Digital Filters

Filters are closely related to spectral analysis since the goal of filtering is to reshape the spectrum to one's advantage. Most noise is broadband (the broadest-band noise being white noise with a flat spectrum) and most signals are narrow-band; hence, filters that appropriately reshape a waveform's spectrum will almost always provide some improvement in SNR. As a general concept, a basic filter can be viewed as a linear process in which the input signal's spectrum is reshaped in some well-defined (and, one hopes, beneficial) manner. Filters differ in the way they achieve this spectral reshaping, and can be classified into two groups based on their approach. These two groups are termed *finite impulse response* (FIR) filters and *infinite impulse response* (IIR) filters, although this terminology is based on characteristics which are secondary to the actual methodology. We will describe these two approaches separately, clarifying the major differences between them. As in preceding chapters, these descriptions will be followed by a presentation of the MATLAB implementation.

THE Z-TRANSFORM

The frequency-based analysis introduced in the last chapter is a most useful tool for analyzing systems or responses in which the waveforms are periodic or aperiodic, but cannot be applied to transient responses of infinite length, such as step functions, or systems with nonzero initial conditions. These shortcomings motivated the development of the *Laplace transform* in the analog domain. Laplace analysis uses the complex variable s ($s = \sigma + j\omega$) as a representation of complex frequency in place of $j\omega$ in the Fourier transform. The *Z-transform* is a digital operation analogous to the Laplace transform in the analog domain, and it is used in a similar manner. The Z-transform is based around the complex variable, z, where z is an arbitrary complex number, $|z|\, e^{j\omega}$. This variable is also termed the complex frequency, and as with its time domain counterpart, the Laplace variable s, it is possible to substitute $e^{j\omega}$ for z to perform a strictly sinusoidal analysis.*

The Z-transform follows the format of the general transform equation (Eq. (7)) and is also similar to the Fourier transform equation (Eq. (6)):

$$X(z) \triangleq Z[x(n)] = \sum_{n=-\infty}^{\infty} x(n)\, Z^{-n} \tag{1}$$

where z = an arbitrary complex variable. Note that the probing function for this transform is simply z^{-n}. In any real application, the limit of the summation will be finite, usually the length of $x(n)$.

When identified with a data sequence, such as $x(n)$ above, z^{-n} represents an interval shift of n samples, or an associated time shift of nT_s seconds. Note that Eq. (1) indicates that every data sample in the sequence $x(n)$ is associated with a unique power of z, and this power of z defines a sample's position in the sequence. This time shifting property of z^{-n} can be formally stated as:

$$Z(x(n - k))] = z^{-k}\, Z(x(n)) \tag{2}$$

For example, the time shifting characteristic of the Z-transform can be used to define a unit delay process, z^{-1}. For such a process, the output is the same as the input, but shifted (or delayed) by one data sample (Figure 4.1).

Digital Transfer Function

As in Laplace transform analysis, one of the most useful applications of the Z-transform lies in its ability to define the digital equivalent of a transfer function.

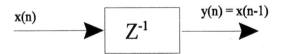

FIGURE 4.1 A *unit delay* process shifts the input by one data sample. Other powers of z could be used to provide larger shifts.

---

*If $|z|$ is set to 1, then $z = e^{j\omega}$. This is called evaluating z on the unit circle. See Bruce (2001) for a thorough discussion of the properties of z and the Z-transform.

By analogy to linear system analysis, the digital transfer function is defined as:

$$H(z) = \frac{Y(z)}{X(z)} \tag{3}$$

For the simple example of Figure 4.1, the digital transfer function would be: $H(z) = z^{-1}$. Of course, most transfer functions will be more complicated, including polynomials of z in both the numerator and denominator, just as analog transfer functions contain polynomials of s:

$$H(z) = \frac{b_0 + b_1 z^{-1} + b_2 z^{-2} + \cdots + b_N z^{-N}}{1 + a_1 z^{-1} + a_2 z^{-2} + \cdots + b_D z^{-D}} \tag{4}$$

While $H(z)$ has a structure similar to the Laplace domain transfer function $H(s)$, there is no simple relationship between them. For example, unlike analog systems, the order of the numerator, N, need not be less than, or equal to, the order of the denominator, D, for stability. In fact, systems that have a denominator order of 1 are more stable that those having higher order denominators.

From the digital transfer function, $H(z)$, it is possible to determine the output given any input. In the Z-transform domain this relationship is simply:

$$Y(z) = H(z)\, X(z) = X(z)\, \frac{\sum\limits_{k=0}^{N-1} b(k)\, z^{-n}}{\sum\limits_{\ell=0}^{D-1} a(\ell)\, z^{-n}} \tag{5}$$

The input–output or difference equation analogous to the time domain equation can be obtained from Eq. (5) by applying the time shift interpretation to the term z^{-n} :

$$y(n) = \sum_{k=0}^{K} b(k)\, x(n-k) - \sum_{\ell=0}^{L} a(\ell)\, y(n-\ell) \tag{6}$$

This equation assumes that a(0) = 1 as specified in Eq. (4). We will find that Eq. (6) is similar to the equation representing other linear processes such as the ARMA model in Chapter 5 (Eq. (3), Chapter 5). This is appropriate as the ARMA model is a linear digital process containing both denominator terms and numerator terms.*

All basic digital filters can be interpreted as linear digital processes, and, in fact, the term digital filter is often used interchangeably with digital systems (Stearns and David, 1996). Filter design, then, is simply the determination of

---

*Borrowing from analog terminology, the terms *poles* is sometimes uses for denominator coefficients and *zeros* for numerator coefficients.

the appropriate filter coefficients, $a(n)$ and $b(n)$, that provide the desired spectral shaping. This design process can be aided by MATLAB routines that can generate the $a(n)$ and $b(n)$ coefficients of Eq. (6) given a desired frequency response.

If the frequency spectrum of $H(z)$ is desired, it can be obtained from a modification of Eq. (5) substituting $z = e^{j\omega}$:

$$H(m) = \frac{Y(m)}{X(m)} = \frac{\sum_{n=0}^{N-1} b(n)\, e^{(-j2\pi mn/N)}}{\sum_{n=0}^{D-1} a(n)\, e^{(-j2\pi mn/N)}} = \frac{\text{fft}(b_n)}{\text{fft}(a_n)} \tag{7}$$

where fft indicates the Fourier transform. As with all Fourier transforms, frequency can be obtained from the variable m by multiplying by f_s/N or $1/(NT_s)$.

MATLAB Implementation

Many MATLAB functions used in filter design and application can also be used in digital transfer function analysis. The MATLAB routine `filter` described below uses Eq. (6) to implement a digital filter, but can be used to implement a linear process given the Z-transform transfer function (see Example 4.1). With regard to implementation, note that if the $a(\ell)$ coefficients in Eq. (6) are zero (with the exception of $a(0) = 1$), Eq. (6) reduces to convolution (see Eq. (15) in Chapter 2).

The function `filter` determines the output, $y(n)$, to an input, $x(n)$, for a linear system with a digital transfer function as specified by the a and b coefficients. Essentially this function implements Eq. (6). The calling structure is:

```
y = filter(b,a,x)
```

where `x` is the input, `y` the output, and `b` and `a` are the coefficients of the transfer function in Eq. (4).

Example 4.1   Find and plot the frequency spectrum and the impulse response of a digital linear process having the digital transfer function:

$$H(z) = \frac{0.2 + 0.5z^{-1}}{1 - 0.2z^{-1} + 0.8z^{-2}}$$

Solution: Find $H(z)$ using MATLAB's `fft`. Then construct an impulse function and determine the output using the MATLAB `filter` routine.

```
% Example 4.1 and Figures 4.2 and 4.3
% Plot the frequency characteristics and impulse response
```

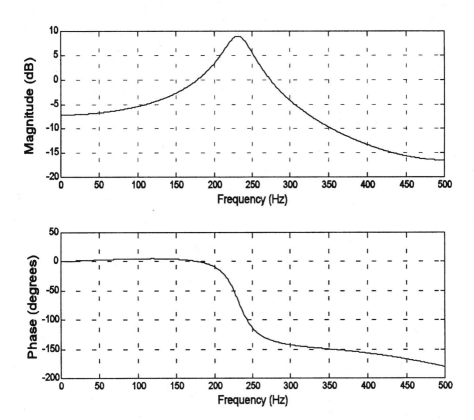

FIGURE 4.2 Plot of frequency characteristic (magnitude and phase) of the digital transfer function given above.

```
%       of a linear digital system with the given digital
%    transfer function
%    Assume a sampling frequency of 1 kHz
%
close all; clear all;
fs = 1000;                      % Sampling frequency
N = 512;                        % Number of points
% Define a and b coefficients based on H(z)
a = [1-.2 .8];                  % Denominator of transfer
                                %   function
b = [.2 .5];                    % Numerator of transfer function
%
% Plot the Frequency characteristic of H(z) using the fft
H = fft(b,N)./fft(a,N);         % Compute H(f)
```

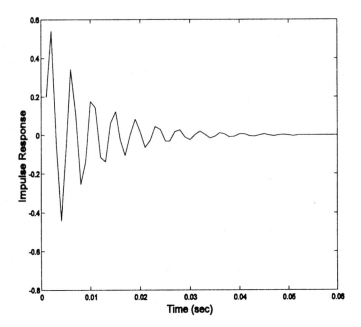

FIGURE 4.3 Impulse response of the digital transfer function described above. Both Figure 4.2 and Figure 4.3 were generated using the MATLAB code given in Example 1.

```
Hm = 20*log10(abs(H));          % Get magnitude in db
Theta = (angle(H)) *2*pi;       % and phase in deg.
f = (1:N/2) *fs/N;              % Frequency vector for plotting
%
subplot(2,1,1);
  plot(f,Hm(1:N/2),'k');        % Plot and label mag H(f)
  xlabel ('Frequency (Hz)'); ylabel('|H(z)| (db)');
  grid on;                      % Plot using grid lines
subplot(2,1,2);
  plot(f,Theta(1:N/2),'k');  % Plot the phase
xlabel ('Frequency (Hz)'); ylabel('Phase (deg)');
grid on;
%
%
% Compute the Impulse Response
x = [1, zeros(1,N-1)];          % Generate an impulse function
y = filter(b,a,x);             % Apply b and a to impulse using
                               % Eq. (6)
```

```
figure;                        % New figure
t = (1:N)/fs;
plot(t(1:60),y(1:60),'k');     % Plot only the first 60 points
                               %  for clarity
    xlabel('Time (sec)'); ylabel ('Impulse Response');
```

The digital filters described in the rest of this chapter use a straightforward application of these linear system concepts. The design and implementation of digital filters is merely a question of determining the $a(n)$ and $b(n)$ coefficients that produce linear processes with the desired frequency characteristics.

FINITE IMPULSE RESPONSE (FIR) FILTERS

FIR filters have transfer functions that have only numerator coefficients, i.e., $H(z) = B(z)$. This leads to an impulse response that is finite, hence the name. They have the advantage of always being stable and having linear phase shifts. In addition, they have initial transients that are of finite durations and their extension to 2-dimensional applications is straightforward. The downside of FIR filters is that they are less efficient in terms of computer time and memory than IIR filters. FIR filters are also referred to as *nonrecursive* because only the input (not the output) is used in the filter algorithm (i.e., only the first term of Eq. (6) is used).

A simple FIR filter was developed in the context of Problem 3 in Chapter 2. This filter was achieved taking three consecutive points in the input array and averaging them together. The filter output was constructed by moving this three-point average along the input waveform. For this reason, FIR filtering has also been referred to as a *moving average* process. (This term is used for any process that uses a moving set of multiplier weights, even if the operation does not really produce an average.) In Problem 4 of Chapter 2, this filter was implemented using a three weight filter, [1/3 1/3 1/3], which was convolved with the input waveform to produce the filtered output. These three numbers are simply the $b(n)$ coefficients of a third-order, or three-weight, FIR filter. All FIR filters are similar to this filter; the only difference between them is the number and value of the coefficients.

The general equation for an FIR filter is a simplification of Eq. (6) and, after changing the limits to conform with MATLAB notation, becomes:

$$y(k) = \sum_{n=1}^{L} b(n)\, x(k - n) \tag{8}$$

where $b(n)$ is the *coefficient function* (also referred to as the *weighting function*) of length L, $x(n)$ is the input, and $y(n)$ is the output. This is identical to the convolution equation in Chapter 2 (Eq. (15)) with the impulse response, $h(n)$, replaced by the filter coefficients, $b(n)$. Hence, FIR filters can be implemented using either convolution or MATLAB's `filter` routine. Eq. (8) indicates that the filter coefficients (or weights) of an FIR filter are the same as the impulse response of the filter. Since the frequency response of a process having an impulse response $h(n)$ is simply the Fourier transform of $h(n)$, the frequency response of an FIR filter having coefficients $b(n)$ is just the Fourier transform of $b(n)$:

$$X(m) = \sum_{n=0}^{N-1} b(n) \, e^{(-j2\pi \, mn/N)} \tag{9}$$

Eq. (9) is a special case of Eq. (5) when the denominator equals one. If $b(n)$ generally consists of a small number of elements, this equation can sometimes be determined manually as well as by computer.

The inverse operation, going from a desired frequency response to the coefficient function, $b(n)$, is known as *filter design*. Since the frequency response is the Fourier transform of the filter coefficients, the coefficients can be found from the inverse Fourier transform of the desired frequency response. This design strategy is illustrated below in the design of a FIR lowpass filter based on the spectrum of an ideal filter. This filter is referred to as a *rectangular window* filter* since its spectrum is ideally a rectangular window.

FIR Filter Design

The ideal lowpass filter was first introduced in Chapter 1 as a rectangular window in the frequency domain (Figure 1.7). The inverse Fourier transform of a rectangular window function is given in Eq. (25) in Chapter 2 and repeated here with a minor variable change:

$$b(n) = \frac{\sin[2\pi f_c T_s(n - L/2)]}{\pi(n - L/2)} \tag{10}$$

where f_c is the cutoff frequency; T_s is the sample interval in seconds; and L is the length of the filter. The argument, $n - L/2$, is used to make the coefficient function symmetrical giving the filter linear phase characteristics. Linear phase characteristics are a desirable feature not easily attainable with IIR filters. The coefficient function, $b(n)$, produced by Eq. (10), is shown for two values of f_c in Figure 4.4. Again, this function is the same as the impulse response. Unfortu-

---

*This filter is sometimes called a *window filter*, but the term *rectangular window* filter will be used in this text so as not to confuse the filter with a *window function* as described in the last chapter. This can be particularly confusing since, as we show later, rectangular window filters also use window functions!

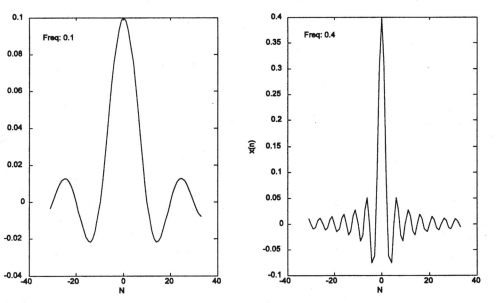

FIGURE 4.4 Symmetrical weighting function of a rectangular filter (Eq. (10)) truncated at 64 coefficients. The cutoff frequencies are given relative to the sampling frequency, f_s, as is often done in discussing digital filter frequencies. Left: Lowpass filter with a cutoff frequency of $0.1 f_s/2$ Hz. Right: Lowpass cutoff frequency of $0.4 f_s/2$ Hz.

nately this coefficient function must be infinitely long to produce the filter characteristics of an ideal filter; truncating it will result in a lowpass filter that is less than ideal. Figure 4.5 shows the frequency response, obtained by taking the Fourier transform of the coefficients for two different lengths. This filter also shows a couple of artifacts associated with finite length: an oscillation in the frequency curve which increases in frequency when the coefficient function is longer, and a peak in the passband which becomes narrower and higher when the coefficient function is lengthened.

Since the artifacts seen in Figure 4.5 are due to truncation of an (ideally) infinite function, we might expect that some of the window functions described in Chapter 3 would help. In discussing window frequency characteristics in Chapter 3, we noted that it is desirable to have a narrow mainlobe and rapidly diminishing sidelobes, and that the various window functions were designed to make different compromises between these two features. When applied to an FIR weight function, the width of the mainlobe will influence the sharpness of the transition band, and the sidelobe energy will influence the oscillations seen

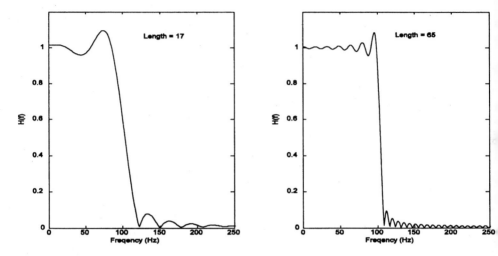

FIGURE 4.5 Freuquency characteristics of an FIR filter based in a weighting function derived from Eq. (10). The weighting functions were abruptly truncated at 17 and 65 coefficients. The artifacts associated with this truncation are clearly seen. The lowpass cutoff frequency is 100 Hz.

in Figure 4.5. Figure 4.6 shows the frequency characteristics that are produced by the same coefficient function used in Figure 4.4 except that a Hamming window has been applied to the filter weights. The artifacts are considerably diminished by the Hamming window: the overshoot in the passband has disappeared and the oscillations are barely visible in the plot. As with the unwindowed filter, there is a significant improvement in the sharpness of the transition band for the filter when more coefficients are used.

The FIR filter coefficients for highpass, bandpass, and bandstop filters can be derived in the same manner from equations generated by applying an inverse FT to rectangular structures having the appropriate associated shape. These equations have the same general form as Eq. (10) except they include additional terms:

$$b(n) = \frac{\sin[\pi(n - L/2)]}{\pi(n - L/2)} - \frac{\sin[2\pi f_c T_s(n - L/2)]}{\pi(n - L/2)} \quad \text{Highpass} \quad (11)$$

$$b(n) = \frac{\sin[2\pi f_H T(n - L/2)]}{\pi(n - L/2)} - \frac{\sin[2\pi f_L T_s(n - L/2)]}{\pi(n - L/2)} \quad \text{Bandpass} \quad (12)$$

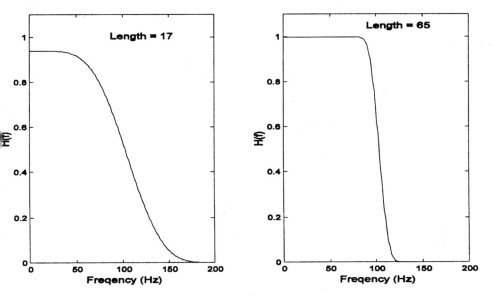

FIGURE 4.6 Frequency characteristics produced by an FIR filter identical to the one used in Figure 4.5 except a Hamming function has been applied to the filter coefficients. (See Example 1 for the MATLAB code.)

$$b(n) = \frac{\sin[2\pi f_L T(n - L/2)]}{\pi(n - L/2)} + \frac{\sin[\pi(n - L/2)]}{\pi(n - L/2)}$$
$$- \frac{\sin[2\pi f_H T_s(n - L/2)]}{\pi(n - L/2)} \quad \text{Bandstop} \tag{13}$$

An FIR bandpass filter designed using Eq. (12) is shown in Figure 4.7 for two different truncation lengths. Implementation of other FIR filter types is a part of the problem set at the end of this chapter. A variety of FIR filters exist that use strategies other than the rectangular window to construct the filter coefficients, and some of these are explored in the section on MATLAB implementation. One FIR filter of particular interest is the filter used to construct the derivative of a waveform since the derivative is often of interest in the analysis of biosignals. The next section explores a popular filter for this operation.

Derivative Operation: The Two-Point Central Difference Algorithm

The derivative is a common operation in signal processing and is particularly useful in analyzing certain physiological signals. Digital differentiation is de-

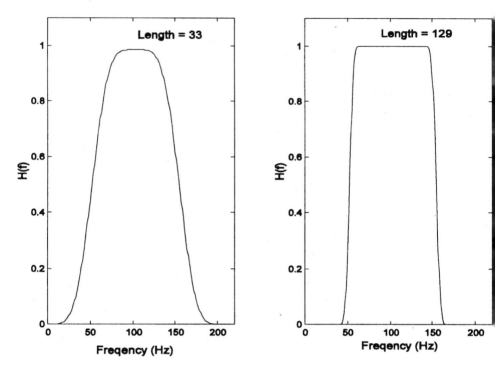

FIGURE 4.7 Frequency characteristics of an FIR Bandpass filter with a coefficient function described by Eq. (12) in conjuction with the Blackman window function. The low and high cutoff frequencies were 50 and 150 Hz. The filter function was truncated at 33 and 129 coefficients. These figures were generated with code similar to that in Example 4.2 below, except modified according to Eq. (12)

fined as $\Delta x/\Delta t$ and can be implemented by taking the difference between two adjacent points, scaling by $1/T_s$, and repeating this operation along the entire waveform. In the context of the FIR filters described above, this is equivalent to a two coefficient filter, $[-1, +1]/T_s$, and this is the approach taken by MATLAB's **derv** routine. The frequency characteristic of the derivative operation is a linear increase with frequency, Figure 4.8 (dashed line) so there is considerable gain at the higher frequencies. Since the higher frequencies frequently contain a greater percentage of noise, this operation tends to produce a noisy derivative curve. Figure 4.9A shows a noisy physiological motor response (vergence eye movements) and the derivative obtained using the **derv** function. Figure 4.9B shows the same response and derivative when the derivative was calculated using the *two-point central difference algorithm*. This algorithm acts

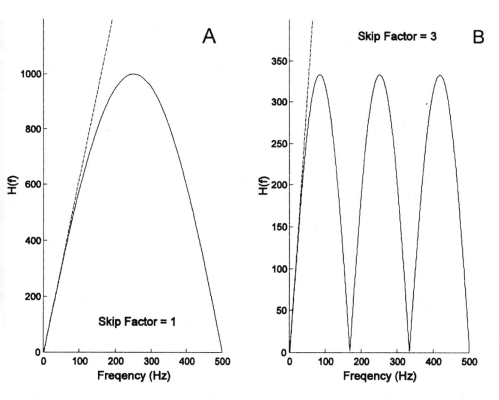

FIGURE 4.8 The frequency response of the two-point central difference algorithm using two different values for the skip factor: (A) $L = 1$; (B) $L = 4$. The sample time was 1 msec.

as a differentiator for the lower frequencies and as an integrator (or lowpass filter) for higher frequencies.

The two-point central difference algorithm uses two coefficients of equal but opposite value spaced L points apart, as defined by the input–output equation:

$$y(n) = \frac{x(n + L) - x(n - L)}{2LT_s} \tag{14}$$

where L is the *skip factor* that influences the effective bandwidth as described below, and T_s is the sample interval. The filter coefficients for the two-point central difference algorithm would be:

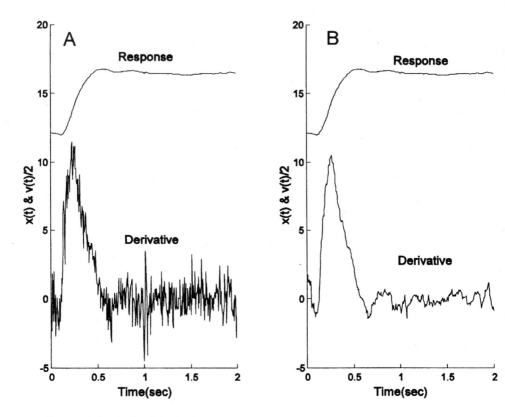

FIGURE 4.9 A physiological motor response to a step input is shown in the upper trace and its derivative is shown in the lower trace. (A) The derivative was calculated by taking the difference in adjacent points and scaling by the sample frequency. (B) The derivative was computed using the two-point central difference algorithm with a skip factor of 4. Derivative functions were scaled by $\frac{1}{2}$ and responses were offset to improve viewing.

$$h(n) = \begin{cases} -0.5/L & n = -L \\ 0.5/L & n = +L \\ 0 & n \neq L \end{cases} \tag{15}$$

The frequency response of this filter algorithm can be determined by taking the Fourier transform of the filter coefficient function. Since this function contains only two coefficients, the Fourier transform can be done either analytically or using MATLAB's `fft` routine. Both methods are presented in the example below.

Example 4.2 Determine the frequency response of the two-point central difference algorithm.

Analytical: Since the coefficient function is nonzero only for $n = \pm L$, the Fourier transform, after adjusting the summation limits for a symmetrical coefficient function with positive and negative n, becomes:

$$X(k) = \sum_{n=-L}^{L} b(n)e^{(-j2\pi\,kn/N)} = \frac{1}{2Lt_s}e^{(-j2\pi\,kL/N)} - \frac{1}{2LT_s}e^{(-j2\pi k(-L)/N)}$$

$$X(k) = \frac{e^{(-j2\pi kL/N)} - e^{(j2\pi kL/N)}}{2LT_s} = \frac{j\sin(2\pi kL/N)}{LT_s} \tag{16}$$

where L is the skip factor and N is the number of samples in the waveform. To put Eq. (16) in terms of frequency, note that $f = m/(NT_s)$; hence, $m = fNT_s$. Substituting:

$$|X(f)| = \left| j\frac{\sin(2\pi fLT_s)}{LT_s} \right| = \frac{\sin(2\pi fLT_s)}{LT_s} \tag{17}$$

Eq. (17) shows that $|X(k)|$ is a sine function that goes to zero at $f = 1/(LT_s)$ or f_s/L. Figure 4.8 shows the frequency characteristics of the two-point central difference algorithm for two different skip factors, and the MATLAB code used to calculate and plot the frequency plot is shown in Example 4.2. A true derivative would have a linear change with frequency (specifically, a line with a slope of $2\pi f$) as shown by the dashed lines in Figure 4.8. The two-point central difference curves approximate a true derivative for the lower frequencies, but has the characteristic of a lowpass filter for higher frequencies. Increasing the skip factor, L, has the effect of lowering the frequency range over which the filter acts like a derivative operator as well as the lowpass filter range. Note that for skip factors >1, the response curve repeats above $f = 1/(LT_s)$. Usually the assumption is made that the signal does not contain frequencies in this range. If this is not true, then these higher frequencies could be altered by the frequency characteristics of this filter above $1/(LT_s)$.

MATLAB Implementation

Since the FIR coefficient function is the same as the impulse response of the filter process, design and application of these filters can be achieved using only FFT and convolution. However, the MATLAB Signal Processing Toolbox has a number of useful FIR filter design routines that greatly facilitate the design of FIR filters, particularly if the desired frequency response is complicated. The

following two examples show the application use of FIR filters using only convolution and the FFT, followed by a discussion and examples of FIR filter
design using MATLAB's Signal Processing Toolbox.

Example 4.2   Generate the coefficient function for the two-point central
difference derivative algorithm and plot the frequency response. This program
was used to generate the plots in Figure 4.8.

```
% Example 4.2 and Figure 4.8
% Program to determine the frequency response
%   of the two point central difference algorithm for
%   differentiation
%
clear all, close all;
Ts = .001                          % Assume a Ts of 1 msec.
N = 1000;                          % Assume 1 sec of data; N =
                                   %   1000

Ln = [1 3];                        % Define two different skip
                                   %   factors
for i = 1:2                        % Repeat for each skip factor
  L = Ln(i);
  bn = zeros((2*L)+1,1);           %Set up b(n). Initialize to
                                   %   zero
  bn(1,1) = -1/(2*L*Ts);           % Put negative coefficient at
                                   %   b(1)
  bn((2*L)+1,1) = 1/(2*L*Ts);      % Put positive coefficient at
                                   %   b(2L+1)
  H = abs(fft(bn,N));              % Cal. frequency response
                                   %   using FFT
  subplot(1,2,i);                  % Plot the result
    hold on;
    plot(H(1:500),'k');            %Plot to fs/2
    axis([0 500 0 max(H)+.2*max(H)]);
    text(100,max(H),['Skip Factor = ',Num2str(L)]);
    xlabel('Frequency (Hz)'); ylabel('H(f)');
  y = (1:500) * 2 * pi;
  plot(y,'--k');                   % Plot ideal derivative
                                   %   function
  end
```

Note that the second to fourth lines of the ***for*** loop are used to build the
filter coefficients, $b(n)$, for the given skip factor, L. The next line takes the
absolute value of the Fourier transform of this function. The coefficient function
is zero-padded out to 1000 points, both to improve the appearance of the result-

ing frequency response curve and to simulate the application of the filter to a 1000 point data array sampled at 1 kHz.

Example 4.3 Develop and apply an FIR bandpass filter to physiological data. This example presents the construction and application of a narrowband filter such as shown in Figure 4.10 (right side) using convolution. The data are from a segment of an EEG signal in the PhysioNet data bank (*http://www. physionet.org*). A spectrum analysis is first performed on both the data and the filter to show the range of the filter's operation with respect to the frequency spectrum of the data. The standard FFT is used to analyze the data without windowing or averaging. As shown in Figure 4.10, the bandpass filter transmits most of the signal's energy, attenuating only a portion of the low frequency and

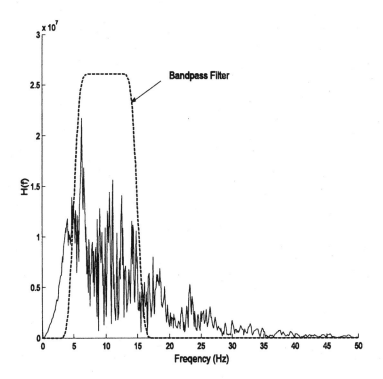

FIGURE 4.10 Frequency spectrum of EEG data shown in Figure 4.11 obtained using the FFT. Also shown is the frequency response of an FIR bandpass filter constructed using Eq. (12). The MATLAB code that generated this figure is presented in Example 4.3.

high frequency components. The result of applying this filter to the EEG signal is shown in Figure 4.11.

```
% Example 4.3 and Figures 4.10 and 4.11
% Application of an FIR bandpass filter based
%   on a rectangular window design as shown in Figure 4.7
%
close all; clear all;
N = 1000;                        % Number of data points
fs = 100;                        % Sample frequency
load sig_2;                      % Get data
```

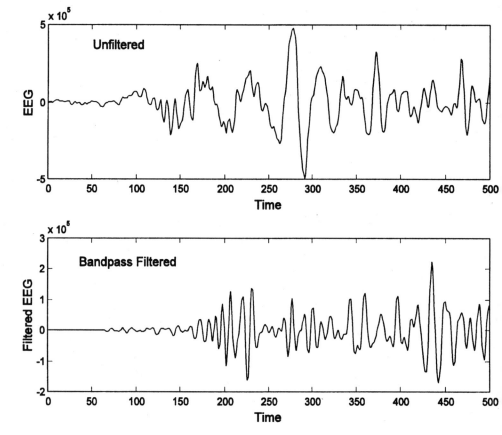

FIGURE 4.11 A segment of unfiltered EEG data (upper trace) and the bandpass filtered version (lower trace). A frequency response of the FIR bandpass filter is given in Figure 4.10.

```
wh = .3 * pi;                           % Set bandpass cutoff
                                        %  frequencies
wl = .1*pi;
L = 128;                                % Number of coeffients
                                        %  equals 128
for i = 1:L+1                           % Generate bandpass
                                        %  coefficient function
  n = i-L/2 ;                           %  and make symmetrical
  if n == 0
    bn(i) = wh/pi-wl/pi;
  else
    bn(i) = (sin(wh*n))/(pi*n)-(sin(wl*n))/(pi*n) ;
                                        % Filter impulse response
  end
end
bn = bn .* blackman(L+1)';              % Apply Blackman window
                                        %  to filter coeffs.
H_data = abs(fft(data));                % Plot data spectrum for
                                        %  comparison
freq = (1:N/2)*fs/N;                    % Frequency vector for
                                        %  plotting
plot(freq,H_data(1:N/2),'k');          % Plot data FFT only to
                                        %  fs/2
hold on;
%
H = abs(fft(bn,N));                     % Find the filter
                                        %  frequency response
H = H*1.2 * (max(H_data)/max(H)); % Scale filter H(z) for
                                        %  comparison
plot(freq,H(1:N/2),'--k');             % Plot the filter
                                        %  frequency response
   xlabel('Frequency (Hz)'); ylabel('H(f)');
y = conv(data,bn);                      % Filter the data using
                                        %  convolution
figure;
t = (1:N)/fs;                           % Time vector for
                                        %  plotting
subplot(2,1,1);
  plot(t(1:N/2),data(1:N/2),'k') % Plot only 1/2 of the
                                        %  data set for clarity
  xlabel('Time (sec)') ;ylabel('EEG');
subplot(2,1,2);                         % Plot the bandpass
                                        %  filtered data
  plot (t(1:N/2), y(1:N/2),'k');
  ylabel('Time'); ylabel('Filtered EEG');
```

In this example, the initial loop constructs the filter weights based on Eq. (12). The filter has high and low cutoff frequencies of 0.1π and 0.3 π radians/sample, or 0.1f_s/2 and 0.3f_s/2 Hz. Assuming a sampling frequency of 100 Hz this would correspond to cutoff frequencies of 5 to 15 Hz. The FFT is also used to evaluate the filter's frequency response. In this case the coefficient function is zero-padded to 1000 points both to improve the appearance of the frequency response curve and to match the data length. A frequency vector is constructed to plot the correct frequency range based on a sampling frequency of 100 Hz. The bandpass filter is applied to the data using convolution. Two adjustments must be made when using convolution to implement an FIR filter. If the filter weighting function is asymmetrical, as with the two-point central difference algorithm, then the filter order should be reversed to compensate for the way in which convolution applies the weights. In all applications, the MATLAB convolution routine generates additional points (N = length(data) + length($b(n)$ − 1) so the output must be shortened to N points. Here the initial N points are taken, but other strategies are mentioned in Chapter 2. In this example, only the first half of the data set is plotted in Figure 4.11 to improve clarity.

Comparing the unfiltered and filtered data in Figure 4.11, note the substantial differences in appearance despite the fact that only a small potion of the signal's spectrum is attenuated. Particularly apparent is the enhancement of the oscillatory component due to the suppression of the lower frequencies. This figure shows that even a moderate amount of filtering can significantly alter the appearance of the data. Also note the 50 msec initial transient and subsequent phase shift in the filtered data. This could be corrected by shifting the filtered data the appropriate number of sample points to the left.

INFINITE IMPULSE RESPONSE (IIR) FILTERS

The primary advantage of IIR filters over FIR filters is that they can usually meet a specific frequency criterion, such as a cutoff sharpness or slope, with a much lower filter order (i.e., a lower number of filter coefficients). The transfer function of IIR filters includes both numerator and denominator terms (Eq. (4)) unlike FIR filters which have only a numerator. The basic equation for the IIR filter is the same as that for any general linear process shown in Eq. (6) and repeated here with modified limits:

$$y(k) = \sum_{n=1}^{L_N} b(n) \, x(k - n) - \sum_{n=1}^{L_D} a(n) \, y(k - n) \tag{18}$$

where $b(n)$ is the numerator coefficients also found in FIR filters, $a(n)$ is the denominator coefficients, $x(n)$ is the input, and $y(n)$ the output. While the $b(n)$ coefficients operate only on values of the input, $x(n)$, the $a(n)$ coefficients operate on passed values of the output, $y(n)$ and are, therefore, sometimes referred to as *recursive* coefficients.

The major disadvantage of IIR filters is that they have nonlinear phase characteristics. However if the filtering is done on a data sequence that totally resides in computer memory, as is often the case, than so-called *noncausal* techniques can be used to produce zero phase filters. Noncausal techniques use both future as well as past data samples to eliminate phase shift irregularities. (Since these techniques use future data samples the entire waveform must be available in memory.) The two-point central difference algorithm with a positive skip factor is a noncausal filter. The Signal Processing Toolbox routine `filt-filt` described in the next section utilizes these noncausal methods to implement IIR (or FIR) filters with no phase distortion.

The design of IIR filters is not as straightforward as FIR filters; however, the MATLAB Signal Processing Toolbox provides a number of advanced routines to assist in this process. Since IIR filters have transfer functions that are the same as a general linear process having both poles and zeros, many of the concepts of analog filter design can be used with these filters. One of the most basic of these is the relationship between the number of poles and the slope, or *rolloff* of the filter beyond the cutoff frequency. As mentioned in Chapter 1, the asymptotic downward slope of a filter increases by 20 db/decade for each filter pole, or filter order. Determining the number of poles required in an IIR filter given the desired attenuation characteristic is a straightforward process.

Another similarity between analog and IIR digital filters is that all of the well-known analog filter types can be duplicated as IIR filters. Specifically the Butterworth, Chebyshev Type I and II, and elliptic (or Cauer) designs can be implemented as IIR digital filters and are supported in the MATLAB Signal Processing Toolbox. As noted in Chapter 1; Butterworth filters provide a frequency response that is maximally flat in the passband and monotonic overall. To achieve this characteristic, Butterworth filters sacrifice rolloff steepness; hence, the Butterworth filter will have a less sharp initial attenuation characteristic than other filters. The Chebyshev Type I filters feature faster rolloff than Butterworth filters, but have ripple in the passband. Chebyshev Type II filters have ripple only in the stopband and a monotonic passband, but they do not rolloff as sharply as Type I. The ripple produced by Chebyshev filters is termed equi-ripple since it is of constant amplitude across all frequencies. Finally, elliptic filters have steeper rolloff than any of the above, but have equi-ripple in both the passband and stopband. In general, elliptic filters meet a given performance specification with the lowest required filter order.

Implementation of IIR filters can be achieved using the `filter` function described above. Design of IIR filters is greatly facilitated by the Signal Processing Toolbox as described below. This Toolbox can also be used to design FIR filters, but is not essential in implementing these filters. However, when filter requirements call for complex spectral characteristics, the use of the Signal Processing Toolbox is of considerable value, irrespective of the filter type. The design of FIR filters using this Toolbox will be covered first, followed by IIR filter design.

FILTER DESIGN AND APPLICATION USING THE MATLAB SIGNAL PROCESSING TOOLBOX

FIR Filters

The MATLAB Signal Processing Toolbox includes routines that can be used to apply both FIR and IIR filters. While they are not necessary for either the design or application of FIR filters, they do ease the design of both filter types, particularly for filters with complex frequency characteristics or demanding attenuation requirements. Within the MATLAB environment, filter design and application occur in either two or three stages, each stage executed by separate, but related routines. In the three-stage protocol, the user supplies information regarding the filter type and desired attenuation characteristics, but not the filter order. The first-stage routines determine the appropriate order as well as other parameters required by the second-stage routines. The second stage routines generate the filter coefficients, $b(n)$, based the arguments produced by the first-stage routines including the filter order. A two-stage design process would start with this stage, in which case the user would supply the necessary input arguments including the filter order. Alternatively, more recent versions of MATLAB's Signal Processing Toolbox provide an interactive filter design package called FDATool (for filter design and analysis tool) which performs the same operations described below, but utilizing a user-friendly graphical user interface (GUI). Another Signal Processing Toolbox package, the SPTool (signal processing tool) is useful for analyzing filters and generating spectra of both signals and filters. New MATLAB releases contain detailed information of the use of these two packages.

The final stage is the same for all filters including IIR filters: a routine that takes the filter coefficients generated by the previous stage and applies them to the data. In FIR filters, the final stage could be implemented using convolution as was done in previous examples, or the MATLAB `filter` routine described earlier, or alternatively the MATLAB Signal Processing Toolbox routine `filtfilt` can be used for improved phase properties.

One useful Signal Processing Toolbox routine determines the frequency response of a filter given the coefficients. Of course, this can be done using the FFT as shown in Examples 4.2 and 4.3, and this is the approach used by the MATLAB routine. However the MATLAB routine `freqz`, also includes frequency scaling and plotting, making it quite convenient. The `freqz` routine plots, or produces, both the magnitude and the phase characteristics of a filter's frequency response:

```
[h,w] = freqz (b,a,n,fs);
```

where again **b** and **a** are the filter coefficients and **n** is the number of points in the desired frequency spectra. Setting **n** as a power of 2 is recommended to speed computation (the default is 512). The input argument, **fs**, is optional and specifies the sampling frequency. Both output arguments are also optional: if **freqz** is called without the output arguments, the magnitude and phase plots are produced. If specified, the output vector **h** is the n-point complex frequency response of the filter. The magnitude would be equal to **abs(h)** while the phase would be equal to **angle(h)**. The second output argument, **w**, is a vector the same length as h containing the frequencies of h and is useful in plotting. If **fs** is given, **w** is in Hz and ranges between 0 and $f_s/2$; otherwise **w** is in rad/sample and ranges between 0 and π.

Two-Stage FIR Filter Design

Two-stage filter design requires that the designer known the filter order, i.e., the number of coefficients in $b(n)$, but otherwise the design procedure is straightforward. The MATLAB Signal Processing Toolbox has two filter design routines based on the rectangular filters described above, i.e., Eqs. (10)–(13). Although implementation of these equations using standard MATLAB code is straightforward (as demonstrated in previous examples), the FIR design routines replace many lines of MATLAB code with a single routine and are seductively appealing. While both routines are based on the same approach, one allows greater flexibility in the specification of the desired frequency curve. The basic rectangular filter is implemented with the routine **fir1** as:

```
b = fir1(n,wn,'ftype' window);
```

where **n** is the filter order, **wn** the cutoff frequency, **ftype** the filter type, and **window** specifies the window function (i.e., Blackman, Hamming, triangular, etc.). The output, **b**, is a vector containing the filter coefficients. The last two input arguments are optional. The input argument **ftype** can be either `'high'` for a highpass filter, or `'stop'` for a stopband filter. If not specified, a lowpass or bandpass filter is assumed depending on the length of **wn**. The argument, **window**, is used as it is in the **pwelch** routine: the function name includes arguments specifying window length (see Example 4.3 below) or other arguments. The window length should equal **n+1**. For bandpass and bandstop filters, **n** must be even and is incremented if not, in which case the window length should be suitably adjusted. Note that MATLAB's popular default window, the Hamming window, is used if this argument is not specified. The cutoff frequency is either a scalar specifying the lowpass or highpass cutoff frequency, or a two-element vector that specifies the cutoff frequencies of a bandpass or bandstop filter. The cutoff frequency(s) ranges between 0 and 1 normalized to $f_s/2$ (e.g., if, wn = 0.5, then $f_c = 0.5 * f_s/2$). Other options are described in the MATLAB Help file on this routine.

A related filter design algorithm, fir2, is used to design rectangular filters when a more general, or arbitrary frequency response curve is desired. The command structure for fir2 is;

```
b = fir2(n,f,A,window)
```

where n is the filter order, f is a vector of normalized frequencies in ascending order, and A is the desired gain of the filter at the corresponding frequency in vector f. (In other words, plot(f,A) would show the desired magnitude frequency curve.) Clearly f and A must be the same length, but duplicate frequency points are allowed, corresponding to step changes in the frequency response. Again, frequency ranges between 0 and 1, normalized to $f_s/2$. The argument window is the same as in fir1, and the output, b, is the coefficient function. Again, other optional input arguments are mentioned in the MATLAB Help file on this routine.

Several other more specialized FIR filters are available that have a two-stage design protocol. In addition, there is a three-stage FIR filter described in the next section.

Example 4.4   Design a window-based FIR bandpass filter having the frequency characteristics of the filter developed in Example 4.3 and shown in Figure 4.12.

```
% Example 4.4 and Figure 4.12 Design a window-based bandpass
% filter with cutoff frequencies of 5 and 15 Hz.
% Assume a sampling frequency of 100 Hz.
% Filter order = 128
%
clear all; close all;
fs = 100;                        % Sampling frequency
order = 128;                     % Filter order
wn = [5*fs/2 15*fs/2];           % Specify cutoff
                                 %  frequencies
b = fir1(order,wn);              % On line filter design,
                                 %  Hamming window
[h,freq] = freqz(b,1,512,100);   % Get frequency response
plot(freq,abs(h),'k');           % Plot frequency response
   xlabel('Frequency (Hz)'); ylabel('H(f)');
```

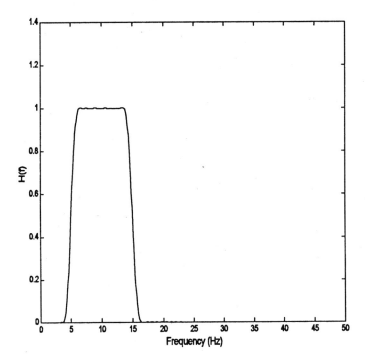

FIGURE 4.12 The frequency response of an FIR filter based in the rectangular filter design described in Eq. (10). The cutoff frequencies are 5 and 15 Hz. The frequency response of this filter is identical to that of the filter developed in Example 4.5 and presented in Figure 4.10. However, the development of this filter required only one line of code.

Three-Stage FIR Filter Design

The first stage in the three-stage design protocol is used to determine the filter order and cutoff frequencies to best approximate a desired frequency response curve. Inputs to these routines specify an ideal frequency response, usually as a piecewise approximation and a maximum deviation from this ideal response. The design routine generates an output that includes the number of stages required, cutoff frequencies, and other information required by the second stage. In the three-stage design process, the first- and second-stage routines work together so that the output of the first stage can be directly passed to the input of the second-stage routine. The second-stage routine generates the filter coefficient function based on the input arguments which include the filter order, the cutoff frequencies, the filter type (generally optional), and possibly other arguments. In cases where the filter order and cutoff frequencies are known, the first stage can be bypassed and arguments assigned directly to the second-stage routines. This design process will be illustrated using the routines that implement Parks–McClellan optimal FIR filter.

The first design stage, the determination of filter order and cutoff frequencies uses the MATLAB routine `remezord`. (First-stage routines end in the letters `ord` which presumably stands for filter order). The calling structure is

```
[n, fo, ao, w] = remezord (f,a,dev,Fs);
```

The input arguments, `f`, `a` and `dev` specify the desired frequency response curve in a somewhat roundabout manner. `Fs` is the sampling frequency and is optional (the default is 2 Hz so that $f_s/2 = 1$ Hz). Vector `f` specifies frequency ranges between 0 and $f_s/2$ as a pair of frequencies while `a` specifies the desired gains within each of these ranges. Accordingly, `f` has a length of `2n-2`, where n is the length of `a`. The `dev` vector specifies the maximum allowable deviation, or ripple, within each of these ranges and is the same length as `a`. For example, assume you desire a bandstop filter that has a passband between 0 and 100 with a ripple of 0.01, a stopband between 300 and 400 Hz with a gain of 0.1, and an upper passband between 500 and 1000 Hz (assuming $f_s/2 = 1000$) with the same ripple as the lower passband. The `f`, `a`, and `dev` vectors would be: `f = [100 300 400 500]`; `a = [1 0 1]`; and `dev = [.01 .1 .01]`. Note that the ideal stopband gain is given as zero by vector `a` while the actual gain is specified by the allowable deviation given in vector `dev`. Vector `dev` requires the deviation or ripple to be specified in linear units not in db. The application of this design routine is shown in Example 4.5 below.

The output arguments include the required filter order, `n`, the normalized frequency ranges, `fo`, the frequency amplitudes for those ranges, `a0`, and a set of weights, `w`, that tell the second stage how to assess the accuracy of the fit in each of the frequency ranges. These four outputs become the input to the second stage filter design routine `remez`. The calling structure to the routine is:

```
b = remez (n, f, a, w, 'ftype');
```

where the first four arguments are supplied by `remezord` although the input argument `w` is optional. The fifth argument, also optional, specifies either a `hilbert` linear-phase filter (most common, and the default) or a `differentiator` which weights the lower frequencies more heavily so they will be the most accurately constructed. The output is the FIR coefficients, `b`.

If the desired filter order is known, it is possible to bypass remezord and input the arguments n, `f`, and `a` directly. The input argument, n, is simply the filter order. Input vectors `f` and `a` specify the desired frequency response curve in a somewhat different manner than described above. The frequency vector still contains monotonically increasing frequencies normalized to $f_s/2$; i.e., ranging between 0 and 1 where 1 corresponds to $f_s/2$. The **a** vector represents desired filter gain at each end of a frequency pair, and the gain between pairs is an unspecified transition region. To take the example above: a bandstop filter that has a passband (gain = 1) between 0 and 100, a stopband between 300 and 400 Hz with a gain of 0.1, and an upper passband between 500 and 700 Hz; assuming $f_s/2 = 1$ kHz, the **f** and a vector would be: **f** = [0 .1 .3 .4 .5 .7]; **a** = [1 1 .1 .1 1 1]. Note that the desired frequency curve is unspecified between 0.1 and 0.3 and also between 0.4 and 0.5.

As another example, assume you wanted a filter that would differentiate a signal up to $0.2f_s/2$ Hz, then lowpass filter the signal above $0.3f_s/2$ Hz. The **f** and **a** vector would be: **f** = [0 .1 .3 1]; **a** = [0 1 0 0].

Another filter that uses the same input structure as `remezord` is the least square linear-phase filter design routine `firls`. The use of this filter in for calculation the derivative is found in the Problems.

The following example shows the design of a bandstop filter using the Parks–McClellan filter in a three-stage process. This example is followed by the design of a differentiator Parks–McClellan filter, but a two-stage design protocol is used.

Example 4.5 Design a bandstop filter having the following characteristics: a passband gain of 1 (0 db) between 0 and 100, a stopband gain of −40 db between 300 and 400 Hz, and an upper passband gain of 1 between 500 and 1000 Hz. Maximum ripple for the passband should be ±1.5 db. Assume $f_s = 2$ kHz. Use the three-stage design process. In this example, specifying the **dev** argument is a little more complicated because the requested deviations are given in db while `remezord` expects linear values.

```
% Example 4.5 and Figure 4.13
% Bandstop filter with a passband gain of 1 between 0 and 100,
% a stopband gain of -40 db between 300 and 400 Hz,
% and an upper passband gain of 1 between 500 and fs/2 Hz (1000
%  Hz).
% Maximum ripple for the passband should be ±1.5 db
%
rp_pass = 3;                    % Specify ripple
                                %  tolerance in passband
rp_stop = 40;                   % Specify error
                                %  tolerance in passband
fs = 2000;                      % Sample frequency: 2
                                %  kHz
f = [100 300 400 500];          % Define frequency
                                %  ranges
a= [1 0 1];                     % Specify gain in
                                %  those regions
%
```

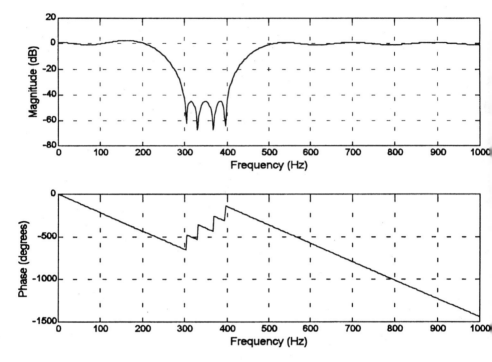

FIGURE 4.13   The magnitude and phase frequency response of a Parks–McClellan bandstop filter produced in Example 4.5. The number of filter coefficients as determined by `remezord` was 24.

```
% Now specify the deviation converting from db to linear
dev = [(10^(rp_pass/20)-1)/(10^(rp_pass/20)+1) 10^
        (-rp_stop/20)....(10^(rp_pass/20)-1)/(10^(rp_pass/
        20)+1)];
%
% Design filter - determine filter order
[n, fo, ao, w] = remezord(f,a,dev,fs)    % Determine filter
                                          %  order, Stage 1
b = remez(n, fo, ao, w);                  % Determine filter
                                          %  weights, Stage 2
freq.(b,1,[ ],fs);                        % Plot filter fre-
                                          %  quency response
```

In Example 4.5 the vector assignment for the a vector is straightforward: the desired gain is given as 1 in the passband and 0 in the stopband. The actual stopband attenuation is given by the vector that specifies the maximum desirable error, the `dev` vector. The specification of this vector, is complicated by the fact that it must be given in linear units while the ripple and stopband gain are specified in db. The db to linear conversion is included in the `dev` assignment. Note the complicated way in which the passband gain must be assigned.

Figure 4.13 shows the plot produced by `freqz` with no output arguments, a = 1, n = 512 (the default), and `b` was the FIR coefficient function produced in Example 4.6 above. The phase plot demonstrates the linear phase characteristics of this FIR filter in the passband. This will be compared with the phase characteristics of IIR filter in the next section.

The frequency response curves for Figure 4.13 were generated using the MATLAB routine `freqz`, which applies the FFT to the filter coefficients following Eq. (7). It is also possible to generate these curves by passing white noise through the filter and computing the spectral characteristics of the output. A comparison of this technique with the direct method used above is found in Problem 1.

Example 4.6 Design a differentiator using the MATLAB FIR filter `remez`. Use a two-stage design process (i.e., select a 28-order filter and bypass the first stage design routine `remezord`). Compare the derivative produced by this signal with that produced by the two-point central difference algorithm. Plot the results in Figure 4.14.

The FIR derivative operator will be designed by requesting a linearly increasing frequency characteristic (slope = 1) up to some f_c Hz, then a sharp drop off within the next $0.1 f_s/2$ Hz. Note that to make the initial magnitude slope equal to 1, the magnitude value at `fc` should be: $f_c * f_s * \pi$.

```
% Example 4.6 and Figure 4.14
% Design a FIR derivative filter and compare it to the
% Two point central difference algorithm
%
close all; clear all;
load sig1;                      % Get data
Ts = 1/200;                     % Assume a Ts of 5 msec.
fs = 1/Ts;                      % Sampling frequency
order = 28;                     % FIR Filter order
L = 4;                          % Use skip factor of 4
fc = .05                        % Derivative cutoff
                                %  frequency
t = (1:length(data))*Ts;
%
% Design filter
f = [ 0 fc fc+.1 .9];           % Construct desired freq.
                                %  characteristic
```

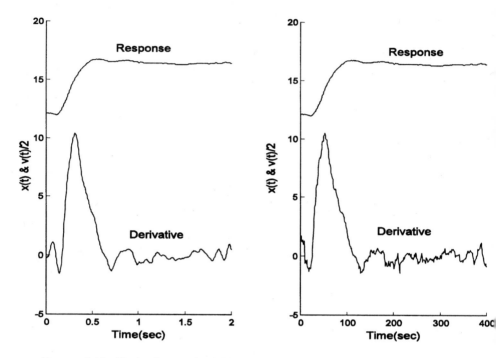

FIGURE 4.14 Derivative produced by an FIR filter (left) and the two-point central difference differentiator (right). Note that the FIR filter does produce a cleaner derivative without reducing the value of the peak velocity. The FIR filter order ($n = 28$) and deriviative cutoff frequency ($f_c = .05\ f_s/2$) were chosen empirically to produce a clean derivative with a maximal velocity peak. As in Figure 4.5 the velocity (i.e., derivative) was scaled by $1/2$ to be more compatible with response amplitude.

```
a = [0 (fc*fs*pi) 0 0];          % Upward slope until .05 fₛ
                                  %   then lowpass
b = remez(order,f,a,             % Design filter coeffi-
    'differentiator');           %   cients and
d_dt1 = filter(b,1,data);        % apply FIR Differentiator
figure;
subplot(1,2,1);
  hold on;
  plot(t,data(1:400)+12,'k');    % Plot FIR filter deriva-
                                  %   tive (data offset)
  plot(t,d_dt1(1:400)/2,'k');    % Scale velocity by 1/2
  ylabel('Time(sec)');
  ylabel('x(t) & v(t)/2');
```

```
%
%
% Now apply two-point central difference algorithm
hn = zeros((2*L)+1,1);              % Set up h(n)
hn(1,1) = 1/(2*L* Ts);
hn((2*L)+1,1) = -1/(2*L*Ts);        % Note filter weight
                                    %  reversed if
d_dt2 = conv(data,hn);              % using convolution
%
subplot(1,2,2);
  hold on;
  plot(data(1:400)+12,'k');         % Plot the two-point cen-
                                    %  tral difference
  plot(d_dt2(1:400)/2,'k');         % algorithm derivative
  ylabel('Time(sec)');
  ylabel('x(t) & v(t)/2');
```

IIR Filters

IIR filter design under MATLAB follows the same procedures as FIR filter design; only the names of the routines are different. In the MATLAB Signal Processing Toolbox, the three-stage design process is supported for most of the IIR filter types; however, as with FIR design, the first stage can be bypassed if the desired filter order is known.

The third stage, the application of the filter to the data, can be implemented using the standard `filter` routine as was done with FIR filters. A Signal Processing Toolbox routine can also be used to implement IIR filters given the filter coefficients:

```
y = filtfilt(b,a,x)
```

The arguments for `filtfilt` are identical to those in `filter`. The only difference is that `filtfilt` improves the phase performance of IIR filters by running the algorithm in both forward and reverse directions. The result is a filtered sequence that has zero-phase distortion and a filter order that is doubled. The downsides of this approach are that initial transients may be larger and the approach is inappropriate for many FIR filters that depend on phase response for proper operations. A comparison between the `filter` and `filtfilt` algorithms is made in the example below.

As with our discussion of FIR filters, the two-stage filter processes will be introduced first, followed by three-stage filters. Again, all filters can be implemented using a two-stage process if the filter order is known. This chapter concludes with examples of IIR filter application.

Two-Stage IIR Filter Design

The Yule–Walker recursive filter is the only IIR filter that is not supported by an order-selection routine (i.e., a three-stage design process). The design routine yulewalk allows for the specification of a general desired frequency response curve, and the calling structure is given on the next page.

```
[b,a] = yulewalk(n,f,m)
```

where n is the filter order, and m and f specify the desired frequency characteristic in a fairly straightforward way. Specifically, m is a vector of the desired filter gains at the frequencies specified in f. The frequencies in f are relative to $f_s/2$: the first point in f must be zero and the last point 1. Duplicate frequency points are allowed and correspond to steps in the frequency response. Note that this is the same strategy for specifying the desired frequency response that was used by the FIR routines fir2 and firls (see Help file).

Example 4.7 Design an 12th-order Yule–Walker bandpass filter with cutoff frequencies of 0.25 and 0.5. Plot the frequency response of this filter and compare with that produced by the FIR filter fir2 of the same order.

```
% Example 4.7 and Figure 4.15
% Design a 12th-order Yulewalk filter and compare
% its frequency response with a window filter of the same
%   order
%
close all; clear all;
n = 12;                     % Filter order
f = [0 .25 .25 .6 .6 1];    % Specify desired frequency re-
                            %   sponse
m = [0 0 1 1 0 0];
[b,a] = yulewalk(n,f,m);    % Construct Yule-Walker IIR Filter
h = freqz(b,a,256);
b1 = fir2(n,f,m);           % Construct FIR rectangular window
                            %   filter
h1 = freqz(b1,1,256);
plot(f,m,'k');              % Plot the ideal "window" freq.
                            %   response
hold on
w = (1:256)/256;
plot(w,abs(h),'--k');       % Plot the Yule-Walker filter
plot(w,abs(h1),':k');       % Plot the FIR filter
   xlabel('Relative Frequency');
```

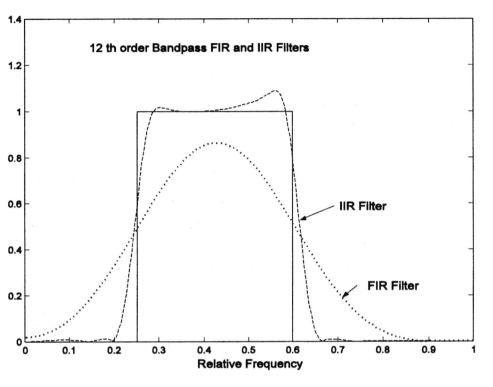

FIGURE 4.15 Comparison of the frequency response of 12th-order FIR and IIR filters. Solid line shows frequency characteristics of an ideal bandpass filter.

Three-Stage IIR Filter Design: Analog Style Filters

All of the analog filter types—Butterworth, Chebyshev, and elliptic—are supported by order selection routines (i.e., first-stage routines). The first-stage routines follow the nomenclature as FIR first-stage routines, they all end in `ord`. Moreover, they all follow the same strategy for specifying the desired frequency response, as illustrated using the Butterworth first-stage routine `buttord`:

```
[n,wn] = buttord(wp, ws, rp, rs); Butterworth filter
```

where `wp` is the passband frequency relative to $f_s/2$, `ws` is the stopband frequency in the same units, `rp` is the passband ripple in db, and `rs` is the stopband ripple also in db. Since the Butterworth filter does not have ripple in either the passband or stopband, `rp` is the maximum attenuation in the passband and `rs` is the minimum attenuation in the stopband. This routine returns the output arguments n, the required filter order and wn, the actual −3 db cutoff frequency. For example, if the maximum allowable attenuation in the passband is set to 3 db, then ws should be a little larger than wp since the gain must be less that 3 db at wp.

As with the other analog-based filters described below, lowpass, highpass, bandpass, and bandstop filters can be specified. For a highpass filter wp is greater than ws. For bandpass and bandstop filters, wp and ws are two-element vectors that specify the corner frequencies at both edges of the filter, the lower frequency edge first. For bandpass and bandstop filters, buttord returns wn as a two-element vector for input to the second-stage design routine, butter.

The other first-stage IIR design routines are:

```
[n,wn] = cheb1ord(wp, ws, rp, rs);     % Chebyshev Type I
                                       % filter
[n,wn] = cheb2ord(wp, ws, rp, rs);     % Chebyshev Type II
                                       %  filter
[n,wn] = ellipord(wp, ws, rp, rs);     % Elliptic filter
```

The second-stage routines follow a similar calling structure, although the Butterworth does not have arguments for ripple. The calling structure for the Butterworth filter is:

```
[b,a] = butter(n,wn,'ftype')
```

where n and wn are the order and cutoff frequencies respectively. The argument ftype should be 'high' if a highpass filter is desired and 'stop' for a bandstop filter. In the latter case wn should be a two-element vector, wn = [w1 w2], where w1 is the low cutoff frequency and w2 the high cutoff frequency. To specify a bandpass filter, use a two-element vector without the ftype argument. The output of butter is the b and a coefficients that are used in the third or application stage by routines filter or filtfilt, or by freqz for plotting the frequency response.

The other second-stage design routines contain additional input arguments to specify the maximum passband or stopband ripple if appropriate:

```
[b,a] = cheb1(n,rp,wn,'ftype')    % Chebyshev Type I filter
```

where the arguments are the same as in butter except for the additional argument, rp, which specifies the maximum desired passband ripple in db.

The Type II Chebyshev filter is:

```
[b,a] = cheb2(n,rs, wn,'ftype')    % Chebyshev Type II filter
```

where again the arguments are the same, except rs specifies the stopband ripple. As we have seen in FIR filters, the stopband ripple is given with respect to passband gain. For example a value of 40 db means that the ripple will not exceed 40 db below the passband gain. In effect, this value specifies the minimum attenuation in the stopband.

The elliptic filter includes both stopband and passband ripple values:

```
[b,a] = ellip(n,rp,rs,wn,'ftype')   % Elliptic filter
```

where the arguments presented are in the same manner as described above, with rp specifying the passband gain in db and rs specifying the stopband ripple relative to the passband gain.

The example below uses the second-stage routines directly to compare the frequency response of the four IIR filters discussed above.

Example 4.8 Plot the frequency response curves (in db) obtained from an 8th-order lowpass filter using the Butterworth, Chebyshev Type I and II, and elliptic filters. Use a cutoff frequency of 200 Hz and assume a sampling frequency of 2 kHz. For all filters, the passband ripple should be less than 3 db and the minimum stopband attenuation should be 60 db.

```
% Example 4.8 and Figure 4.16
% Frequency response of four 8th-order lowpass filters
%
N = 256;                  % Spectrum number of points
fs = 2000;                % Sampling filter
n = 8;                    % Filter order
wn = 200/fs/2;            % Filter cutoff frequency
rp = 3;                   % Maximum passband ripple in db
rs = 60;                  % Stopband attenuation in db
%
%
%Butterworth
[b,a] = butter(n,wn);     % Determine filter coefficients
[h,f] = freqz(b,a,N,fs);  % Determine filter spectrum
subplot(2,2,1);
  h = 20*log10(abs(h));   % Convert to db
  semilogx(f,h,'k');      % Plot on semilog scale
  axis([100 1000 -80 10]); % Adjust axis for better visi-
                          % bility
  xlabel('Frequency (Hz)'); ylabel('X(f)(db)');
  title('Butterworth');
%
```

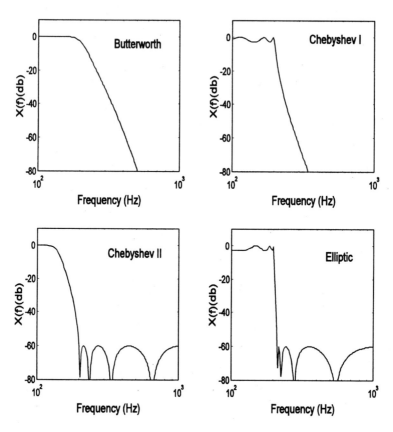

FIGURE 4.16 Four different 8th-order IIR lowpass filters with a cutoff frequency of 200 Hz. Sampling frequency was 2 kHz.

```
%
%Chebyshev Type I
[b,a] = cheby1(n,rp,wn);        % Determine filter coefficients
[h,f] = freqz(b,a,N,fs);        % Determine filter spectrum
subplot(2,2,2);
  h = 20*log10(abs(h));         % Convert to db
  semilogx(f,h,'k');            % Plot on semilog scale
  axis([100 1000-80 10]);       % Adjust axis for better visi-
                                  bility
  xlabel('Frequency (Hz)');  ylabel('X(f)(db)');
  title('Chebyshev I');
%
%
```

```
% Chebyshev Type II
[b,a] = cheby2(n,rs,wn);      % Determine filter coefficients
[h,f] = freqz(b,a,N,fs);      % Determine filter spectrum
subplot(2,2,3);
h = 20*log10(abs(h));         % Convert to db
   semilogx(f,h,'k');         % Plot on semilog scale
   axis([100 1000-80 10]);    % Adjust axis for better visi-
                              % bility
   xlabel('Frequency (Hz)');  ylabel('X(f)(db)');
   title('Chebyshev II');


% Elliptic
[b,a] = ellip(n,rp,rs,wn);    % Determine filter coefficients
[h,f] = freqz(b,a,N,fs);      % Determine filter spectrum
subplot(2,2,4);
   h = 20*log10(abs(h));      % Convert to db
   semilogx(f,h,'k');         % Plot on semilog scale
   axis([100 1000-80 10]);    % Adjust axis for better visi-
                              % bility
   xlabel('Frequency (Hz)');  ylabel('X(f)(db)');
   title('Elliptic');
```

PROBLEMS

1. Find the frequency response of a FIR filter with a weighting function of bn = [.2 .2 .2 .2 .2] in three ways: apply the FFT to the weighting function, use freqz, and pass white noise through the filter and plot the magnitude spectra of the output. In the third method, use a 1024-point array; i.e., y = filter (bn,1,randn(1024,1)). Note that you will have to scale the frequency axis differently to match the relative frequencies assumed by each method.

2. Use sig_noise to construct a 512-point array consisting of two closely spaced sinusoids of 200 and 230 Hz with SNR of −8 db and −12 db respectively. Plot the magnitude spectrum using the FFT. Now apply an 24 coefficient FIR bandpass window type filter to the data using either the approach in Example 4.2 or the fir1 MATLAB routine. Replot the bandpass filter data.

3. Use sig_noise to construct a 512-point array consisting of a single sinusoid of 200 Hz at an SNR of −20 db. Narrowband filter the data with an FIR rectangular window type filter, and plot the FFT spectra before and after filtering. Repeat using the Welch method to obtain the power spectrum before and after filtering.

4. Construct a 512-point array consisting of a step function. Filter the step by four different FIR lowpass filters and plot the first 150 points of the resultant

step response: a 15th order Parks–McClellan; a 15th-order rectangular window; a 30th-order rectangular window; and a 15th-order least squares `firls`. Use a bandwidth of 0.15 $f_s/2$.

5. Repeat Problem 4 for four different IIR 12th-order lowpass filters: Butterworth, Chebyshev Type I, Chebyshev Type II, and an elliptic. Use a passband ripple of 0.5 db and a stopband ripple of 80 db where appropriate. Use the same bandwidth as in Problem 4.

6. Load the data file `ensemble_data` used in Problem 1 in Chapter 2. Calculate the ensemble average of the ensemble `data`, then filter the average with a 12th-order Butterworth filter. Select a cutoff frequency that removes most of the noise, but does not unduly distort the response dynamics. Implement the Butterworth filter using `filter` and plot the data before and after filtering. Implement the same filter using `filtfilt` and plot the resultant filter data. How do the two implementations of the Butterworth compare? Display the cutoff frequency on the one of the plots containing the filtered data.

7. Determine the spectrum of the Butterworth filter used in the above problem. Then use the three-stage design process to design and equivalent Parks–McClellan FIR filter. Plot the spectrum to confirm that they are similar and apply to the data of Problem 4 comparing the output of the FIR filter with the IIR Butterworth filter in Problem 4. Display the order of both filters on their respective data plots.

8. Differentiate the ensemble average data of Problems 6 and 7 using the two-point central difference operator with a *skip factor* of 10. Construct a differentiator using a 16th-order least square linear phase `firls` FIR with a constant upward slope until some frequency f_c, then rapid attenuation to zero. Adjust f_c to minimize noise and still maintain derivative peaks. Plots should show data and derivative for each method, scaled for reasonable viewing. Also plot the filter's spectral characteristic for the best value of f_c.

9. Use the first stage IIR design routines, `buttord, chebylord, cheby2ord,` and `elliptord` to find the filter order required for a lowpass filter that attenuates 40 db/octave. (An octave is a doubling in frequency: a slope of 6 db/octave = a slope of 20 db/decade). Assume a cutoff frequency of 200 Hz and a sampling frequency of 2 kHz.

10. Use `sig_noise` to construct a 512-point array consisting of two widely separated sinusoids: 150 and 350 Hz, both with SNR of -14 db. Use a 16-order Yule–Walker filter to generate a double bandpass filter with peaks at the two sinusoidal frequencies. Plot the filter's frequency response as well as the FFT spectrum before and after filtering.

5

Spectral Analysis: Modern Techniques

PARAMETRIC MODEL-BASED METHODS

The techniques for determining the power spectra described in Chapter 3 are all based on the Fourier transform and are referred to as classical methods. These methods are the most robust of the spectral estimators. They require little in the way of assumptions regarding the origin or nature of the data, although some knowledge of the data could be useful for window selection and averaging strategies. In these classical approaches, the waveform outside the data window is implicitly assumed to be zero. Since this is rarely true, such an assumption can lead to distortion in the estimate (Marple, 1987). In addition, there are distortions due to the various data windows (including the rectangular window) as described in Chapter 3.

Modern approaches to spectral analysis are designed to overcome some of the distortions produced by the classical approach and are particularly effective if the data segments are short. Modern techniques fall into two broad classes: parametric, model-based* or eigen decomposition, and nonparametric. These techniques attempt to overcome the limitations of traditional methods by taking advantage of something that is known, or can be assumed, about the source signal. For example, if something is known about the process that gener-

---

*In some semantic contexts, all spectral analysis approaches can be considered model-based. For example, classic Fourier transform spectral analysis could be viewed as using a model consisting of harmonically related sinusoids. Here the term *parametric* is used to avoid possible confusion.

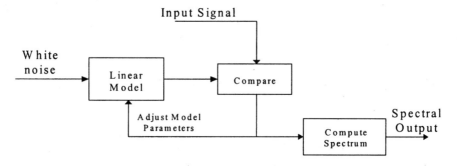

FIGURE 5.1 Schematic representation of model-based methods of spectral estimation.

ated the waveform of interest, then model-based, or parametric, methods can make assumptions about the waveform outside the data window. This eliminates the need for windowing and can improve spectral resolution and fidelity, particularly when the waveform contains a large amount of noise. Any improvement in resolution and fidelity will depend strongly on the appropriateness of the model selected (Marple, 1987). Accordingly, modern approaches, particularly parametric spectral methods, require somewhat more judgement in their application than classical methods. Moreover, these methods provide only magnitude information in the form of the power spectrum.

Parametric methods make use of a linear process, commonly referred to as a model* to estimate the power spectrum. The basic strategy of this approach is shown in Figure 5.1. The linear process or model is assumed to be driven by white noise. (Recall that white noise contains equal energy at all frequencies; its power spectrum is a constant over all frequencies.) The output of this model is compared with the input waveform and the model parameters adjusted for the best match between model output and the waveform of interest. When the best match is obtained, the model's frequency characteristics provide the best estimate of the waveform's spectrum, given the constraints of the model. This is because the input to the model is spectrally flat so that the spectrum at the output is a direct reflection of the model's magnitude transfer function which, in turn, reflects the input spectrum. This method may seem roundabout, but it permits well-defined constraints, such as model type and order, to be placed on the type of spectrum that can be found.

---

*To clarify the terminology, a *linear process* is referred to as a *model* in parametric spectral analysis, just as it is termed a *filter* when it is used to shape a signal's spectral characteristics. Despite the different terms, linear models, filters, or processes are all described by the basic equations given at the beginning of Chapter 4.

A number of different model types are used in this approach, differentiated by the nature of their transfer functions. Three models types are the most popular: *autoregressive* (AR), *moving average* (MA), and *autoregressive moving average* (ARMA). Selection of the most appropriate model selection requires some knowledge of the probable shape of the spectrum. The AR model is particularly useful for estimating spectra that have sharp peaks but no deep valleys. The AR model has a transfer function with only a constant in the numerator and a polynomial in the denominator; hence, this model is sometimes referred to as an *all-pole* model. This gives rise to a time domain equation similar to Eq. (6) in Chapter 4, but with only a single numerator coefficient, $b(0)$, which is assumed to be 1:

$$y(n) = -\sum_{k=1}^{p} a(k) \, y(n - k) + u(n) \tag{1}$$

where $u(n)$ is the input or noise function and p is the model order. Note that in Eq. (1), the output is obtained by convolving the model weight function, $a(k)$, with past versions of the output (i.e., $y(n-k)$). This is similar to an IIR filter with a constant numerator.

The *moving average* model is useful for evaluating spectra with the valleys, but no sharp peaks. The transfer function for this model has only a numerator polynomial and is sometimes referred to as an *all-zero* model. The equation for an MA model is the same as for an FIR filter, and is also given by Eq. (6) in Chapter 4 with the single denominator coefficient $a(0)$ set to 1:

$$y(n) = -\sum_{k=1}^{q} b(k) \, u(n - k) \tag{2}$$

where again $x(n)$ is the input function and q is the model order*.

If the spectrum is likely to contain bold sharp peaks and the valleys, then a model that combines both the AR and MA characteristics can be used. As might be expected, the transfer function of an ARMA model contains both numerator and denominator polynomials, so it is sometimes referred to as a pole–zero model. The ARMA model equation is the same as Chapter 4's Eq. (6) which describes a general linear process:

$$y(n) = -\sum_{k=1}^{p} a(k) \, y(n - k) + \sum_{k=1}^{q} b(k) \, u(n - k) \tag{3}$$

In addition to selecting the type of model to be used, it is also necessary to select the model order, p and/or q. Some knowledge of the process generating

---

*Note p and q are commonly used symbols for the order of AR and MA models, respectively.

the data would be helpful in this task. A few schemes have been developed to assist in selecting model order and are described briefly below. The general approach is based around the concept that model order should be sufficient to allow the model spectrum to fit the signal spectrum, but not so large that it begins fitting the noise as well. In many practical situations, model order is derived on a trial-and-error basis. The implications of model order are discussed below.

While many techniques exist for evaluating the parameters of an AR model, algorithms for MA and ARMA are less plentiful. In general, these algorithms involve significant computation and are not guaranteed to converge, or may converge to the wrong solution. Most ARMA methods estimate the AR and MA parameters separately, rather than jointly, as required for optimal solution. The MA approach cannot model narrowband spectra well: it is not a high-resolution spectral estimator. This shortcoming limits its usefulness in power spectral estimation of biosignals. Since only the AR model is implemented in the MATLAB Signal Processing Toolbox, the rest of this description of model-based power spectral analysis will be restricted to autoregressive spectral estimation. For a more comprehensive implementation of these and other models, the MATLAB Signal Identification Toolbox includes both MA and ARMA models along with a number of other algorithms for AR model estimation, in addition to other more advanced model-based approaches.

AR spectral estimation techniques can be divided into two categories: algorithms that process block data and algorithms that process data sequentially. The former are appropriate when the entire waveform is available in memory, while the latter are effective when incoming data must be evaluated rapidly for real-time considerations. Here we will consider only block-processing algorithms as they find the largest application in biomedical engineering and are the only algorithms implemented in the MATLAB Signal Processing Toolbox.

As with the concept of power spectral density introduced in the last chapter, the AR spectral approach is usually defined with regard to estimation based on the autocorrelation sequence. Nevertheless, better results are obtained, particularly for short data segments, by algorithms that operate directly on the waveform without estimating the autocorrelation sequence.

There are a number of different approaches for estimating the AR model coefficients and related power spectrum directly from the waveform. The four approaches that have received the most attention are: the Yule-Walker, the Burg, the covariance, and the modified covariance methods. All of these approaches to spectral estimation are implemented in the MATLAB Signal Processing Toolbox.

The most appropriate method will depend somewhat on the expected (or desired) shape of the spectrum, since the different methods theoretically enhance different spectral characteristics. For example, the Yule-Walker method is thought to produce spectra with the least resolution among the four, but provides the most smoothing, while the modified covariance method should produce the sharpest peaks, useful for identifying sinusoidal components in the data (Marple, 1987). The Burg and covariance methods are known to produce similar spectra. In reality, the MATLAB implementations of the four methods all produce similar spectra, as show below.

Figure 5.2 illustrates some of the advantages and disadvantages of using AR as a spectral analysis tool. A test waveform is constructed consisting of a low frequency broader-band signal, four sinusoids at 100, 240, 280, and 400 Hz, and white noise. A classically derived spectrum (Welch) is shown without the added noise in Figure 5.2A and with noise in Figure 5.2B. The remaining plots show the spectra obtained with an AR model of differing model orders. Figures 5.2C–E show the importance of model order on the resultant spectrum. Using the Yule-Walker method and a relatively low-order model (p = 17) produces a smooth spectrum, particularly in the low frequency range, but the spectrum combines the two closely spaced sinusoids (240 and 280 Hz) and does not show the 100 Hz component (Figure 5.2C). The two higher order models (p = 25 and 35) identify all of the sinusoidal components with the highest order model showing sharper peaks and a better defined peak at 100 Hz (Figure 5.2D and E). However, the highest order model (p = 35) also produces a less accurate estimate of the low frequency spectral feature, showing a number of low frequency peaks that are not present in the data. Such artifacts are termed *spurious peaks* and occur most often when high model orders are used. In Figure 5.2F, the spectrum produced by the covariance method is shown to be nearly identical to the one produced by the Yule-Walker method with the same model order.

The influence of model order is explored further in Figure 5.3. Four spectra are obtained from a waveform consisting of 3 sinusoids at 100, 200, and 300 Hz, buried in a fair amount of noise (SNR = -8 db). Using the traditional Welch method, the three sinusoidal peaks are well-identified, but other lesser peaks are seen due to the noise (Figure 5.3A). A low-order AR model, Figure 5.3B, smooths the noise very effectively, but identifies only the two outermost peaks at 100 and 300 Hz. Using a higher order model results in a spectrum where the three peaks are clearly identified, although the frequency resolution is moderate as the peaks are not very sharp. A still higher order model improves the frequency resolution (the peaks are sharper), but now a number of spurious peaks can be seen. In summary, the AR along with other model-based methods can be useful spectral estimators if the nature of the signal is known, but considerable care must be taken in selecting model order and model type. Several problems at the end of this chapter further explore the influence of model order.

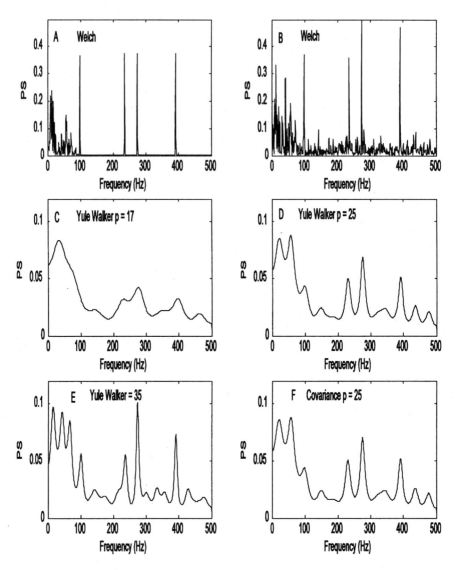

FIGURE 5.2 Comparison of AR and classical spectral analysis on a complex spectrum. (A) Spectrum obtained using classical methods (Welch) of a waveform consisting of four sinusoids (100, 240, 280, and 400 Hz) and a low frequency region generated from lowpass filtered noise. (B) Spectrum obtained using the Welch method applied to the same waveform after white noise has been added (SNR = -8 db). (C, D and E) Spectra obtained using AR models (Yule-Walker) having three different model orders. The lower order model (p = 17) cannot distinguish the two closely spaced sinusoids (240 and 280 Hz). The highest order model (p = 35) better identifies the 100 Hz signal and shows sharper peaks, but shows spurious peaks in the low frequency range. (F) AR spectral analysis using the covariance method produces results nearly identical to the Yule-Walker method.

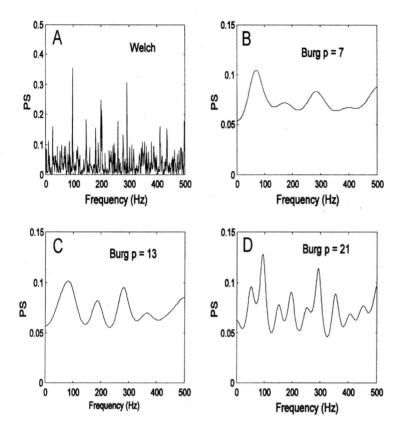

FIGURE 5.3 Spectra obtained from a waveform consisting of equal amplitude sinusoids at 100, 200, and 300 Hz with white noise ($N = 1024$; SNR = -12 db). (A) The traditional Welch method shows the 3 sinusoids, but also lesser peaks due solely to the noise. (B) The AR method with low model order ($p = 7$) shows the two outside peaks with a hint of the center peak. (C) A higher order AR model ($p = 13$) shows the three peaks clearly. (D) An even higher order model ($p = 21$) shows the three peaks with better frequency resolution, but also shows a number of spurious peaks.

MATLAB Implementation

The four AR-based spectral analysis approaches described above are available in the MATLAB Signal Processing Toolbox. The AR routines are implemented though statements very similar in format to that used for the Welsh power spectral analysis described in Chapter 3. For example, to implement the Yule-Walker AR method the MATLAB statement would be:

```
[PS, freq] = pyulear(x,p,nfft,Fs);
```

Only the first two input arguments, x and p, are required as the other two have default values. The input argument, x, is a vector containing the input waveform, and p is the order of the AR model to be used. The input argument nfft specifies the length of the data segment to be analyzed, and if nfft is less than the length of x, averages will be taken as in pwelch. The default value for nfft is 256*. As in pwelch, Fs is the sampling frequency and if specified is used to appropriately fill the frequency vector, freq, in the output. This output variable can be used in plotting to obtain a correctly scaled frequency axis (see Example 5.1). In the AR spectral approach, Fs is also needed to scale the horizontal axis of the output spectrum correctly. If Fs is not specified, the output vector freq varies in the range of 0 to π.

As in routine pwelch, only the first output argument, PS, is required, and it contains the resultant power spectrum. Similarly, the length of PS is either (nfft/2)+1 if nfft is even, or (nfft+1)/2 if nfft is odd since additional points would be redundant. An exception is made if x is complex, in which case the length of PS is equal to nfft. Other optional arguments are available and are described in the MATLAB help file.

The other AR methods are implemented using similar MATLAB statements, differing only in the function name.

```
[Pxx, freq] = pburg(x,p,nfft,Fs);
[Pxx, freq] = pcov(x,p,nfft,Fs);
[Pxx, freq] = pmcov(x,p,nfft,Fs);
```

The routine pburg, uses the Burg method, pcov the covariance method and pmcov the modified covariance method. As we will see below, this general format is followed in other MATLAB spectral methods.

Example 5.1   Generate a signal combining lowpass filtered noise, four sinusoids, two of which are closely spaced, and white noise (SNR = -3 db). This example is used to generate the plots in Figure 5.2.

```
% Example 5.1 and Figure 5.2
% Program to evaluate different modern spectral methods
% Generate a spectra of lowpass filtered noise, sinusoids, and
% noise that applies classical and AR sprectral analysis methods
%
```

---

*Note the use of the term nfft is somewhat misleading since it implies an FFT is taken, and this is not the case in AR spectral analysis. We use it here to be consistent with MATLAB's terminology.

```
N = 1024;                        % Size of arrays
fs = 1000;                       % Sampling frequency
n1 = 8;                          % Filter order
w = pi/20;                       % Filter cutoff frequency
                                 % (25 Hz)
%
% Generate the low frequency broadband process
% Compute the impulse response of a Butterworth lowpass filter
noise = randn(N,1);              % Generate noise
[b,a] = butter(n1,w);            % Filter noise with Butter-
                                 % worth filter
out = 5 * filter(b,a,noise);
%
% Generate the sinusoidal data and add to broadband signal
[x,f,sig] = sig_noise([100 240 280 400],-8,N);
data = data + out(1:1024,1)';    % Construct data set with added
                                 % noise
sig = sig + out(1:1024,1)';      % Construct data set without
                                 % noise
%
% Estimate the Welch spectrum using all points, no window, and no
% overlap
% Plot noiseless signal
[PS,f] = pwelch(sig,N,[ ],[ ],fs);
subplot(3,2,1);
    plot(f,PS,'k');              % Plot PS
.......labels, text, and axis .......
%
% Apply Welch method to noisy data set
[PS,f] = pwelch(x, N,[ ],[ ],fs);
subplot(3,2,2);
    plot(f,PS,'k');                    .......labels, text, and axis
                                       .......
%
% Apply AR to noisy data set at three different weights
[PS,f] = pyulear(x,17,N,fs);     % Yule-Walker; p = 17
subplot(3,2,3);
    plot(f,PS,'k');                    .......labels, text, and axis
                                       .......
%
[PS,f] = pyulear(x,25,N,fs);     % Yule-Walker; p = 25
subplot(3,2,4);
    plot(f,PS,'k');                    .......labels, text, and axis
                                       .......
%
[PS,f] = pyulear(x,35,N,fs);     % Yule-Walker; p = 35
```

```
subplot(3,2,5);
   plot(f,PS,'k');              .......labels, text, and axis
                                .......
%
% Apply Covariance method to data set
[PS,f] = pmcov(x,25,N,fs);      % Covariance; p = 25
subplot(3,2,6);
   plot(f,PS,'k');              .......labels, text, and axis
                                .......
```

In this example, the waveform is constructed by combining filtered low-pass noise with sinusoids in white noise. The filtered lowpass noise is constructed by applying an FIR filter to white noise. A similar approach to generating colored noise was used in Example 2 in Chapter 2. The routine sig_noise was then used to construct a waveform containing four sinusoids at 100, 240, 280, and 400 Hz with added white noise (SNR = -8 db). This waveform was then added to the colored noise after the latter was scaled by 5.0. The resultant waveform was then analyzed using different power spectral methods: the Welch FFT-based method for reference (applied to the signal with and without added noise); the Yule-Walker method with a model orders of 17, 25, and 35; and the modified covariance method with a model order of 25. The sampling frequency was 1000 Hz, the frequency assumed by the waveform generator routine, sig_noise.

Example 5.2   Explore the influence of noise on the AR spectrum specifically with regard to the ability to detect two closely related sinusoids.

Solution The program defines a vector, noise, that specifies four different levels of SNR (0, -4, -9, and -15 db). A loop is used to run through waveform generation and power spectrum estimation for the four noise levels. The values in noise are used with routine sig_noise to generate white noise of different levels along with two closely spaced sin waves at 240 and 280 Hz. The Yule-Walker AR method is used to determine the power spectrum, which is then plotted. A 15th-order model is used.

```
% Example 5.2 and Figure 5.4
% Program to evaluate different modern spectral methods
%    with regard to detecting a narrowband signal in various
%    amounts of noise
clear all; close all;
N = 1024;                  % Size of arrays
fs = 1000;                 % Sample frequency
order = 15;                % Model order
noise = [0 -4 -9 -15];     % Define SNR levels in db
for i = 1:4
```

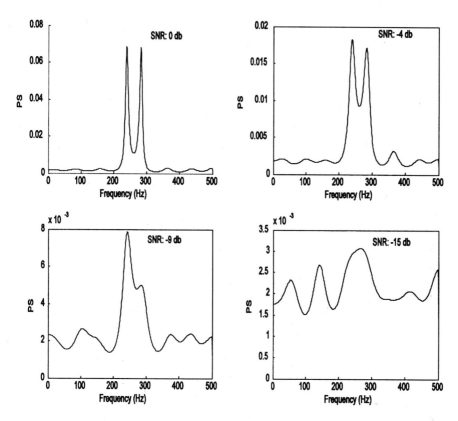

FIGURE 5.4 Power spectra obtained using the AR Yule-Walker method with a 15th-order model. The waveform consisted of two sinusoids at 240 and 280 Hz with various levels of noise. At the lowest noise levels, the two sinusoids are clearly distinguished, but appear to merge into one at the higher noise levels.

```
% Generate two closely space sine waves in white noise
x = sig_noise([240 280],noise(i),N);
[PS,f] = pyulear(data,order,N,fs);
subplot(2,2,i);            % Select subplot
  plot(f,PS,'k');          % Plot power spectrum and label
  text(200,max(PS),['SNR: ',num2str(noise(i)), 'db']);
  xlabel('Frequency (Hz)'); ylabel('PS ');
end
```

The output of this Example is presented in Figure 5.4. Note that the sinusoids are clearly identified at the two lower noise levels, but appear to merge together for the higher noise levels. At the highest noise level, only a single, broad peak can be observed at a frequency that is approximately the average of the two sine wave frequencies. The number of points used will also strongly influence the resolution of all spectral methods. This behavior is explored in the problems at the end of this chapter.

NON-PARAMETRIC EIGENANALYSIS FREQUENCY ESTIMATION

Eigenanalysis spectral methods are promoted as having better resolution and better frequency estimation characteristics, especially at high noise levels.* They are particularly effective in identifying sinusoidal, exponential, or other narrow-band processes in white noise as these methods can eliminate much of the noise contribution. However, if the noise is not white, but contains some spectral features (i.e., *colored noise*), performance can be degraded. The key feature of eigenvector approaches is to divide the information contained in the data waveform (or autocorrelation function) into two subspaces: a signal subspace and a noise subspace. The eigen-decomposition produces eigenvalues of decreasing order, and, most importantly, eigenvectors that are orthonormal. Since all the eigenvectors are orthonormal, if those eigenvectors that are deemed part of the noise subspace are eliminated, the influence of that noise is effectively eliminated. Functions can be computed based on either signal or noise subspace and can be plotted in the frequency domain. Such plots generally show sharp peaks where sinusoids or narrowband processes exist. Unlike parametric methods discussed above, these techniques are not considered true power spectral estimators, since they do not preserve signal power, nor can the autocorrelation sequence be reconstructed by applying the Fourier transform to these estimators. Better termed frequency estimators, they provide spectra in relative units.

The most problematic aspect of applying eigenvector spectral analysis is selecting the appropriate dimension of the signal (or noise) subspace. If the number of narrowband processes is known, then the signal subspace can be dimensioned on this basis; since each real sinusoid is the sum of two complex exponentials, the signal subspace dimension should be twice the number of sinusoids, or narrowband processes present. In some applications the signal subspace can be determined by the size of the eigenvalues; however, this method does not often work in practice, particularly with short data segments† [Marple,

---

*Another application of eigen-decomposition, principal component analysis, will be presented in Chapter 9.

†A similar use of eigenvalues is the determination of dimension in multivariate data as shown in Chapter 9. The *Scree plot*, a plot of eigenvalue against eigenvalue numbers is sometime used to estimate signal subspace dimension (see Figure 9.7). This plot is also found in Example 5.3.

1987]. As with the determination of the order of an AR model, the determination of the signal subspace often relies the on trial-and-error approach.

Figure 5.5 shows the importance of subspace dimension and illustrates both the strength and weaknesses of eigenvector spectral analysis. All four spectra were obtained from the same small data set ($N = 32$) consisting of two closely spaced sinusoids (320 and 380 Hz) in white noise (SNR = -7 db). Figure 5.5A shows the spectrum obtained using the classical, FFT-based Welch method. The other three plots show spectra obtained using eigenvector analysis, but with different partitions between the signal and noise subspaces. In Figure 5.5B, the spectrum was obtained using a signal subspace dimension of three. In this case, the size of the signal subspace is not large enough to differentiate

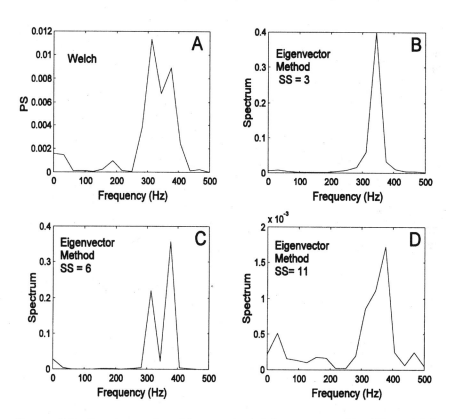

FIGURE 5.5 Spectra produced from a short data sequence (N = 32) containing two closely spaced sinusoids (320 and 380 Hz) in white noise (SNR = 7 db). The upper-left plot was obtained using the classical Welch method while the other three use eigenvector analysis with different partitions between the signal and noise subspace.

between the two closely spaced sinusoids, and, indeed, only a single peak is shown. When the signal subspace dimension is increased to 6 (Figure 5.5C) the two sinusoidal peaks are clearly distinguished and show better separation than with the classical method. However, when the signal subspace is enlarged further to a dimension of 11 (Figure 5.5D), the resulting spectrum contains small spurious peaks, and the two closely spaced sinusoids can no longer be distinguished. Hence, a signal subspace that is too large can be even more detrimental than one that is too small.

MATLAB Implementation

Two popular versions of frequency estimation based on eigenanalysis are the *Pisarenko* harmonic decomposition (PHP) and the MUltiple SIgnal Classifications (*MUSIC*) algorithms. These two eigenvector spectral analysis methods are available in the MATLAB Signal Processing Toolbox. Both methods have the same calling structure, a structure similar to that used by the AR routines. The command to evoke MUSIC algorithm is:

```
[PS, f,v,e] = pmusic(x, [p thresh], nfft, Fs, window, noverlap);
```

The last four input arguments are optional and have the same meaning as in `pwelch`, except that if `window` is a scalar or omitted, a rectangular window is used (as opposed to a Hamming window). The second argument is used to control the dimension of the signal (or noise) subspace. Since this parameter is critical to the successful application of the eigenvector approach, extra flexibility is provided. This argument can be either a scalar or vector. If only a single number is used, it will be taken as `p`, the dimension of the signal subspace. If the optional `thresh` is included, then eigenvalues below `thresh` times the minimum eigenvalue (i.e., `thresh` $\times \lambda_{min}$) will be assigned to the noise subspace; however, `p` still specifies the maximum signal subspace. Thus, `thresh` can be used to reduce the signal subspace dimension below that specified by `p`. To be meaningful, `thresh` must be > 1, otherwise the noise threshold would be < λ_{min} and its subspace dimension would be 0 (hence, if `thresh` < 1 it is ignored). Similarly `p` must be < n, the dimension of the eigenvectors. The dimension of the eigenvectors, n, is either `nfft`, or if not specified, the default value of 256. Alternatively, n is the size of the data matrix if the `corr` option is used, and the input is the correlation matrix as described below.

As suggested above, the data argument, `x`, is also more flexible. If `x` is a vector, then it is taken as one observation of the signal as in previous AR and Welch routines. However, `x` can also be a matrix in which case the routine assumes that each row of `x` is a separate observation of the signal. For example, each row could be the output of an array of sensors or a single response in a response ensemble. Such data are termed *multivariate* and are discussed in Chapter 9. Finally, the input argument x could be the correlation matrix. In this case, x must be a square matrix and the argument `'corr'` should be added to the input sequence anywhere after the argument p. If the input is the correlation matrix, then the arguments `window` and `noverlap` have no meaning and are ignored.

The only required output argument is PS, which contains the power spectrum (more appropriately termed the *pseudospectrum* due to the limitation described previously). The second output argument, f, is the familiar frequency vector useful in plotting. The output argument, v, following f, is a matrix of eigenvectors spanning the noise subspace (one per column) and the final output argument, e, is either a vector of singular values (squared) or a vector of eigenvalues of the correlation matrix when the input argument `'corr'` is used. An example of the use of the pmusic routine is given in the example below. An alternative eigenvector method can be implemented using the call peig. This routine has a calling structure identical to that of pmusic.

Example 5.3 This example compares classical, autoregressive and eigenanalysis spectral analysis methods, plots the singular values, generates Figure 5.6, and uses an optimum value for AR model order and eigenanalysis subspace dimension.

```
% Example 5.3 and Figure 5.6
% Compares FFT-based, AR, and eigenanalysis spectral methods
%
close all; clear all;
N = 1024;                    % Size of arrays
fs = 1000;                   % Sampling frequency
%
% Generate a spectra of sinusoids and noise
[data,t] = sig_noise([50 80 240 400],-10,N);
%
% Estimate the Welch spectrum for comparison, no window and
% no overlap
[PS,f] = pwelch(x,N,[],[],fs);
subplot(2,2,1);              % Plot spectrum and label
  plot(f,PS,'k');
    .......axis, labels, title.......
% Calculate the modified covariance spectrum for comparison
subplot(2,2,2);              % Plot spectrum and label
[PS,f] = pmcov(x,15,N,fs);
  plot(f,PS,'k');
    .......labels, title.......
% Generate the eigenvector spectrum using the MUSIC method
```

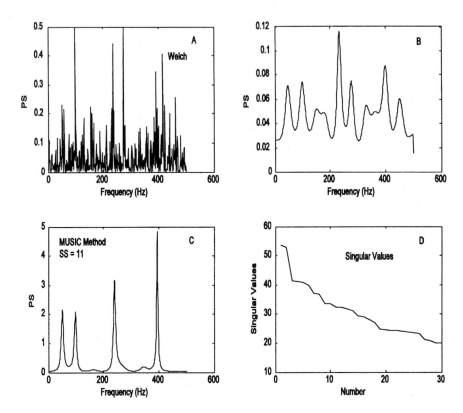

FIGURE 5.6 Spectrum obtained using 3 different methods applied to a waveform containing 4 equal amplitude sinusoids at frequencies of 50, 80, 240, and 400 Hz and white noise (SNR = -10 db; N = 1024). The eigenvector method (C) most clearly identifies the four components. The singular values determined from the eigenvalues (D) show a possible break or change in slope around n = 4 and another at n = 9, the latter being close to the actual signal subspace of 8.

```
% no window and no overlap
subplot(2,2,3);
[PS,f] = pmusic(x,11,N,fs);
  plot(f,PS,'k');                % Plot spectrum and label
  .......labels, title.......
%
% Get the singular values from the eigenvector routine
%   and plot. Use high subspace dimension to get many singular
%   values
subplot(2,2,4);
```

```
[PS,f,evects,svals] =          % Get eigenvalues (svals)
   pmusic(x,30,N, fs);
plot(svals,'k');               % Plot singular values
......labels, title.......
```

The plots produced by Example 5.3 are shown in Figure 5.6, and the strength of the eigenvector method for this task is apparent. In this example, the data length was quite long ($N = 1024$), but the SNR was low (-10 db). The signal consists of four equal amplitude sinusoids, two of which are closely spaced (50 and 80 Hz). While the spectrum produced by the classical Welch method does detect the four peaks, it also shows a number of other peaks in response to the noise. It would be difficult to determine, definitively and uniquely, the signal peaks from this spectrum. The AR method also detects the four peaks and greatly smooths the noise, but like the Welch method it shows spurious peaks related to the noise, and the rounded spectral shapes make it difficult to accurately determine the frequencies of the peaks. The eigenvector method not only resolves the four peaks, but provides excellent frequency resolution.

Figure 5.6 also shows a plot of the singular values as determined by pmusic. This plot can be used to estimate the dimensionality of multivariate data as detailed in Chapter 9. Briefly, the curve is examined for a break point between a steep and gentle slope, and this break point is taken as the dimensionality of the signal subspace. The idea is that a rapid decrease in the singular values is associated with the signal while a slower decrease indicates that the singular values are associated with the noise. Indeed, a slight break is seen around 9, approximately the correct value of the signal subspace. Unfortunately, well-defined break points are not always found when real data are involved.

The eigenvector method also performs well with short data sets. The behavior of the eigenvector method with short data sets and other conditions is explored in the problems.

Most of the examples provided evaluate the ability of the various spectral methods to identify sinusoids or narrowband processes in the presence of noise, but what of a more complex spectrum? Example 5.4 explores the ability of the classical (FFT), model-based, and eigenvalue methods in estimating a more complicated spectrum. In this example, we use a linear process (one of the filters described in Chapter 4) driven by white noise to create a complicated broadband spectrum. Since the filter is driven by white noise, the spectrum of its output waveform should be approximately the same as the transfer function of the filter itself. The various spectral analysis techniques are applied to this waveform and their ability to estimate the actual filter Transfer Function is evaluated. The *derivative* FIR filter of Example 4.6 will be used, and its transfer function will be evaluated directly from the filter coefficients using the FFT.

Example 5.4   This example is designed to compare the ability of several spectral analysis approaches, classical, model-based, and eigenvalue, to estimate a complex, broadband spectrum. The filter is the same as that used in Example 4.6 except that the derivative cutoff frequency has been increased to 0.25 $f_s/2$.

```
% Example 5.4 and Figure 5.7
% Construct a spectrum for white noise passed through
% a FIR derivative filter. Use the filter in Example 4.6.
% Compare classical, model-based, and eigenvector methods
```

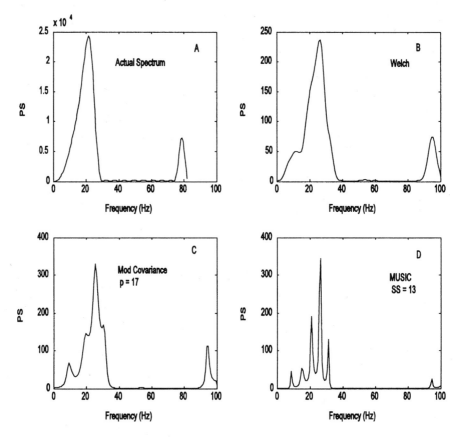

FIGURE 5.7 Estimation of a complex, broader-band spectrum using classical, model-based, and eigenvalue methods. (A) Transfer function of filter used to generate the data plotted a magnitude squared. (B) Estimation of the data spectrum using the Welch (FFT) method with 2 averages and maximum overlap. (C) Estimation of data spectrum using AR model, $p = 17$. (D) Estimation of data spectrum using an eigenvalue method with a subspace dimension of 13.

```
%
close all; clear all;
Ts = 1/200;                  % Assume a Ts of 5 msec
fs = 1/Ts;                   % Sampling frequency
fc = .25                     % Derivative cutoff frequency
N = 256;                     % Data length
%
% The initial code is the same as Example 4.6
x = randn(N,1);              % Generate white noise
%
% Design filter and plot magnitude characteristics
f1 = [ 0 fc fc+.1 .9];       % Specify desired frequency curve
a = [0 (fc*fs*pi) 0 0];      % Upward slope until 0.25 fs then
                             % lowpass
b = remez(28,f1,a,'differentiator');
x = filter(b,1,x);           % Apply FIR filter
%
% Calculate and plot filter transfer function
PS = (abs(fft(b,N))).^2;     % Calculate filter's transfer
                             % function
subplot(2,2,1);              %
  f = (1:N/2)*N/(2*fs);      % Generate freq. vector for
                             % plotting
  plot(f,PS(1:N/2),'k');     % Plot filter frequency response
  ......labels and text.......
%
[PS,f] = pwelch(x,N/4,       % Use 99% overlap
  (N/4)-1,[ ],fs);
subplot(2,2,2);              % Classical method (Welch)
  plot(f,PS,'k');
  ......labels and text.......
%
[PS,f] = pmcov(x,17,N,fs);
subplot(2,2,3);              % Model-based (AR-Mod.
                             % Covariance)
  plot(f,PS,'k');
  ......labels and text.......
%
[PS,f] = music(x,13,N,fs);
subplot(2,2,4);              % Eigenvector method (Music)
  plot(f,PS,'k');
  ......labels and text.......
```

The plots produced by this program are shown in Figure 5.7. In Figure 5.7A, the filter's transfer function is plotted as the magnitude squared so that it can be directly compared with the various spectral techniques that estimate the power spectrum of the filter's output waveform. The parameters associated with the various approaches have been adjusted to produce as close a match to the filter transfer function as possible. The influence of some of these parameters is explored in the problems. The power spectrum produced by the classical approach is shown in Figure 5.7B and roughly approximates the spectral characteristics of the filter. The classical approach used the Welch method and averaged four segments with a maximum overlap. The model-based approach used the modified covariance method and a model order of 17, and produced a spectrum similar to that produced by the Welch method. The eigenvalue approach used a subspace of 13 and could only approximate the actual spectrum as a series of narrowband processes. This demonstrates that eigenvalue methods, while well-suited to identifying sinusoids in noise, are not good at estimating spectra that contain broader-band features.

PROBLEMS

1. Use `sig_noise` to generate a 254-point data segment containing two closely spaced sinusoids at 200 and 220 Hz both with SNR of -5 db. Find the best model order to distinguish these two peaks with a minimum of spurious peaks. Use the Burg method. Repeat with an SNR of -10 db.

2. Repeat Problem 1 above, but using a shorter data segment ($N = 64$), and a higher SNR: -1 db. Now lower the SNR to -5 db as in Problem 1 and note the severe degradation in performance.

3. Use `sig_noise` to generate a moderately long ($N = 128$) data segment consisting of a moderate (SNR = -5 db) sinusoid at 200 Hz and weak (SNR = -9 db) sinusoid at 230 Hz. Compare the spectrum generated by Welch, AR, and eigenvector methods.

4. Use the data in Problem 1 (SNR $= -10$db) to compare the operation of the `pmusic` and `peig` MATLAB algorithms. Use a signal space of 7 and 13 for each case. Plot power spectrum in db.

5. Use `sig_noise` to generate a short data segment ($N = 64$) containing two closely spaced sinusoids in white noise (300 and 330 Hz). Both have SNR's of -3 db. Compare the spectra obtained with the Welch, AR–Burg, and eigenvalue methods. For the AR model and eigenvector method chose a model or subspace order ranging between 5 to 19. Show the best case frequency plots.

6. Construct a broadband spectrum by passing white noise through a filter as in Example 5.4. Use the IIR bandpass filter of Example 4.7 (and Figure 4.16). Generate the filter's transfer function directly from the coefficients, as in Exam-

ple 5.4. (Note you will have to take the FFT of both numerator and denominator coefficients and divide, or use `freqz`.) Next compare the spectrum produced by the three methods, as in Example 5.4. Adjust the parameters for the best relationship between the filter's actual spectrum and that produced by the various methods.

6

Time–Frequency Analysis

BASIC APPROACHES

The spectral analysis techniques developed thus far represent powerful signal processing tools if one is not especially concerned with signal timing. Classical or modern spectral methods provide a complete and appropriate solution for waveforms that are stationary; that is, waveforms that do not change in their basic properties over the length of the analysis (strictly speaking, that do not change in their statistical properties). Yet many waveforms—particularly those of biological origin–are not stationary, and change substantially in their properties over time. For example, the EEG signal changes considerably depending on various internal states of the subject: i.e., meditation, sleep, eyes closed. Moreover, it is these changes with time that are often of primary interest. Fourier analysis provides a good description of the frequencies in a waveform, but not their timing. The Fourier transform "of a musical passage tells us what notes are played, but it is extremely different to figure out when they are played" (Hubbard, 1998). Such information must be embedded in the frequency spectrum since the Fourier transform is bilateral, and the musical passage can be uniquely reconstructed using the inverse Fourier transform. However, timing is encoded in the phase portion of the transform, and this encoding is difficult to interpret and recover. In the Fourier transform, specific events in time are distributed across all of the phase components. In essence, a local feature in time has been transformed into a global feature in phase.

Timing information is often of primary interest in many biomedical signals, and this is also true for medical images where the analogous information is localized in space. A wide range of approaches have been developed to try to extract both time and frequency information from a waveform. Basically they can be divided into two groups: time–frequency methods and time–scale methods. The latter are better known as *Wavelet* analyses, a popular new approach described in the next chapter. This chapter is dedicated to time–frequency methods.

Short-Term Fourier Transform: The Spectrogram

The first time–frequency methods were based on the straightforward approach of slicing the waveform of interest into a number of short segments and performing the analysis on each of these segments, usually using the standard Fourier transform. A window function similar to those described in Chapter 3 is applied to a segment of data, effectively isolating that segment from the overall waveform, and the Fourier transform is applied to that segment. This is termed the *spectrogram* or "short-term Fourier transform" (STFT)* since the Fourier Transform is applied to a segment of data that is shorter, often much shorter, than the overall waveform. Since abbreviated data segments are used, selecting the most appropriate window length can be critical. This method has been successfully applied in a number of biomedical applications.

The basic equation for the spectrogram in the continuous domain is:

$$X(t,f) = \int_{-\infty}^{\infty} x(\tau)w(t - \tau)e^{-j\pi f\tau}d\tau \tag{1}$$

where $w(t\text{-}\tau)$ is the window function and τ is the variable that slides the window across the waveform, $x(t)$.

The discrete version of Eq. (1) is the same as was given in Chapter 2 for a general probing function (Eq. (11), Chapter 2) where the probing function is replaced by a family of sinusoids represented in complex format (i.e., $e^{-jnm/N}$):

$$X(m,k) = \sum_{n=1}^{N} x(n) \ [W(n - k)e^{-jnm/N}] \tag{2}$$

There are two main problems with the spectrogram: (1) selecting an optimal window length for data segments that contain several different features may not be possible, and (2) the time–frequency tradeoff: shortening the data length, N, to improve time resolution will reduce frequency resolution which is approximately $1/(NT_s)$. Shortening the data segment could also result in the loss of low frequencies that are no longer fully included in the data segment. Hence, if the

---

*The terms STFT and spectrogram are used interchangeably and we will follow the same, slightly confusing convention here. Essentially the reader should be familiar with both terms.

window is made smaller to improve the time resolution, then the frequency resolution is degraded and visa versa. This time–frequency tradeoff has been equated to an *uncertainty principle* where the product of frequency resolution (expressed as bandwidth, *B*) and time, *T*, must be greater than some minimum. Specifically:

$$BT \geq \frac{1}{4\pi} \tag{3}$$

The trade-off between time and frequency resolution inherent in the STFT, or spectrogram, has motivated a number of other time–frequency methods as well as the time–scale approaches discussed in the next chapter. Despite these limitations, the STFT has been used successfully in a wide variety of problems, particularly those where only high frequency components are of interest and frequency resolution is not critical. The area of speech processing has benefitted considerably from the application of the STFT. Where appropriate, the STFT is a simple solution that rests on a well understood classical theory (i.e., the Fourier transform) and is easy to interpret. The strengths and weaknesses of the STFT are explored in the examples in the section on MATLAB Implementation below and in the problems at the end of the chapter.

Wigner-Ville Distribution: A Special Case of Cohen's Class

A number of approaches have been developed to overcome some of the shortcomings of the spectrogram. The first of these was the *Wigner-Ville distribution** which is also one of the most studied and best understood of the many time–frequency methods. The approach was actually developed by Wigner for use in physics, but later applied to signal processing by Ville, hence the dual name. We will see below that the Wigner-Ville distribution is a special case of a wide variety of similar transformations known under the heading of *Cohen's class of distributions*. For an extensive summary of these distributions see Boudreaux-Bartels and Murry (1995).

The Wigner-Ville distribution, and others of Cohen's class, use an approach that harkens back to the early use of the autocorrelation function for calculating the power spectrum. As noted in Chapter 3, the classic method for determining the power spectrum was to take the Fourier transform of the autocorrelation function (Eq. (14), Chapter 3). To construct the autocorrelation function, the waveform is compared with itself for all possible relative shifts, or lags (Eq. (16), Chapter 2). The equation is repeated here in both continuous and discrete form:

---

*The term *distribution* in this usage should more properly be *density* since that is the equivalent statistical term (Cohen, 1990).

$$r_{xx}(\tau) = \int_{-\infty}^{\infty} x(t) \, x(t + \tau) \, dt \tag{4}$$

and

$$r_{xx}(n) = \sum_{k=1}^{M} x(k) \, x(k + n) \tag{5}$$

where τ and n are the shift of the waveform with respect to itself.

In the standard autocorrelation function, time is integrated (or summed) out of the result, and this result, $r_{xx}(\tau)$, is only a function of the lag, or shift, τ. The Wigner-Ville, and in fact all of Cohen's class of distributions, use a variation of the autocorrelation function where time remains in the result. This is achieved by comparing the waveform with itself for all possible lags, but instead of integrating over time, the comparison is done for all possible values of time. This comparison gives rise to the defining equation of the so-called *instantaneous autocorrelation* function:

$$R_{xx}(t,\tau) = x(t + \tau/2)x^*(t - \tau/2) \tag{6}$$

$$R_{xx}(n,k) = x(k + n)x^*(k - n) \tag{7}$$

where τ and n are the time lags as in autocorrelation, and $*$ represents the complex conjugate of the signal, x. Most actual signals are real, in which case Eq. (4) can be applied to either the (real) signal itself, or a complex version of the signal known as the *analytic signal*. A discussion of the advantages of using the analytic signal along with methods for calculating the analytic signal from the actual (i.e., real) signal is presented below.

The instantaneous autocorrelation function retains both lags and time, and is, accordingly, a two-dimensional function. The output of this function to a very simple sinusoidal input is shown in Figure 6.1 as both a three-dimensional and a contour plot. The standard autocorrelation function of a sinusoid would be a sinusoid of the same frequency. The instantaneous autocorrelation function output shown in Figure 6.1 shows a sinusoid along both the time and τ axis as expected, but also along the diagonals as well. These *cross products* are particularly apparent in Figure 6.1B and result from the multiplication in the instantaneous autocorrelation equation, Eq. (7). These cross products are a source of problems for all of the methods based on the instantaneous autocorrelation function.

As mentioned above, the classic method of computing the power spectrum was to take the Fourier transform of the standard autocorrelation function. The Wigner-Ville distribution echoes this approach by taking the Fourier transform

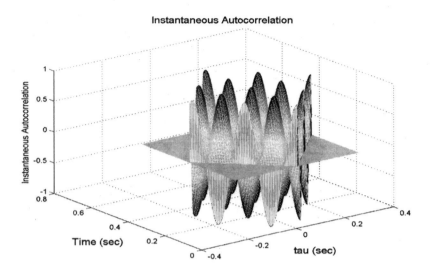

FIGURE 6.1A The instantaneous autocorrelation function of a two-cycle cosine wave plotted as a three-dimensional plot.

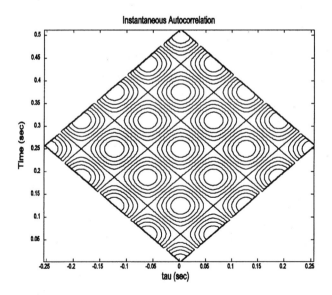

FIGURE 6.1B The instantaneous autocorrelation function of a two-cycle cosine wave plotted as a contour plot. The sinusoidal peaks are apparent along both axes as well as along the diagonals.

of the instantaneous autocorrelation function, but only along the τ (i.e., lag) dimension. The result is a function of both frequency and time. When the one-dimensional power spectrum was computed using the autocorrelation function, it was common to filter the autocorrelation function before taking the Fourier transform to improve features of the resulting power spectrum. While no such filtering is done in constructing the Wigner-Ville distribution, all of the other approaches apply a filter (in this case a two-dimensional filter) to the instantaneous autocorrelation function before taking the Fourier transform. In fact, the primary difference between many of the distributions in Cohen's class is simply the type of filter that is used.

The formal equation for determining a time–frequency distribution from Cohen's class of distributions is rather formidable, but can be simplified in practice. Specifically, the general equation is:

$$\rho(t,f) = \iiint g(v,\tau)e^{j2\pi v(u-\tau)}x(u+\tfrac{1}{2}\tau)x^*(u-\tfrac{1}{2}\tau)e^{-j2\pi fr}dv\,du\,d\tau \tag{8}$$

where $g(v,\tau)$ provides the two-dimensional filtering of the instantaneous autocorrelation and is also know as a *kernel*. It is this filter-like function that differentiates between the various distributions in Cohen's class. Note that the rest of the integrand is the Fourier transform of the instantaneous autocorrelation function.

There are several ways to simplify Eq. (8) for a specific kernel. For the Wigner-Ville distribution, there is no filtering, and the kernel is simply 1 (i.e., $g(v,\tau) = 1$) and the general equation of Eq. (8), after integration by dv, reduces to Eq. (9), presented in both continuous and discrete form.

$$W(t,f) = \int_{-\infty}^{\infty} e^{-j2\pi f\tau}x(t-\tfrac{\tau}{2})x(t-\tfrac{\tau}{2})d\tau \tag{9a}$$

$$W(n,m) = 2\sum_{k=-\infty}^{\infty} e^{-2\pi nm/N}x(n+k)x^*(n-k) \tag{9b}$$

$$W(n,m) = \sum_{m=-\infty}^{\infty} e^{-2\pi nm/N}R_x(n,k) = \text{FFT}_k[R_x(n,k)] \tag{9c}$$

Note that $t = nT_s$, and $f = m/(NT_s)$

The Wigner-Ville has several advantages over the STFT, but also has a number of shortcomings. It greatest strength is that produces "a remarkably good picture of the time-frequency structure" (Cohen, 1992). It also has favorable marginals and conditional moments. The marginals relate the summation over time or frequency to the signal energy at that time or frequency. For example, if we sum the Wigner-Ville distribution over frequency at a fixed time, we get a value equal to the energy at that point in time. Alternatively, if we fix frequency and sum over time, the value is equal to the energy at that frequency. The conditional moment of the Wigner-Ville distribution also has significance:

$$f_{\text{inst}} = \frac{1}{p(t)} \int\limits_{-\infty}^{\infty} f\rho(f,t)df \tag{10}$$

where $p(t)$ is the marginal in time.

This conditional moment is equal to the so-called *instantaneous frequency*. The instantaneous frequency is usually interpreted as the average of the frequencies at a given point in time. In other words, treating the Wigner-Ville distribution as an actual probability density (it is not) and calculating the mean of frequency provides a term that is logically interpreted as the mean of the frequencies present at any given time.

The Wigner-Ville distribution has a number of other properties that may be of value in certain applications. It is possible to recover the original signal, except for a constant, from the distribution, and the transformation is invariant to shifts in time and frequency. For example, shifting the signal in time by a delay of T seconds would produce the same distribution except shifted by T on the time axis. The same could be said of a frequency shift (although biological processes that produce shifts in frequency are not as common as those that produce time shifts). These characteristics are also true of the STFT and some of the other distributions described below. A property of the Wigner-Ville distribution not shared by the STFT is *finite support* in time and frequency. Finite support in time means that the distribution is zero before the signal starts and after it ends, while finite support in frequency means the distribution does not contain frequencies beyond the range of the input signal. The Wigner-Ville does contain nonexistent energies due to the cross products as mentioned above and observed in Figure 6.1, but these are contained within the time and frequency boundaries of the original signal. Due to these cross products, the Wigner-Ville distribution is not necessarily zero whenever the signal is zero, a property Cohen called *strong finite support*. Obviously, since the STFT does not have finite support it does not have strong finite support. A few of the other distributions do have strong finite support. Examples of the desirable attributes of the Wigner-Ville will be explored in the MATLAB Implementation section, and in the problems.

The Wigner-Ville distribution has a number of shortcomings. Most serious of these is the production of cross products: the demonstration of energies at time–frequency values where they do not exist. These phantom energies have been the prime motivator for the development of other distributions that apply various filters to the instantaneous autocorrelation function to mitigate the damage done by the cross products. In addition, the Wigner-Ville distribution can have negative regions that have no meaning. The Wigner-Ville distribution also has poor noise properties. Essentially the noise is distributed across all time and frequency including cross products of the noise, although in some cases, the cross products and noise influences can be reduced by using a window. In such cases, the desired window function is applied to the lag dimension of the instantaneous autocorrelation function (Eq. (7)) similar to the way it was applied to the time function in Chapter 3. As in Fourier transform analysis, windowing will reduce frequency resolution, and, in practice, a compromise is sought between a reduction of cross products and loss of frequency resolution. Noise properties and the other weaknesses of the Wigner-Ville distribution along with the influences of windowing are explored in the implementation and problem sections.

The Choi-Williams and Other Distributions

The existence of cross products in the Wigner-Ville transformation has motived the development of other distributions. These other distributions are also defined by Eq. (8); however, now the kernel, $g(v,\tau)$, is no longer 1. The general equation (Eq. (8)) can be simplified two different ways: for any given kernel, the integration with respect to the variable v can be performed in advance since the rest of the transform (i.e., the signal portion) is not a function of v; or use can be made of an intermediate function, called the *ambiguity function*.

In the first approach, the kernel is multiplied by the exponential in Eq. (9) to give a new function, $G(u,\tau)$:

$$G(u,\tau) = \int_{-\infty}^{\infty} g(v,\tau)e^{j\pi vu}dv \tag{11}$$

where the new function, $G(u,\tau)$ is referred to as the *determining function* (Boashash and Reilly, 1992). Then Eq. (9) reduces to:

$$\rho(t,f) = \iint G(u - t,\tau)x(u + \tfrac{1}{2}\tau)x^*(u - \tfrac{1}{2}\tau)e^{-2\pi ft}dudt \tag{12}$$

Note that the second set of terms under the double integral is just the instantaneous autocorrelation function given in Eq. (7). In terms of the determining function and the instantaneous autocorrelation function, the discrete form of Eq. (12) becomes:

$$\rho(t,f) = \sum_{\tau=0}^{M} R_x(t,\tau)G(t,\tau)e^{-j2\pi f\tau} \tag{13}$$

where $t = u/f_s$. This is the approach that is used in the section on MATLAB implementation below. Alternatively, one can define a new function as the inverse Fourier transform of the instantaneous autocorrelation function:

$$A_x(\theta,\tau) \triangleq \mathrm{IFT}_t[x(t + \tau/2)x^*(t - \tau/2)] = \mathrm{IFT}_t[R_x(t,\tau)] \tag{14}$$

where the new function, $A_x(\theta,\tau)$, is termed the *ambiguity function*. In this case, the convolution operation in Eq. (13) becomes multiplication, and the desired distribution is just the double Fourier transform of the product of the ambiguity function times the instantaneous autocorrelation function:

$$\rho(t,f) = \text{FFT}_t\{\text{FFT}_f[A_x(\theta,\tau)R_x(t,\tau)]\} \tag{15}$$

One popular distribution is the *Choi-Williams*, which is also referred to as an *exponential distribution* (ED) since it has an exponential-type kernel. Specifically, the kernel and determining function of the Choi-Williams distribution are:

$$g(v,\tau) = e^{-v^2\tau^2/\sigma} \tag{16}$$

After integrating the equation above as in Eq. (11), $G(t,\tau)$ becomes:

$$G(t,\tau) = \frac{\sqrt{\sigma/\pi}}{2\tau} e^{-\sigma t^2/4\tau^2} \tag{17}$$

The Choi-Williams distribution can also be used in a modified form that incorporates a window function and in this form is considered one of a class of reduced interference distributions (RID) (Williams, 1992). In addition to having reduced cross products, the Choi-Williams distribution also has better noise characteristics than the Wigner-Ville. These two distributions will be compared with other popular distributions in the section on implementation.

Analytic Signal

All of the transformations in Cohen's class of distributions produce better results when applied to a modified version of the waveform termed the *Analytic signal*, a complex version of the real signal. While the real signal can be used, the analytic signal has several advantages. The most important advantage is due to the fact that the analytic signal does not contain negative frequencies, so its use will reduce the number of cross products. If the real signal is used, then both the positive and negative spectral terms produce cross products. Another benefit is that if the analytic signal is used the sampling rate can be reduced. This is because the instantaneous autocorrelation function is calculated using evenly spaced values, so it is, in fact, undersampled by a factor of 2 (compare the discrete and continuous versions of Eq. (9)). Thus, if the analytic function is not used, the data must be sampled at twice the normal minimum; i.e., twice the Nyquist frequency or four times f_{MAX}.* Finally, if the instantaneous frequency

---

*If the waveform has already been sampled, the number of data points should be doubled with intervening points added using interpolation.

is desired, it can be determined from the first moment (i.e., mean) of the distribution only if the analytic signal is used.

Several approaches can be used to construct the analytic signal. Essentially one takes the real signal and adds an imaginary component. One method for establishing the imaginary component is to argue that the negative frequencies that are generated from the Fourier transform are not physical and, hence, should be eliminated. (Negative frequencies are equivalent to the redundant frequencies above $f_s/2$. Following this logic, the Fourier transform of the real signal is taken, the negative frequencies are set to zero, or equivalently, the redundant frequencies above $f_s/2$, and the (now complex) signal is reconstructed using the inverse Fourier transform. This approach also multiplies the positive frequencies, those below $f_s/2$, by 2 to keep the overall energy the same. This results in a new signal that has a real part identical to the real signal and an imaginary part that is the *Hilbert Transform* of the real signal (Cohen, 1989). This is the approach used by the MATLAB routine `hilbert` and the routine `hilber` on the disk, and the approach used in the examples below.

Another method is to perform the Hilbert transform directly using the Hilbert transform filter to produce the complex component:

$$z(n) = x(n) + j\ \mathcal{H}[x(n)] \tag{18}$$

where $\mathcal{H}$ denotes the Hilbert transform, which can be implemented as an FIR filter (Chapter 4) with coefficients of:

$$h(n) = \begin{cases} \dfrac{2\ \sin^2(\pi n/2)}{\pi n} & \text{for } n \neq 0 \\ 0 & \text{for } n = 0 \end{cases} \tag{19}$$

Although the Hilbert transform filter should have an infinite impulse response length (i.e., an infinite number of coefficients), in practice an FIR filter length of approximately 79 samples has been shown to provide an adequate approximation (Bobashash and Black, 1987).

MATLAB IMPLEMENTATION

The Short-Term Fourier Transform

The implementation of the time–frequency algorithms described above is straightforward and is illustrated in the examples below. The spectrogram can be generated using the standard `fft` function described in Chapter 3, or using a special function of the Signal Processing Toolbox, `specgram`. The arguments for `specgram` (given on the next page) are similar to those use for `pwelch` described in Chapter 3, although the order is different.

```
[B,f,t] = specgram(x,nfft,fs,window,noverlap)
```

where the output, **B**, is a complex matrix containing the magnitude and phase of the STFT time–frequency spectrum with the rows encoding the time axis and the columns representing the frequency axis. The optional output arguments, **f** and **t**, are time and frequency vectors that can be helpful in plotting. The input arguments include the data vector, **x**, and the size of the Fourier transform window, **nfft**. Three optional input arguments include the sampling frequency, **fs**, used to calculate the plotting vectors, the window function desired, and the number of overlapping points between the windows. The window function is specified as in **pwelch**: if a scalar is given, then a Hanning window of that length is used.

The output of all MATLAB-based time–frequency methods is a function of two variables, time and frequency, and requires either a three-dimensional plot or a two-dimensional *contour* plot. Both plotting approaches are available through MATLAB standard graphics and are illustrated in the example below.

Example 6.1 Construct a time series consisting of two sequential sinusoids of 10 and 40 Hz, each active for 0.5 sec (see Figure 6.2). The sinusoids should be preceded and followed by 0.5 sec of no signal (i.e., zeros). Determine the magnitude of the STFT and plot as both a three-dimensional grid plot and as a contour plot. Do not use the Signal Processing Toolbox routine, but develop code for the STFT. Use a Hanning window to isolate data segments.

Example 6.1 uses a function similar to MATLAB's **specgram**, except that the window is fixed (Hanning) and all of the input arguments must be specified. This function, **spectog**, has arguments similar to those in **specgram**. The code for this routine is given below the main program.

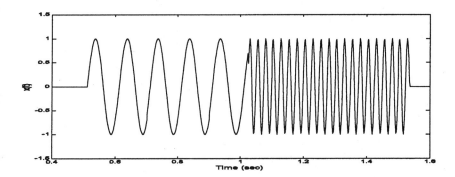

FIGURE 6.2 Waveform used in Example 6.1 consisting of two sequential sinusoids of 10 and 40 Hz. Only a portion of the 0.5 sec endpoints are shown.

```
% Example 6.1 and Figures 6.2, 6.3, and 6.4
% Example of the use of the spectrogram
%   Uses function spectog given below
%
clear all; close all;
% Set up constants
fs = 500;                   % Sample frequency in Hz
N = 1024;                   % Signal length
f1 = 10;                    % First frequency in Hz
f2 = 40;                    % Second frequency in Hz
nfft = 64;                  % Window size
noverlap = 32;              % Number of overlapping points (50%)
%
% Construct a step change in frequency
tn = (1:N/4)/fs;            % Time vector used to create sinusoids
x = [zeros(N/4,1); sin(2*pi*f1*tn)'; sin(2*pi*f2*tn)'...
  zeros(N/4,1)];
t = (1:N)/fs;               % Time vector used to plot
plot(t,x,'k');
  ....labels....
% Could use the routine specgram from the MATLAB Signal Processing
%   Toolbox: [B,f,t] = specgram(x,nfft,fs,window,noverlap),
%   but in this example, use the "spectog" function shown below.
```

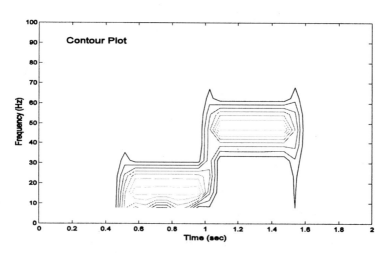

FIGURE 6.3 Contour plot of the STFT of two sequential sinusoids. Note the broad time and frequency range produced by this time–frequency approach. The appearance of energy at times and frequencies where no energy exists in the original signal is evident.

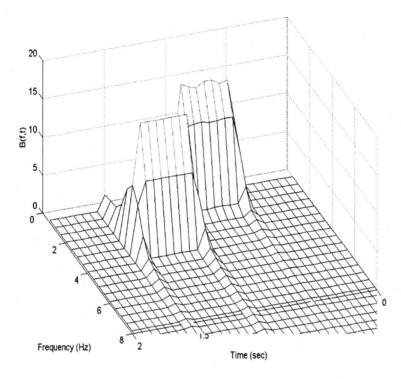

FIGURE 6.4 Time–frequency magnitude plot of the waveform in Figure 6.3 using the three-dimensional grid technique.

```
%
[B,f,t] = spectog(x,nfft,fs,noverlap);
B = abs(B);                  % Get spectrum magnitude
figure;
  mesh(t,f,B);               % Plot Spectrogram as 3-D mesh
  view(160,40);              % Change 3-D plot view
  axis([0 2 0 100 0 20]);    % Example of axis and
  xlabel('Time (sec)');      % labels for 3-D plots
  ylabel('Frequency (Hz)');
figure
  contour(t,f,B);            % Plot spectrogram as contour plot
  ....labels and axis....
```

The function spectog is coded as:

```
function [sp,f,t] = spectog(x,nfft,fs,noverlap);
% Function to calculate spectrogram
```

```
% Output arguments
%   sp spectrogram
%   t time vector for plotting
%   f frequency vector for plotting
% Input arguments
%   x data
%   nfft window size
%   fs sample frequency
%   noverlap number of overlapping points in adjacent segments
% Uses Hanning window
%
[N xcol] = size(x);
if N < xcol
   x = x';                      % Insure that the input is a row
   N = xcol;                    %   vector (if not already)
end
incr = nfft-noverlap;          % Calculate window increment
hwin = fix(nfft/2);            % Half window size
f = (1:hwin)*(fs/nfft);        % Calculate frequency vector
% Zero pad data array to handle edge effects
x_mod = [zeros(hwin,1); x; zeros(hwin,1)];
%
j = 1;                          % Used to index time vector
% Calculate spectra for each window position
% Apply Hanning window
for i = 1:incr:N
   data = x_mod(i:i+nfft-1) .* hanning(nfft);
   ft = abs(fft(data));         % Magnitude data
   sp(:,j) = ft(1:hwin);        % Limit spectrum to meaningful
                                %   points
   t(j) = i/fs;                 % Calculate time vector
   j = j + 1;                   % Increment index
end
```

Figures 6.3 and 6.4 show that the STFT produces a time–frequency plot with the step change in frequency at approximately the correct time, although neither the step change nor the frequencies are very precisely defined. The lack of finite support in either time or frequency is evidenced by the appearance of energy slightly before 0.5 sec and slightly after 1.5 sec, and energies at frequencies other than 10 and 40 Hz. In this example, the time resolution is better than the frequency resolution. By changing the time window, the compromise between time and frequency resolution could be altered. Exploration of this tradeoff is given as a problem at the end of this chapter.

A popular signal used to explore the behavior of time–frequency methods is a sinusoid that increases in frequency over time. This signal is called a *chirp* signal because of the sound it makes if treated as an audio signal. A sample of such a signal is shown in Figure 6.5. This signal can be generated by multiplying the argument of a sine function by a linearly increasing term, as shown in Example 6.2 below. Alternatively, the Signal Processing Toolbox contains a special function to generate a chip that provides some extra features such as logarithmic or quadratic changes in frequency. The MATLAB `chirp` routine is used in a latter example. The output of the STFT to a chirp signal is demonstrated in Figure 6.6.

Example 6.2 Generate a linearly increasing sine wave that varies between 10 and 200 Hz over a 1sec period. Analyze this chirp signal using the STFT program used in Example 6.1. Plot the resulting spectrogram as both a 3-D grid and as a contour plot. Assume a sample frequency of 500 Hz.

```
% Example 6.2 and Figure 6.6
% Example to generate a sine wave with a linear change in frequency
% Evaluate the time-frequency characteristic using the STFT
% Sine wave should vary between 10 and 200 Hz over a 1.0 sec period
% Assume a sample rate of 500 Hz
%
clear all; close all;
% Constants
N = 512;                            % Number of points
```

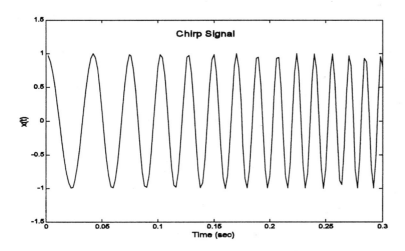

FIGURE 6.5 Segment of a *chirp* signal, a signal that contains a single sinusoid that changes frequency over time. In this case, signal frequency increases linearly with time.

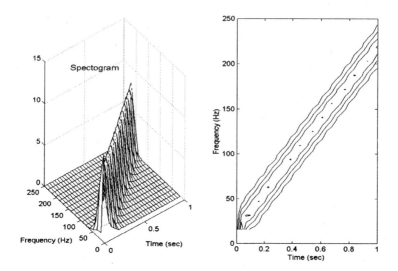

FIGURE 6.6 The STFT of a chirp signal, a signal linearly increasing in frequency from 10 to 200 Hz, shown as both a 3-D grid and a contour plot.

```
fs = 500;                              % Sample freq;
f1 = 10;                               % Minimum frequency
f2 = 200;                              % Maximum frequency
nfft = 32;                             % Window size
t = (1:N)/fs;                          % Generate a time
                                       %   vector for chirp
% Generate chirp signal (use a linear change in freq)
fc = ((1:N)*((f2-f1)/N)) + f1;
x = sin(pi*t.*fc);
%
% Compute spectrogram using the Hanning window and 50% overlap
[B,f,t] = spectog(x,nfft,fs,nfft/2);   % Code shown above
%
subplot(1,2,1);                        % Plot 3-D and contour
                                       %   side-by-side
   mesh(t,f,abs(B));                   % 3-D plot
   ....labels, axis, and title....
subplot(1,2,2);
   contour(t,f,abs(B));                % Contour plot
   ....labels, axis, and title....
```

The Wigner-Ville Distribution

The Wigner-Ville distribution will provide a much more definitive picture of the time–frequency characteristics, but will also produce cross products: time–

frequency energy that is not in the original signal, although it does fall within the time and frequency boundaries of the signal. Example 6.3 demonstrates these properties on a signal that changes frequency abruptly, the same signal used in Example 6.1 with the STFT. This will allow a direct comparison of the two methods.

Example 6.3   Apply the Wigner-Ville distribution to the signal of Example 6.1. Use the analytic signal and provide plots similar to those of Example 6.1.

```
% Example 6.3 and Figures 6.7 and 6.8
% Example of the use of the Wigner-Ville distribution
%  Applies the Wigner-Ville to data similar to that of Example
%    6.1, except that the data has been shortened from 1024 to 512
%    to improve run time.
%
clear all; close all;
% Set up constants (same as Example 6-1)
fs = 500;              % Sample frequency
N = 512;               % Signal length
f1 = 10;               % First frequency in Hz
f2 = 40;               % Second frequency in Hz
```

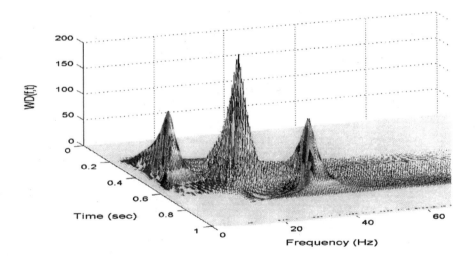

FIGURE 6.7 Wigner-Ville distribution for the two sequential sinusoids shown in Figure 6.3. Note that while both the frequency ranges are better defined than in Figure 6.2 produced by the STFT, there are large cross products generated in the region between the two actual signals (central peak). In addition, the distributions are sloped inward along the time axis so that onset time is not as precisely defined as the frequency range.

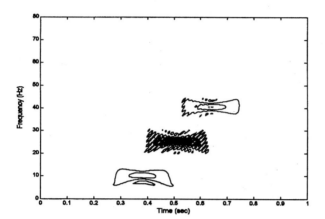

FIGURE 6.8 Contour plot of the Wigner-Ville distribution of two sequential sinusoids. The large cross products are clearly seen in the region between the actual signal energy. Again, the slope of the distributions in the time domain make it difficult to identify onset times.

```
%
% Construct a step change in frequency as in Ex. 6-1
tn = (1:N/4)/fs;
x = [zeros(N/4,1); sin(2*pi*f1*tn)'; sin(2*pi*f2*tn)';
  zeros(N/4,1)];
%
% Wigner-Ville analysis
x = hilbert(x);        % Construct analytic function
[WD,f,t] = wvd(x,fs);  % Wigner-Ville transformation
WD = abs(WD);          % Take magnitude
mesh(t,f,WD);          % Plot distribution
view(100,40);          % Use different view
....Labels and axis....
figure
contour(t,f,WD);       % Plot as contour plot
....Labels and axis....
```

The function wwd computes the Wigner-Ville distribution.

```
function [WD,f,t] = wvd(x,fs)
% Function to compute Wigner-Ville time-frequency distribution
% Outputs
%    WD Wigner-Ville distribution
%    f Frequency vector for plotting
%    t Time vector for plotting
```

```
% Inputs
%    x    Complex signal
%    fs Sample frequency
%
[N, xcol] = size(x);
if N < xcol                    % Make signal a column vector if necessary
   x = x!;                     % Standard (non-complex) transpose
   N = xcol;
end
WD = zeros(N,N);               % Initialize output
t = (1:N)/fs;                  % Calculate time and frequency vectors
f = (1:N)*fs/(2*N);
%
%
%Compute instantaneous autocorrelation: Eq. (7)
for ti = 1:N % Increment over time
   taumax = min([ti-1,N-ti,round(N/2)-1]);
   tau = -taumax:taumax;
   % Autocorrelation: tau is in columns and time is in rows
   WD(tau-tau(1)+1,ti) = x(ti+tau) .* conj(x(ti-tau));
end
%
WD = fft(WD);
```

The last section of code is used to compute the instantaneous autocorrelation function and its Fourier transform as in Eq. (9c). The `for` loop is used to construct an array, `WD`, containing the instantaneous autocorrelation where each column contains the correlations at various lags for a given time, `ti`. Each column is computed over a range of lags, ± `taumax`. The first statement in the loop restricts the range of `taumax` to be within signal array: it uses all the data that is symmetrically available on either side of the time variable, `ti`. Note that the phase of the lag signal placed in array `WD` varies by column (i.e., time). Normally this will not matter since the Fourier transform will be taken over each set of lags (i.e., each column) and only the magnitude will be used. However, the phase was properly adjusted before plotting the instantaneous autocorrelation in Figure 6.1. After the instantaneous autocorrelation is constructed, the Fourier transform is taken over each set of lags. Note that if an array is presented to the MATLAB `fft` routine, it calculates the Fourier transform for each column; hence, the Fourier transform is computed for each value in time producing a two-dimensional function of time and frequency.

The Wigner-Ville is particularly effective at detecting single sinusoids that change in frequency with time, such as the chirp signal shown in Figure 6.5 and used in Example 6.2. For such signals, the Wigner-Ville distribution produces very few cross products, as shown in Example 6.4.

Example 6.4 Apply the Wigner-Ville distribution to a chirp signal the ranges linearly between 20 and 200 Hz over a 1 second time period. In this example, use the MATLAB `chirp` routine.

```
% Example 6.4 and Figure 6.9
% Example of the use of the Wigner-Ville distribution applied to
%    a chirp
% Generates the chirp signal using the MATLAB chirp routine
%
clear all; close all;
% Set up constants           % Same as Example 6.2
fs = 500;                     % Sample frequency
N = 512;                      % Signal length
f1 = 20;                      % Starting frequency in Hz
f2 = 200;                     % Frequency after 1 second (end)
                              %   in Hz
%
% Construct "chirp" signal
tn = (1:N)/fs;
```

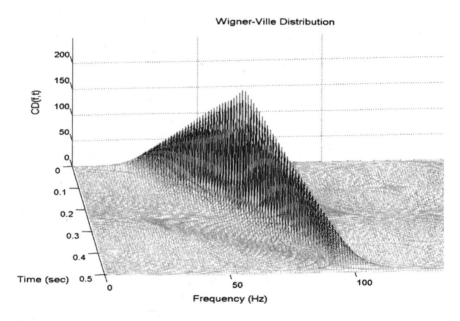

FIGURE 6.9 Wigner-Ville of a chirp signal in which a single sine wave increases linearly with time. While both the time and frequency of the signal are well-defined, the amplitude, which should be constant, varies considerably.

```
x = chirp(tn,f1,1,f2)';      % MATLAB routine
%
% Wigner-Ville analysis
x = hilbert(x);              % Get analytic function
[WD,f,t] = wvd(x,fs);        % Wigner-Ville—see code above
WD = abs(WD);                % Take magnitude
mesh(t,f,WD);                % Plot in 3-D

   .......3D labels, axis, view.......
```

If the analytic signal is not used, then the Wigner-Ville generates considerably more cross products. A demonstration of the advantages of using the analytic signal is given in Problem 2 at the end of the chapter.

Choi-Williams and Other Distributions

To implement other distributions in Cohen's class, we will use the approach defined by Eq. (13). Following Eq. (13), the desired distribution can be obtained by convolving the related determining function (Eq. (17)) with the instantaneous autocorrelation function ($R_x(t,\tau)$; Eq. (7)) then taking the Fourier transform with respect to τ. As mentioned, this is simply a two-dimensional filtering of the instantaneous autocorrelation function by the appropriate filter (i.e., the determining function), in this case an exponential filter. Calculation of the instantaneous autocorrelation function has already been done as part of the Wigner-Ville calculation. To facilitate evaluation of the other distributions, we first extract the code for the instantaneous autocorrelation from the Wigner-Ville function, **wvd** in Example 6.3, and make it a separate function that can be used to determine the various distributions. This function has been termed **int_autocorr**, and takes the data as input and produces the instantaneous autocorrelation function as the output. These routines are available on the CD.

```
function Rx = int_autocorr(x)
% Function to compute the instantenous autocorrelation
% Output
%    Rx instantaneous autocorrelation
% Input
%    x signal
%
[N, xcol] = size(x);
Rx = zeros(N,N);             % Initialize output
%
% Compute instantaneous autocorrelation
for ti = 1:N % Increment over time
  taumax = min([ti-1,N-ti,round(N/2)-1]);
  tau = -taumax:taumax;
```

```
Rx(tau-tau(1)+1,ti) = x(ti+tau) .* conj(x(ti-tau));
end
```

The various members of Cohen's class of distributions can now be implemented by a general routine that starts with the instantaneous autocorrelation function, evaluates the appropriate determining function, filters the instantaneous autocorrelation function by the determining function using convolution, then takes the Fourier transform of the result. The routine described below, cohen, takes the data, sample interval, and an argument that specifies the type of distribution desired and produces the distribution as an output along with time and frequency vectors useful for plotting. The routine is set up to evaluate four different distributions: Choi-Williams, Born-Jorden-Cohen, Rihaczek-Margenau, with the Wigner-Ville distribution as the default. The function also plots the selected determining function.

```
function [CD,f,t] = cohen(x,fs,type)
% Function to compute several of Cohen's class of time-frequencey
%   distributions
%
% Outputs
%    CD Desired distribution
%    f  Frequency vector for plotting
%    t  Time vector for plotting
%Inputs
%    x  Complex signal
%    fs  Sample frequency
%    type of distribution. Valid arguements are:
%       'choi' (Choi-Williams), 'BJC' (Born-Jorden-Cohen);
%       and 'R_M' (Rihaczek-Margenau) Default is Wigner-Ville
%
% Assign constants and check input
sigma = 1;                    % Choi-Williams constant
L = 30;                       % Size of determining function
%
[N, xcol] = size(x);
if N < xcol                   % Make signal a column vector if
  x = x';                     %  necessary
  N = xcol;
end
t = (1:N)/fs;                 % Calculate time and frequency
f = (1:N) *(fs/(2*N));        %  vectors for plotting
%
% Compute instantaneous autocorrelation: Eq. (7)
```

```
CD = int_autocorr(x);
if type(1) == 'c'              % Get appropriate determining
                              %  function
  G = choi(sigma,L);          % Choi-Williams
elseif type(1) == 'B'
  G = BJC(L);                 % Born-Jorden-Cohen
elseif type(1) == 'R'
  G = R_M(L);                 % Rihaczek-Margenau
else
  G = zeros(N,N);             % Default Wigner-Ville
  G(N/2,N/2) = 1;
end
%
figure
  mesh(1:L-1,1:L-1,G);        % Plot determining function
  xlabel('N'); ylabel('N');   %  and label axis
  zlabel('G(,N,N)');
%
% Convolve determining function with instantaneous
%  autocorrelation
CD = conv2(CD,G);             % 2-D convolution
CD = CD(1:N,1:N);             % Truncate extra points produced
                              %  by convolution
%
% Take FFT again, FFT taken with respect to columns
CD = flipud(fft(CD));         % Output distribution
```

The code to produce the Choi-Williams determining function is a straight-forward implementation of $G(t,\tau)$ in Eq. (17) as shown below. The function is generated for only the first quadrant, then duplicated in the other quadrants. The function itself is plotted in Figure 6.10. The code for other determining functions follows the same general structure and can be found in the software accompanying this text.

```
function G = choi(sigma,N)
% Function to calculate the Choi-Williams distribution function
%  (Eq. (17)
G(1,1) = 1;                   % Compute one quadrant then expand
for j = 2:N/2
  wt = 0;
  for i = 1:N/2
    G(i,j) = exp(-(sigma*(i-1)^2)/(4*(j-1)^2));
    wt = wt + 2*G(i,j);
  end
```

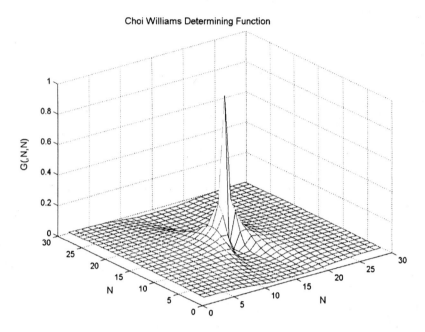

Choi Williams Determining Function

FIGURE 6.10 The Choi-Williams determining function generated by the code below.

```
wt = wt-G(1,j);              % Normalize array so that
                             %  G(n,j) = 1
  for i = 1:N/2
    G(i,j) = G(i,j)/wt;
  end
end
%
% Expand to 4 quadrants
G = [ fliplr(G(:,2:end)) G]; % Add 2nd quadrant
G = [flipud(G(2:end,:)); G]; % Add 3rd and 4th quadrants
```

To complete the package, Example 6.5 provides code that generates the data (either two sequential sinusoids or a chirp signal), asks for the desired distributions, evaluates the distribution using the function cohen, then plots the result. Note that the code for implementing Cohen's class of distributions is written for educational purposes only. It is not very efficient, since many of the operations involve multiplication by zero (for example, see Figure 6.10 and Figure 6.11), and these operations should be eliminated in more efficient code.

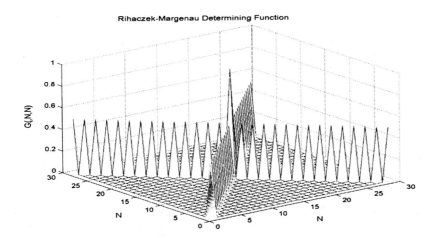

FIGURE 6.11 The determining function of the Rihaczek-Margenau distribution.

Example 6.5 Compare the Choi-Williams and Rihaczek-Margenau distributions for both a double sinusoid and chirp stimulus. Plot the Rihaczek-Margenau determining function* and the results using 3-D type plots.

```
% Example 6.5 and various figures
% Example of the use of Cohen's class distributions applied to
%    both sequential sinusoids and a chirp signal
%
clear all; close all;
global G;
% Set up constants. (Same as in previous examples)
fs = 500;                          % Sample frequency
N = 256;                           % Signal length
f1 = 20;                           % First frequency in Hz
f2 = 100;                          % Second frequency in Hz
%
% Construct a step change in frequency
signal_type = input ('Signal type (1 = sines; 2 = chirp):');
if signal_type == 1
   tn = (1:N/4)/fs;
   x = [zeros(N/4,1); sin(2*pi*f1*tn)'; sin(2*pi*f2*tn)';
```

*Note the code for the Rihaczek-Margenau determining function and several other determining functions can be found on disk with the software associated with this chapter.

```
    zeros(N/4,1)];
else
  tn = (1:N)/fs;
  x = chirp(tn,f1,.5,f2)';
end
%
%
% Get desired distribution
type = input('Enter type (choi,BJC,R_M,WV):','s');
%
x = hilbert(x);                          % Get analytic function
[CD,f,t] = cohen(x,fs,type);             % Cohen's class of
                                         %  transformations
CD = abs(CD);                            % Take magnitude
%                                        % Plot distribution in
figure;                                  %  3-D
  mesh(t,f,CD);
  view([85,40]);                         % Change view for better
                                         %  display
  .......3D labels and scaling.......
  heading = [type ' Distribution'];      % Construct appropriate
  eval(['title(','heading', ');']);      %  title and add to plot
%
%
figure;
  contour(t,f,CD);                       % Plot distribution as a
                                         % contour plot
  xlabel('Time (sec)');
  ylabel('Frequency (Hz)');
  eval(['title(','heading', ');']);
```

This program was used to generate Figures 6.11–6.15.

In this chapter we have explored only a few of the many possible time–frequency distributions, and, necessarily, covered only the very basics of this extensive subject. Two of the more important topics that were not covered here are the estimation of instantaneous frequency from the time–frequency distribution, and the effect of noise on these distributions. The latter is covered briefly in the problem set below.

PROBLEMS

1. Construct a chirp signal similar to that used in Example 6.2. Evaluate the analysis characteristics of the STFT using different window filters and sizes. Specifically, use window sizes of 128, 64, and 32 points. Repeat this analysis

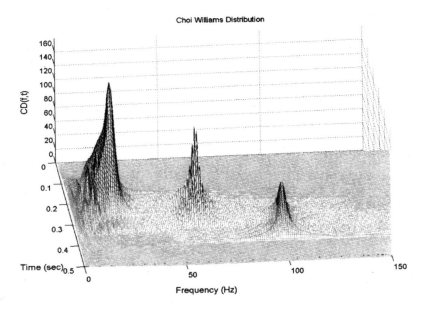

FIGURE 6.12 Choi-Williams distribution for the two sequential sinusoids shown in Figure 6.3. Comparing this distribution with the Wigner-Ville distribution of the same stimulus, Figure 6.7, note the decreased cross product terms.

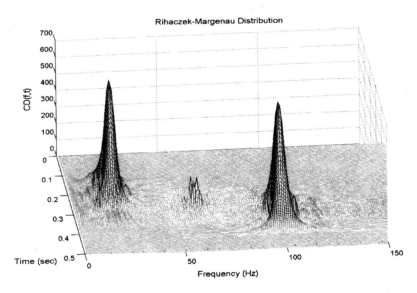

FIGURE 6.13 The Rihaczek-Margenau distribution for the sequential sinusoid signal. Note the very low value of cross products.

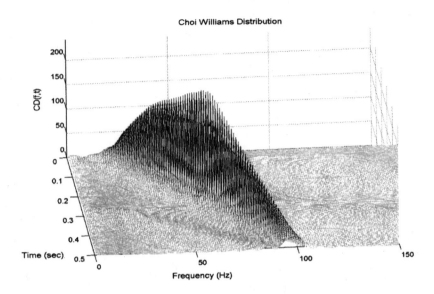

FIGURE 6.14   The Choi-Williams distribution from the chirp signal. Compared to the Wigner-Ville distribution (Figure 6.9), this distribution has a flatter ridge, but neither the Choi-Williams nor the the Wigner-Ville distributions show significant cross products to this type of signal.

using a Chebyshev window. (Modify `spectog` to apply the Chebyshev window, or else use MATLAB's `specgram`.) Assume a sample frequency of 500 Hz and a total time of one second.

2.   Rerun the two examples that involve the Wigner-Ville distribution (Examples 6.3 and 6.4), but use the real signal instead of the analytic signal. Plot the results as both 3-D mesh plots and contour plots.

3.   Construct a signal consisting of two components: a continuous sine wave of 20 Hz and a chirp signal that varies from 20 Hz to 100 Hz over a 0.5 sec time period. Analyze this signal using two different distributions: Wigner-Ville and Choi-Williams. Assume a sample frequency of 500 Hz, and use analytical signal.

4.   Repeat Problem 3 above using the Born-Jordan-Cohen and Rihaczek-Margenau distributions.

5.   Construct a signal consisting of two sine waves of 20 and 100 Hz. Add to this signal Gaussian random noise having a variance equal to 1/4 the amplitude of the sinusoids. Analyze this signal using the Wigner-Ville and Choi-Williams

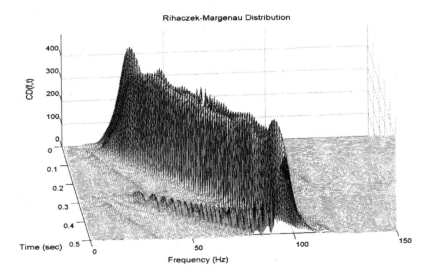

FIGURE 6.15 The Rihaczek-Margenau distribution to a chirp signal. Note that this distribution shows the most constant amplitude throughout the time-frequency plot, but does show some small cross products that diagonal away from the side. In addition, the frequency peak is not as well-defined as in the other distributions.

distributions. Assume a sample frequency of 300 Hz and a 2 sec time period. Use analytical signal.

6. Repeat Problem 5 above using a chirp signal that varies between 20 and 100 Hz, with the same amplitude of added noise.

7. Repeat Problem 6 with twice the amount of added noise.

8. Repeat Problems 6 and 7 using the Rihaczek-Margenau distribution.

7

Wavelet Analysis

INTRODUCTION

Before introducing the wavelet transform we review some of the concepts regarding transforms presented in Chapter 2. A transform can be thought of as a
remapping of a signal that provides more information than the original. The
Fourier transform fits this definition quite well because the frequency information it provides often leads to new insights about the original signal. However,
the inability of the Fourier transform to describe both time and frequency characteristics of the waveform led to a number of different approaches described
in the last chapter. None of these approaches was able to completely solve the
time–frequency problem. The wavelet transform can be used as yet another way
to describe the properties of a waveform that changes over time, but in this case
the waveform is divided not into sections of time, but segments of scale.

In the Fourier transform, the waveform was compared to a sine function—in fact, a whole family of sine functions at harmonically related frequencies. This comparison was carried out by multiplying the waveform with the
sinusoidal functions, then averaging (using either integration in the continuous
domain, or summation in the discrete domain):

$$X(\omega_m) = \int_{-\infty}^{\infty} x(t)e^{-j\omega_m t}dt \tag{1}$$

Eq. (1) is the continuous form of Eq. (6) in Chapter 3 used to define the
discrete Fourier transform. As discussed in Chapter 2, almost any family of func-

tions could be used to probe the characteristics of a waveform, but sinusoidal functions are particularly popular because of their unique frequency characteristics: they contain energy at only one specific frequency. Naturally, this feature makes them ideal for probing the frequency makeup of a waveform, i.e., its frequency spectrum.

Other probing functions can be used, functions chosen to evaluate some particular behavior or characteristic of the waveform. If the probing function is of finite duration, it would be appropriate to translate, or slide, the function over the waveform, $x(t)$, as is done in convolution and the short-term Fourier transform (STFT), Chapter 6's Eq. (1), repeated here:

$$\text{STFT}(t, f) = \int_{-\infty}^{\infty} x(\tau)(w(t - \tau)e^{-2j\pi f\tau})d\tau \tag{2}$$

where f, the frequency, also serves as an indication of family member, and $w(t - \tau)$ is some sliding window function where t acts to translate the window over x. More generally, a translated probing function can be written as:

$$X(t,m) = \int_{-\infty}^{\infty} x(\tau) f(t - \tau)_m d\tau \tag{3}$$

where $f(t)_m$ is some family of functions, with m specifying the family number. This equation was presented in discrete form in Eq. (10), Chapter 2.

If the family of functions, $f(t)_m$, is sufficiently large, then it should be able to represent all aspects the waveform $x(t)$. This would then allow $x(t)$ to be reconstructed from $X(t,m)$ making this transform *bilateral* as defined in Chapter 2. Often the family of basis functions is so large that $X(t,m)$ forms a redundant set of descriptions, more than sufficient to recover $x(t)$. This redundancy can sometimes be useful, serving to reduce noise or acting as a control, but may be simply unnecessary. Note that while the Fourier transform is not redundant, most transforms represented by Eq. (3) (including the STFT and all the distributions in Chapter 6) would be, since they map a variable of one dimension (t) into a variable of two dimensions (t,m).

THE CONTINUOUS WAVELET TRANSFORM

The wavelet transform introduces an intriguing twist to the basic concept defined by Eq. (3). In wavelet analysis, a variety of different probing functions may be used, but the family always consists of enlarged or compressed versions of the basic function, as well as translations. This concept leads to the defining equation for the continuous wavelet transform (CWT):

$$W(a,b) = \int_{-\infty}^{\infty} x(t)\frac{1}{\sqrt{|a|}}\psi^*\left(\frac{t - b}{a}\right)dt \tag{4}$$

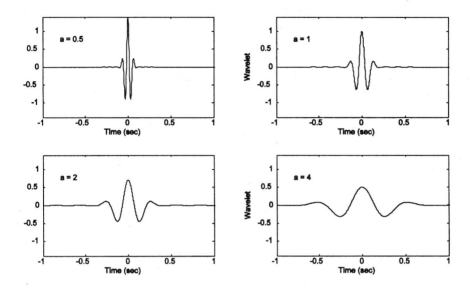

FIGURE 7.1 A *mother* wavelet ($a = 1$) with two dilations ($a = 2$ and 4) and one contraction ($a = 0.5$).

where b acts to translate the function across $x(t)$ just as t does in the equations above, and the variable a acts to vary the time scale of the probing function, ψ. If a is greater than one, the wavelet function, ψ, is stretched along the time axis, and if it is less than one (but still positive) it contacts the function. Negative values of a simply flip the probing function on the time axis. While the probing function ψ could be any of a number of different functions, it always takes on an oscillatory form, hence the term "wavelet." The $*$ indicates the operation of complex conjugation, and the normalizing factor $1/\sqrt{a}$ ensures that the energy is the same for all values of a (all values of b as well, since translations do not alter wavelet energy). If $b = 0$, and $a = 1$, then the wavelet is in its natural form, which is termed the *mother* wavelet;* that is, $\psi_{1,0}(t) \equiv \psi(t)$. A mother wavelet is shown in Figure 7.1 along with some of its family members produced by dilation and contraction. The wavelet shown is the popular *Morlet* wavelet, named after a pioneer of wavelet analysis, and is defined by the equation:

$$\psi(t) = e^{-t^2} \cos(\pi \sqrt{\tfrac{2}{\ln 2}}\, t) \tag{5}$$

---

*Individual members of the wavelet family are specified by the subscripts a and b; i.e., $\psi_{a,b}$. The mother wavelet, $\psi_{1,0}$, should not be confused with the *mother of all Wavelets* which has yet to be discovered.

The wavelet coefficients, $W(a,b)$, describe the correlation between the waveform and the wavelet at various translations and scales: the similarity between the waveform and the wavelet at a given combination of scale and position, a,b. Stated another way, the coefficients provide the amplitudes of a series of wavelets, over a range of scales and translations, that would need to be added together to reconstruct the original signal. From this perspective, wavelet analysis can be thought of as a search over the waveform of interest for activity that most clearly approximates the shape of the wavelet. This search is carried out over a range of wavelet sizes: the time span of the wavelet varies although its shape remains the same. Since the net area of a wavelet is always zero by design, a waveform that is constant over the length of the wavelet would give rise to zero coefficients. Wavelet coefficients respond to changes in the waveform, more strongly to changes on the same scale as the wavelet, and most strongly, to changes that resemble the wavelet. Although a redundant transformation, it is often easier to analyze or recognize patterns using the CWT. An example of the application of the CWT to analyze a waveform is given in the section on MATLAB implementation.

If the wavelet function, $\psi(t)$, is appropriately chosen, then it is possible to reconstruct the original waveform from the wavelet coefficients just as in the Fourier transform. Since the CWT decomposes the waveform into coefficients of two variables, a and b, a double summation (or integration) is required to recover the original signal from the coefficients:

$$x(t) = \frac{1}{C} \int_{a=-\infty}^{\infty} \int_{b=-\infty}^{\infty} W(a,b)\psi_{a,b}(t) \, da \, db \qquad (6)$$

where:

$$C = \int_{-\infty}^{\infty} \frac{|\Psi(\omega)|^2}{|\omega|} \, d\omega$$

and $0 < C < \infty$ (the so-called *admissibility condition*) for recovery using Eq. (6).

In fact, reconstruction of the original waveform is rarely performed using the CWT coefficients because of the redundancy in the transform. When recovery of the original waveform is desired, the more parsimonious discrete wavelet transform is used, as described later in this chapter.

Wavelet Time–Frequency Characteristics

Wavelets such as that shown in Figure 7.1 do not exist at a specific time or a specific frequency. In fact, wavelets provide a compromise in the battle between time and frequency localization: they are well localized in both time and frequency, but not precisely localized in either. A measure of the time range of a specific wavelet, Δt_ψ, can be specified by the square root of the second moment of a given wavelet about its time center (i.e., its first moment) (Akansu & Haddad, 1992):

$$\Delta t_\psi = \sqrt{\frac{\int\limits_{-\infty}^{\infty} (t - t_0)^2 |\psi(t/a)|^2 dt}{\int\limits_{-\infty}^{\infty} |\psi(t/a)|^2 dt}} \tag{7}$$

where t_0 is the center time, or first moment of the wavelet, and is given by:

$$t_0 = \frac{\int\limits_{-\infty}^{\infty} t |\psi(t/a)|^2 dt}{\int\limits_{-\infty}^{\infty} |\psi(t/a)|^2 dt} \tag{8}$$

Similarly the frequency range, $\Delta \omega_\psi$, is given by:

$$\Delta \omega t_\psi = \sqrt{\frac{\int\limits_{-\infty}^{\infty} (\omega - \omega_0)^2 |\Psi(\omega)|^2 d\omega}{\int\limits_{-\infty}^{\infty} |\Psi(\omega)|^2 d\omega}} \tag{9}$$

where $\Psi(\omega)$ is the frequency domain representation (i.e., Fourier transform) of $\psi(t/a)$, and ω_0 is the center frequency of $\Psi(\omega)$. The center frequency is given by an equation similar to Eq. (8):

$$\omega_0 = \frac{\int\limits_{-\infty}^{\infty} \omega |\Psi(\omega)|^2 d\omega}{\int\limits_{-\infty}^{\infty} |\Psi(\omega)|^2 d\omega} \tag{10}$$

The time and frequency ranges of a given family can be obtained from the mother wavelet using Eqs. (7) and (9). Dilation by the variable a changes the time range simply by multiplying Δt_ψ by a. Accordingly, the time range of $\psi_{a,0}$ is defined as $\Delta t_\psi(a) = |a| \Delta t_\psi$. The inverse relationship between time and frequency is shown in Figure 7.2, which was obtained by applying Eqs. (7–10) to the *Mexican hat wavelet*. (The code for this is given in Example 7.2.) The Mexican hat wavelet is given by the equation:

$$\psi(t) = (1 - 2t^2)e^{-t^2} \tag{11}$$

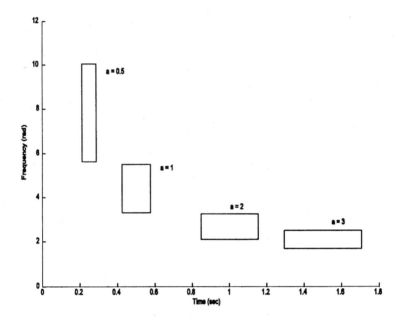

FIGURE 7.2 Time–frequency boundaries of the Mexican hat wavelet for various values of a. The area of each of these boxes is constant (Eq. (12)). The code that generates this figure is based on Eqs. (7–10) and is given in Example 7.2.

The frequency range, or bandwidth, would be the range of the mother Wavelet divided by a: $\Delta\omega_\psi(a) = \Delta\omega_\psi / |a|$. If we multiply the frequency range by the time range, the a's cancel and we are left with a constant that is the product of the constants produced by Eq. (7) and (9):

$$\Delta\omega_\psi(a)\Delta t_\psi(a) = \Delta\omega_\psi\Delta t_\psi = \text{constant}_\psi \tag{12}$$

Eq. (12) shows that the product of the ranges is invariant to dilation* and that the ranges are inversely related; increasing the frequency range, $\Delta\omega_\psi(a)$, decreases the time range, $\Delta t_\psi(a)$. These ranges correlate to the time and frequency resolution of the CWT. Just as in the short-term Fourier transform, there is a time–frequency trade-off (recall Eq. (3) in Chapter 6): decreasing the wavelet time range (by decreasing a) provides a more accurate assessment of time characteristics (i.e., the ability to separate out close events in time) at the expense of frequency resolution, and vice versa.

---

*Translations (changes in the variable b), do alter either the time or frequency resolution; hence, both time and frequency resolution, as well as their product, are independent of the value of b.

Since the time and frequency resolutions are inversely related, the CWT will provide better frequency resolution when a is large and the length of the wavelet (and its effective time window) is long. Conversely, when a is small, the wavelet is short and the time resolution is maximum, but the wavelet only responds to high frequency components. Since a is variable, there is a built-in trade-off between time and frequency resolution, which is key to the CWT and makes it well suited to analyzing signals with rapidly varying high frequency components superimposed on slowly varying low frequency components.

MATLAB Implementation

A number of software packages exist in MATLAB for computing the continuous wavelet transform, including MATLAB's Wavelet Toolbox and *Wavelab* which is available free over the Internet: (www.stat.stanford.edu/~wavelab/). However, it is not difficult to implement Eq. (4) directly, as illustrated in the example below.

Example 7.1   Write a program to construct the CWT of a signal consisting of two sequential sine waves of 10 and 40 Hz. (i.e. the signal shown in Figure 6.1). Plot the wavelet coefficients as a function of a and b. Use the Morlet wavelet.

The signal waveform is constructed as in Example 6.1. A time vector, `ti`, is generated that will be used to produce the positive half of the wavelet. This vector is initially scaled so that the mother wavelet ($a = 1$) will be $\pm$ 10 sec long. With each iteration, the value of a is adjusted (128 different values are used in this program) and the wavelet time vector is it then scaled to produce the appropriate wavelet family member. During each iteration, the positive half of the Morlet wavelet is constructed using the defining equation (Eq. (5)), and the negative half is generated from the positive half by concatenating a time reversed (flipped) version with the positive side. The wavelet coefficients at a given value of a are obtained by convolution of the scaled wavelet with the signal. Since convolution in MATLAB produces extra points, these are removed symmetrically (see Chapter 2), and the coefficients are plotted three-dimensionally against the values of a and b. The resulting plot, Figure 7.3, reflects the time–frequency characteristics of the signal which are quantitatively similar to those produced by the STFT and shown in Figure 6.2.

```
% Example 7.1 and Figure 7.3
% Generate 2 sinusoids that change frequency in a step-like
%  manner
% Apply the continuous wavelet transform and plot results
%
clear all; close all;
% Set up constants
```

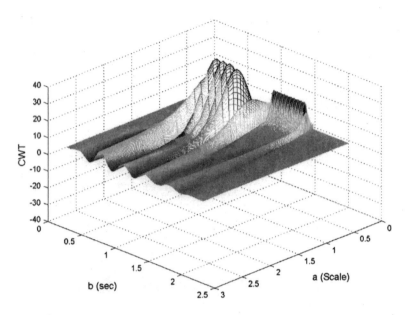

FIGURE 7.3 Wavelet coefficients obtained by applying the CWT to a waveform consisting of two sequential sine waves of 10 and 40 Hz, as shown in Figure 6.1. The Morlet wavelet was used.

```
fs = 500                          % Sample frequency
N = 1024;                         % Signal length
N1 = 512;                         % Wavelet number of points
f1 = 10;                          % First frequency in Hz
f2 = 40;                          % Second frequency in Hz
resol_level = 128;                % Number of values of a
decr_a = .5;                      % Decrement for a
a_init = 4;                       % Initial a
wo = pi * sqrt(2/log2(2));        % Wavelet frequency scale
                                  %  factor
%
% Generate the two sine waves. Same as in Example 6.1
tn = (1:N/4)/fs;                  % Time vector to create
                                  %  sinusoids
b = (1:N)/fs;                     % Time vector for plotting
x = [zeros(N/4,1); sin(2*pi*f1*tn)'; sin(2*pi*f2*tn)';
   zeros(N/4,1)];
ti = ((1:N1/2)/fs)*10;            % Time vector to construct
                                  %  ± 10 sec. of wavelet
```

```
% Calculate continuous Wavelet transform
% Morlet wavelet, Eq. (5)
for i = 1:resol_level
  a(i) = a_init/(1+i*decr_a);      % Set scale
  t = abs(ti/a(i));                % Scale vector for wavelet
  mor = (exp(-t.^2).* cos(wo*t))/ sqrt(a(i));
  Wavelet = [fliplr(mor) mor];     % Make symmetrical about
                                   %  zero
  ip = conv(x,Wavelet);            % Convolve wavelet and
                                   %  signal
  ex = fix((length(ip)-N)/2);      % Calculate extra points /2
  CW_Trans(:,i) =ip(ex+1:N+ex,1);  % Remove extra points
                                   %  symmetrically
end
%
% Plot in 3 dimensions
d = fliplr(CW_Trans);
mesh(a,b,CW_Trans);
   ***** labels and view angle *****
```

In this example, a was modified by division with a linearly increasing value. Often, wavelet scale is modified based on octaves or fractions of octaves.

A determination of the time–frequency boundaries of a wavelet though MATLAB implementation of Eqs. (7–10) is provided in the next example.

Example 7.2 Find the time–frequency boundaries of the Mexican hat wavelet.

For each of 4 values of a, the scaled wavelet is constructed using an approach similar to that found in Example 7.1. The magnitude squared of the frequency response is calculated using the FFT. The center time, t_0, and center frequency, w_0, are constructed by direct application of Eqs. (8) and (10). Note that since the wavelet is constructed symmetrically about $t = 0$, the center time, t_0, will always be zero, and an appropriate offset time, t_1, is added during plotting. The time and frequency boundaries are calculated using Eqs. (7) and (9), and the resulting boundaries as are plotted as a rectangle about the appropriate time and frequency centers.

```
% Example 7.2 and Figure 7.2
% Plot of wavelet boundaries for various values of 'a'
% Determines the time and scale range of the Mexican wavelet.
% Uses the equations for center time and frequency and for time
% and frequency spread given in Eqs. (7-10)
%
```

```
clear all; close all;
N = 1000;                              % Data length
fs = 1000;                             % Assumed sample frequency
wo1 = pi * sqrt(2/log2(2));            % Const. for wavelet time
                                       %   scale
a = [.5 1.0 2.0 3.0];                  % Values of a
xi = ((1:N/2)/fs)*10;                  % Show ± 10 sec of the wavelet
t = (1:N)/fs;                          % Time scale
omaga = (1:N/2) * fs/N;                % Frequency scale
%
for i = 1:length(a)
  t1 = xi./a(i);                       % Make time vector for
                                       %   wavelet
  mex = exp(-t1./\2).* (1-2*t1./\2);   %% Generate Mexican hat
                                       %   wavelet
  w = [fliplr(mex) mex];               % Make symmetrical about zero
  wsq = abs(w)./\2                     % Square wavelet;
  W = fft(w);                          % Get frequency representa-
  Wsq = abs(W(1:N/2))./\2;             %   tion and square. Use only
                                       %   fs/2 range
  t0 = sum(t.* wsq)/sum(wsq);          % Calculate center time
  d_t = sqrt(sum((t-to)./\2 .*wsq)/sum(wsq));
                                       % Calculate time spread
  w0 = sum(omaga.*Wsq)/sum(Wsq);       % Calculate center frequency
  d_w0 = sqrt(sum((omaga-w0)./\2 .* Wsq)/sum(Wsq));
  t1 = t0*a(i);                        % Adjust time position to
                                       %   compensate for symmetri-
                                       %   cal waveform
hold on;
% Plot boundaries
  plot([t1-d_t t1-d_t],[w0-d_w0 w0+d_w0],'k');
  plot([t1+d_t t1+d_t],[w0-d_w0 w0+d_w0],'k');
  plot([t1-d_t t1+d_t],[w0-d_w0 w0-d_w0],'k');
  plot([t1-d_t t1+d_t],[w0+d_w0 w0+d_w0],'k');
end
% ***** lables*****
```

THE DISCRETE WAVELET TRANSFORM

The CWT has one serious problem: it is highly redundant.* The CWT provides an oversampling of the original waveform: many more coefficients are generated than are actually needed to uniquely specify the signal. This redundancy is

---

*In its continuous form, it is actually infinitely redundant!

usually not a problem in analysis applications such as described above, but will be costly if the application calls for recovery of the original signal. For recovery, all of the coefficients will be required and the computational effort could be excessive. In applications that require bilateral transformations, we would prefer a transform that produces the minimum number of coefficients required to recover accurately the original signal. The *discrete wavelet transform* (DWT) achieves this parsimony by restricting the variation in translation and scale, usually to powers of 2. When the scale is changed in powers of 2, the discrete wavelet transform is sometimes termed the *dyadic wavelet transform* which, unfortunately, carries the same abbreviation (DWT). The DWT may still require redundancy to produce a bilateral transform unless the wavelet is carefully chosen such that it leads to an orthogonal family (i.e., a orthogonal basis). In this case, the DWT will produce a nonredundant, bilateral transform.

The basic analytical expressions for the DWT will be presented here; however, the transform is easier to understand, and easier to implement using filter banks, as described in the next section. The theoretical link between filter banks and the equations will be presented just before the MATLAB Implementation section. The DWT is often introduced in terms of its recovery transform:

$$x(t) = \sum_{k=-\infty}^{\infty} \sum_{\ell=-\infty}^{\infty} d(k,\ell) 2^{-k/2} \psi(2^{-k}t - \ell) \tag{13}$$

Here k is related to a as: $a = 2^k$; b is related to ℓ as $b = 2^k \ell$; and $d(k,\ell)$ is a sampling of $W(a,b)$ at discrete points k and ℓ.

In the DWT, a new concept is introduced termed the *scaling function*, a function that facilitates computation of the DWT. To implement the DWT efficiently, the finest resolution is computed first. The computation then proceeds to coarser resolutions, but rather than start over on the original waveform, the computation uses a smoothed version of the fine resolution waveform. This smoothed version is obtained with the help of the scaling function. In fact, the scaling function is sometimes referred to as the *smoothing function*. The definition of the scaling function uses a *dilation* or a *two-scale difference equation*:

$$\phi(t) = \sum_{n=-\infty}^{\infty} \sqrt{2} c(n) \phi(2t - n) \tag{14}$$

where $c(n)$ is a series of scalars that defines the specific scaling function. This equation involves two time scales (t and $2t$) and can be quite difficult to solve.

In the DWT, the wavelet itself can be defined from the scaling function:

$$\psi(t) = \sum_{n=-\infty}^{\infty} \sqrt{2} d(n) \phi(2t - n) \tag{15}$$

where $d(n)$ is a series of scalars that are related to the waveform $x(t)$ (Eq. (13)) and that define the discrete wavelet in terms of the scaling function. While the DWT can be implemented using the above equations, it is usually implemented using filter bank techniques.

Filter Banks

For most signal and image processing applications, DWT-based analysis is best described in terms of filter banks. The use of a group of filters to divide up a signal into various spectral components is termed *subband coding*. The most basic implementation of the DWT uses only two filters as in the filter bank shown in Figure 7.4.

The waveform under analysis is divided into two components, $y_{lp}(n)$ and $y_{hp}(n)$, by the digital filters $H_0(\omega)$ and $H_1(\omega)$. The spectral characteristics of the two filters must be carefully chosen with $H_0(\omega)$ having a lowpass spectral characteristic and $H_1(\omega)$ a highpass spectral characteristic. The highpass filter is analogous to the application of the wavelet to the original signal, while the lowpass filter is analogous to the application of the scaling or smoothing function. If the filters are *invertible filters*, then it is possible, at least in theory, to construct complementary filters (filters that have a spectrum the inverse of $H_0(\omega)$ or $H_1(\omega)$) that will recover the original waveform from either of the subband signals, $y_{lp}(n)$ or $y_{hp}(n)$. The original signal can often be recovered even if the filters are not invertible, but both subband signals will need to be used. Signal recovery is illustrated in Figure 7.5 where a second pair of filters, $G_0(\omega)$ and $G_1(\omega)$, operate on the high and lowpass subband signals and their sum is used

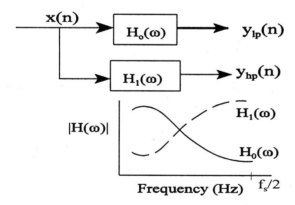

FIGURE 7.4 Simple filter bank consisting of only two filters applied to the same waveform. The filters have lowpass and highpass spectral characteristics. Filter outputs consist of a lowpass subband, $y_{lp}(n)$, and a highpass subband, $y_{hp}(n)$.

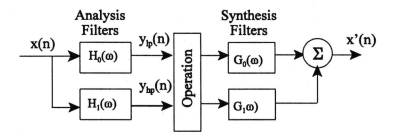

FIGURE 7.5 A typical wavelet application using filter banks containing only two filters. The input waveform is first decomposed into subbands using the *analysis filter* bank. Some process is applied to the filtered signals before reconstruction. Reconstruction is performed by the *synthesis filter* bank.

to reconstruct a close approximation of the original signal, $x'(t)$. The Filter Bank that decomposes the original signal is usually termed the *analysis filters* while the filter bank that reconstructs the signal is termed the *syntheses filters*. FIR filters are used throughout because they are inherently stable and easier to implement.

Filtering the original signal, $x(n)$, only to recover it with inverse filters would be a pointless operation, although this process may have some instructive value as shown in Example 7.3. In some analysis applications only the subband signals are of interest and reconstruction is not needed, but in many wavelet applications, some operation is performed on the subband signals, $y_{lp}(n)$ and $y_{hp}(n)$, before reconstruction of the output signal (see Figure 7.5). In such cases, the output will no longer be exactly the same as the input. If the output is essentially the same, as occurs in some data compression applications, the process is termed *lossless*, otherwise it is a *lossy* operation.

There is one major concern with the general approach schematized in Figure 7.5: it requires the generation of, and operation on, twice as many points as are in the original waveform $x(n)$. This problem will only get worse if more filters are added to the filter bank. Clearly there must be redundant information contained in signals $y_{lp}(n)$ and $y_{hp}(n)$, since they are both required to represent $x(n)$, but with twice the number of points. If the analysis filters are correctly chosen, then it is possible to reduce the length of $y_{lp}(n)$ and $y_{hp}(n)$ by one half and still be able to recover the original waveform. To reduce the signal samples by one half and still represent the same overall time period, we need to eliminate every other point, say every odd point. This operation is known as *downsampling* and is illustrated schematically by the symbol $\downarrow 2$. The downsampled version of $y(n)$ would then include only the samples with even indices [$y(2), y(4), y(6), \ldots$] of the filtered signal.

If downsampling is used, then there must be some method for recovering the missing data samples (those with odd indices) in order to reconstruct the original signal. An operation termed *upsampling* (indicated by the symbol ↑ 2) accomplishes this operation by replacing the missing points with zeros. The recovered signal ($x'(n)$ in Figure 7.5) will not contain zeros for these data samples as the synthesis filters, $G_0(\omega)$ or $G_1(\omega)$, 'fill in the blanks.' Figure 7.6 shows a wavelet application that uses three filter banks and includes the downsampling and upsampling operations. Downsampled amplitudes are sometimes scaled by $\sqrt{2}$, a normalization that can simplify the filter calculations when matrix methods are used.

Designing the filters in a wavelet filter bank can be quite challenging because the filters must meet a number of criteria. A prime concern is the ability to recover the original signal after passing through the analysis and synthesis filter banks. Accurate recovery is complicated by the downsampling process. Note that downsampling, removing every other point, is equivalent to sampling the original signal at half the sampling frequency. For some signals, this would lead to aliasing, since the highest frequency component in the signal may no

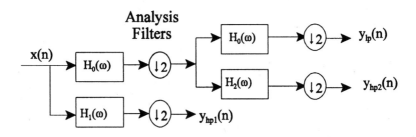

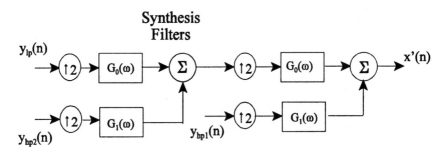

FIGURE 7.6 A typical wavelet application using three filters. The downsampling (↓ 2) and upsampling (↑ 2) processes are shown. As in Figure 7.5, some process would be applied to the filtered signals, $y_{lp}(n)$ and $y_{hp}(n)$, before reconstruction.

longer be twice the now reduced sampling frequency. Appropriately chosen filter banks can essentially cancel potential aliasing. If the filter bank contains only two filter types (highpass and lowpass filters) as in Figure 7.5, the criterion for aliasing cancellation is (Strang and Nguyen, 1997):

$$G_0(z)H_0(-z) + G_1(z)H_1(-z) = 0 \tag{16}$$

where $H_0(z)$ is the transfer function of the analysis lowpass filter, $H_1(z)$ is the transfer function of the analysis highpass filter, $G_0(z)$ is the transfer function of the synthesis lowpass filter, and $G_1(z)$ is the transfer function of the synthesis highpass filter.

The requirement to be able to recover the original waveform from the subband waveforms places another important requirement on the filters which is satisfied when:

$$G_0(z)H_0(z) + G_1(z)H_1(z) = 2z^{-N} \tag{17}$$

where the transfer functions are the same as those in Eq. (16). N is the number of filter coefficients (i.e., the filter order); hence z^{-N} is just the delay of the filter.

In many analyses, it is desirable to have subband signals that are orthogonal, placing added constraints on the filters. Fortunately, a number of filters have been developed that have most of the desirable properties.* The examples below use filters developed by Daubechies, and named after her. This is a family of popular wavelet filters having 4 or more coefficients. The coefficients of the lowpass filter, $h_0(n)$, for the 4-coefficient Daubechies filter are given as:

$$h(n) = \frac{[(1 + \sqrt{3}), (3 + \sqrt{3}), (3 - \sqrt{3}), (1 - \sqrt{3})]}{8} \tag{18}$$

Other, higher order filters in this family are given in the MATLAB routine `daub` found in the routines associated with this chapter. It can be shown that orthogonal filters with more than two coefficients must have asymmetrical coefficients.† Unfortunately this precludes these filters from having linear phase characteristics; however, this is a compromise that is usually acceptable. More complicated *biorthogonal filters* (Strang and Nguyen, 1997) are required to produce minimum phase and orthogonality.

In order for the highpass filter output to be orthogonal to that of the lowpass output, the highpass filter frequency characteristics must have a specific relationship to those of the lowpass filter:

---

*Although no filter yet exists that has all of the desirable properties.

†The two-coefficient, orthogonal filter is: $h(n) = [\frac{1}{2}; \frac{1}{2}]$, and is known as the *Haar* filter. Essentially a two-point moving average, this filter does not have very strong filter characteristics. See Problem 3.

$$H_1(z) = -z^{-N}H_0(-z^{-1}) \tag{19}$$

The criterion represented by Eq. (19) can be implemented by applying the *alternating flip* algorithm to the coefficients of $h_0(n)$:

$$h_1(n) = [h_0(N), -h_0(N-1), h_0(N-2), -h_0(N-3), \ldots] \tag{20}$$

where N is the number of coefficients in $h_0(n)$. Implementation of this alternating flip algorithm is found in the `analyze` program of Example 7.3.

Once the analyze filters have been chosen, the synthesis filters used for reconstruction are fairly constrained by Eqs. (14) and (15). The conditions of Eq. (17) can be met by making $G_0(z) = H_1(-z)$ and $G_1(z) = -H_0(-z)$. Hence the synthesis filter transfer functions are related to the analysis transfer functions by the Eqs. (21) and (22):

$$G_0(z) = H_1(z) = z^{-N}H_0(z^{-1}) \tag{21}$$

$$G_1(z) = -H_0(-z) = z^{-N}H_1(z^{-1}) \tag{22}$$

where the second equality comes from the relationship expressed in Eq. (19). The operations of Eqs. (21) and (22) can be implemented several different ways, but the easiest way in MATLAB is to use the second equalities in Eqs. (21) and (22), which can be implemented using the *order flip* algorithm:

$$g_0(n) = [h_0(N), h_0(N-1), h_0(N-2), \ldots] \tag{23}$$

$$g_1(n) = [h_1(N), h_1(N-1), h_1(N-2), \ldots] \tag{24}$$

where, again, N is the number of filter coefficients. (It is assumed that all filters have the same order; i.e., they have the same number of coefficients.)

An example of constructing the syntheses filter coefficients from only the analysis filter lowpass filter coefficients, $h_0(n)$, is shown in Example 7.3. First the alternating flip algorithm is used to get the highpass analysis filter coefficients, $h_1(n)$, then the order flip algorithm is applied as in Eqs. (23) and (24) to produce both the synthesis filter coefficients, $g_0(n)$ and $g_1(n)$.

Note that if the filters shown in Figure 7.6 are causal, each would produce a delay that is dependent on the number of filter coefficients. Such delays are expected and natural, and may have to be taken into account in the reconstruction process. However, when the data are stored in the computer it is possible to implement FIR filters without a delay. An example of the use of *periodic convolution* to eliminate the delay is shown in Example 7.4 (see also Chapter 2).

The Relationship Between Analytical Expressions and Filter Banks

The filter bank approach and the discrete wavelet transform represented by Eqs. (14) and (15) were actually developed separately, but have become linked both theoretically and practically. It is possible, at least in theory, to go between the two approaches to develop the wavelet and scaling function from the filter coefficients and vice versa. In fact, the coefficients $c(n)$ and $d(n)$ in Eqs. (14) and (15) are simply scaled versions of the filter coefficients:

$$c(n) = \sqrt{2}\, h_0(n); \quad d(n) = \sqrt{2}\, h_1(n) \tag{25}$$

With the substitution of $c(n)$ in Eq. (14), the equation for the scaling function (the dilation equation) becomes:

$$\phi(t) = \sum_{n=-\infty}^{\infty} 2\, h_0(n) \phi(2t - n) \tag{26}$$

Since this is an equation with two time scales (t and $2t$), it is not easy to solve, but a number of approximation approaches have been worked out (Strang and Nguyen, 1997, pp. 186–204). A number of techniques exist for solving for $\phi(t)$ in Eq. (26) given the filter coefficients, $h_1(n)$. Perhaps the most straightforward method of solving for ϕ in Eq. (26) is to use the frequency domain representation. Taking the Fourier transform of both sides of Eq. (26) gives:

$$\Phi(\omega) = H_0\!\left(\frac{\omega}{2}\right)\Phi\!\left(\frac{\omega}{2}\right) \tag{27}$$

Note that $2t$ goes to $\omega/2$ in the frequency domain. The second term in Eq. (27) can be broken down into $H_0(\omega/4)\,\Phi(\omega/4)$, so it is possible to rewrite the equation as shown below.

$$\Phi(\omega) = H_0\!\left(\frac{\omega}{2}\right)\!\left[H_0\!\left(\frac{\omega}{4}\right)\Phi\!\left(\frac{\omega}{4}\right)\right] \tag{28}$$

$$= H_0\!\left(\frac{\omega}{2}\right)H_0\!\left(\frac{\omega}{4}\right)H_0\!\left(\frac{\omega}{8}\right) \cdots H_0\!\left(\frac{\omega}{2^N}\right)\Phi\!\left(\frac{\omega}{2^N}\right) \tag{29}$$

In the limit as $N \to \infty$, Eq. (29) becomes:

$$\Phi(\omega) = \prod_{j=1}^{\infty} H_0\!\left(\frac{\omega}{2^j}\right) \tag{30}$$

The relationship between $\phi(t)$ and the lowpass filter coefficients can now be obtained by taking the inverse Fourier transform of Eq. (30). Once the scaling function is determined, the wavelet function can be obtained directly from Eq. (16) with $2h_1(n)$ substituted for $d(n)$:

$$\psi(t) = \sum_{n=-\infty}^{\infty} 2\, h_1(n) \phi(2t - n) \tag{31}$$

Eq. (30) also demonstrates another constraint on the lowpass filter coefficients, $h_0(n)$, not mentioned above. In order for the infinite product to converge (or any infinite product for that matter), $H_0(\omega/2^j)$ must approach 1 as $j \to \infty$. This implies that $H_0(0) = 1$, a criterion that is easy to meet with a lowpass filter. While Eq. (31) provides an explicit formula for determining the scaling function from the filter coefficients, an analytical solution is challenging except for very simple filters such as the two-coefficient Haar filter. Solving this equation numerically also has problems due to the short data length ($H_0(\omega)$ would be only 4 points for a 4-element filter). Nonetheless, the equation provides a theoretical link between the filter bank and DWT methodologies.

These issues described above, along with some applications of wavelet analysis, are presented in the next section on implementation.

MATLAB Implementation

The construction of a filter bank in MATLAB can be achieved using either routines from the Signal Processing Toolbox, `filter` or `filtfilt`, or simply convolution. All examples below use convolution. Convolution does not conserve the length of the original waveform: the MATLAB `conv` produces an output with a length equal to the data length plus the filter length minus one. Thus with a 4-element filter the output of the convolution process would be 3 samples longer than the input. In this example, the extra points are removed by simple truncation. In Example 7.4, circular or periodic convolution is used to eliminate phase shift. Removal of the extraneous points is followed by downsampling, although these two operations could be done in a single step, as shown in Example 7.4.

The main program shown below makes use of 3 important subfunctions. The routine `daub` is available on the disk and supplies the coefficients of a Daubechies filter using a simple list of coefficients. In this example, a 6-element filter is used, but the routine can also generate coefficients of 4-, 8-, and 10-element Daubechies filters.

The waveform is made up of 4 sine waves of different frequencies with added noise. This waveform is decomposed into 4 subbands using the routine `analysis`. The subband signals are plotted and then used to reconstruct the original signal in the routine `synthesize`. Since no operation is performed on the subband signals, the reconstructed signal should match the original except for a phase shift.

Example 7.3 Construct an analysis filter bank containing `L` decompositions; that is, a lowpass filter and `L` highpass filters. Decompose a signal consisting of 4 sinusoids in noise and the recover this signal using an `L`-level syntheses filter bank.

```
% Example 7.3 and Figures 7.7 and 7.8
% Dyadic wavelet transform example
% Construct a waveform of 4 sinusoids plus noise
% Decompose the waveform in 4 levels, plot each level, then
%   reconstruct
% Use a Daubechies 6-element filter
%
clear all; close all;
%
fs = 1000;                        % Sample frequency
N = 1024;                         % Number of points in
                                  %  waveform
freqsin = [.63 1.1 2.7 5.6];      % Sinusoid frequencies
                                  %  for mix
ampl = [1.2 1 1.2 .75 ];          % Amplitude of sinusoid
h0 = daub(6);                     % Get filter coeffi-
                                  %  cients: Daubechies 6
```

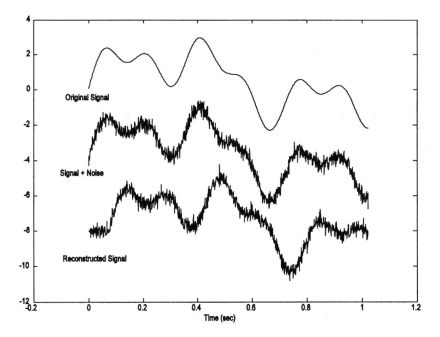

FIGURE 7.7   Input (middle) waveform to the four-level analysis and synthesis filter banks used in Example 7.3. The lower waveform is the reconstructed output from the synthesis filters. Note the phase shift due to the causal filters. The upper waveform is the original signal before the noise was added.

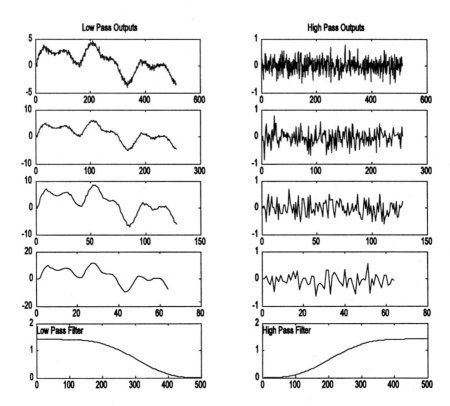

FIGURE 7.8 Signals generated by the analysis filter bank used in Example 7.3 with the top-most plot showing the outputs of the first set of filters with the finest resolution, the next from the top showing the outputs of the second set of set of filters, etc. Only the lowest (i.e., smoothest) lowpass subband signal is included in the output of the filter bank; the rest are used only in the determination of highpass subbands. The lowest plots show the frequency characteristics of the high- and lowpass filters.

```
%
[x t] = signal(freqsin,ampl,N);      % Construct signal
x1 = x + (.25 * randn(1,N));         % Add noise
an = analyze(x1,h0,4);               % Decompose signal,
                                     %   analytic filter bank
sy = synthesize(an,h0,4);            % Reconstruct original
                                     %   signal
figure(fig1);
plot(t,x,'k',t,x1-4,'k',t,sy-8,'k');% Plot signals separated
```

This program uses the function `signal` to generate the mixtures of sinusoids. This routine is similar to `sig_noise` except that it generates only mixtures of sine waves without the noise. The first argument specifies the frequency of the sines and the third argument specifies the number of points in the waveform just as in `sig_noise`. The second argument specifies the amplitudes of the sinusoids, not the SNR as in `sig_noise`.

The `analysis` function shown below implements the analysis filter bank. This routine first generates the highpass filter coefficients, `h1`, from the lowpass filter coefficients, `h`, using the *alternating flip* algorithm of Eq. (20). These FIR filters are then applied using standard convolution. All of the various subband signals required for reconstruction are placed in a single output array, `an`. The length of `an` is the same as the length of the input, $N = 1024$ in this example. The only *lowpass signal* needed for reconstruction is the smoothest lowpass subband (i.e., final lowpass signal in the lowpass chain), and this signal is placed in the first data segment of `an` taking up the first $N/16$ data points. This signal is followed by the last stage highpass subband which is of equal length. The next $N/8$ data points contain the second to last highpass subband followed, in turn, by the other subband signals up to the final, highest resolution highpass subband which takes up all of the second half of `an`. The remainder of the `analyze` routine calculates and plots the high- and lowpass filter frequency characteristics.

```
% Function to calculate analyze filter bank
% an = analyze(x,h,L)
% where
%  x = input waveform in column form which must be longer than
%     2^L + L and power of two.
%  h0 = filter coefficients (lowpass)
%  L = decomposition level (number of highpass filter in bank)
%
function an = analyze(x,h0,L)

lf = length(h0);              % Filter length
lx = length(x);              % Data length
an = x;                      % Initialize output
% Calculate High pass coefficients from low pass coefficients
for i = 0:(lf-1)
  h1(i+1) = (-1)^i * h0(lf-i);  % Alternating flip, Eq. (20)
end
%
% Calculate filter outputs for all levels
for i = 1:L
  a_ext = an;
```

```
lpf = conv(a_ext,h0);          % Lowpass FIR filter
hpf = conv(a_ext,h1);          % Highpass FIR filter
lpf = lpf(1:lx);               % Remove extra points
hpf = hpf(1:lx);
lpfd = lpf(1:2:end);           % Downsample
hpfd = hpf(1:2:end);
an(1:lx) = [lpfd hpfd];        % Low pass output at beginning
                               %  of array, but now occupies
                               %  only half the data
                               %  points as last pass
lx = lx/2;
subplot(L+1,2,2*i-1);          % Plot both filter outputs
  plot(an(1:lx));              % Lowpass output
  if i == 1
    title('Low Pass Outputs'); % Titles
  end
subplot(L+1,2,2*i);
  plot(an(lx+1:2*lx));         % Highpass output
  if i == 1
    title('High Pass Outputs')
  end
end
%
HPF = abs(fft(h1,256));        % Calculate and plot filter
LPF = abs(fft(h0,256));        %  transfer fun of high- and
                               %  lowpass filters
freq = (1:128)* 1000/256;      % Assume fs = 1000 Hz
subplot(L+1,2,2*i+1);
  plot(freq, LPF(1:128));      % Plot from 0 to fs/2 Hz
  text(1,1.7,'Low Pass Filter');
  xlabel('Frequency (Hz.)')'
subplot(L+1,2,2*i+2);
  plot(freq, HPF(1:128));
  text(1,1.7,'High Pass Filter');
  xlabel('Frequency (Hz.)')'
```

The original data are reconstructed from the analyze filter bank signals in the program **synthesize**. This program first constructs the synthesis lowpass filter, g0, using order flip applied to the analysis lowpass filter coefficients (Eq. (23)). The analysis highpass filter is constructed using the alternating flip algorithm (Eq. (20)). These coefficients are then used to construct the synthesis highpass filter coefficients through order flip (Eq. (24)). The synthesis filter loop begins with the course signals first, those in the initial data segments of a with the shortest segment lengths. The lowpass and highpass signals are upsampled, then filtered using convolution, the additional points removed, and the signals added together. This loop is structured so that on the next pass the recently combined segment is itself combined with the next higher resolution highpass signal. This iterative process continues until all of the highpass signals are included in the sum.

```
% Function to calculate synthesize filter bank
% y = synthesize(a,h0,L)
% where
%  a = analyze filter bank outputs (produced by analyze)
%  h = filter coefficients (lowpass)
%  L = decomposition level (number of highpass filters in bank)
%
function y = synthesize(a,h0,L)
lf = length(h0);              % Filter length
lx = length(a);              % Data length
lseg = lx/(2^L);             % Length of first low- and
                             %  highpass segments
y = a;                       % Initialize output
g0 = h0(lf:-1:1);            % Lowpass coefficients using
                             %  order flip, Eq. (23)
% Calculate High pass coefficients, h1(n), from lowpass
% coefficients use Alternating flip Eq. (20)
  for i = 0:(lf-1)
  h1(i+1) = (-1)^i * h0(lf-i);
end
g1 = h1(lf:-1:1);           % Highpass filter coeffi-
                            %  cients using order
                            %  flip, Eq. (24)
% Calculate filter outputs for all levels
for i = 1:L
  lpx = y(1:lseg);          % Get lowpass segment
  hpx = y(lseg+1:2*lseg);   % Get highpass outputs
  up_lpx = zeros(1,2*lseg); % Initialize for upsampling
  up_lpx(1:2:2*lseg) = lpx; % Upsample lowpass (every
                            %  odd point)
  up_hpx = zeros(1,2*lseg); % Repeat for highpass
  up_hpx(1:2:2*lseg) = hpx;
  syn = conv(up_lpx,g0) + conv(up_hpx,g1); % Filter and
                                           %  combine
  y(1:2*lseg) = syn(1:(2*lseg)); % Remove extra points from
                                 %  end
  lseg = lseg * 2;          % Double segment lengths for
                            %  next pass
end
```

The subband signals are shown in Figure 7.8. Also shown are the frequency characteristics of the Daubechies high- and lowpass filters. The input and reconstructed output waveforms are shown in Figure 7.7. The original signal before the noise was added is included. Note that the reconstructed waveform closely matches the input except for the phase lag introduced by the filters. As shown in the next example, this phase lag can be eliminated by using circular or periodic convolution, but this will also introduce some artifact.

Denoising

Example 7.3 was not particularly practical since the reconstructed signal was the same as the original, except for the phase shift. A more useful application of wavelets is shown in Example 7.4, where some processing is done on the subband signals before reconstruction—in this example, nonlinear filtering. The basic assumption in this application is that the noise is coded into small fluctuations in the higher resolution (i.e., more detailed) highpass subbands. This noise can be selectively reduced by eliminating the smaller sample values in the higher resolution highpass subbands. In this example, the two highest resolution highpass subbands are examined and data points below some threshold are zeroed out. The threshold is set to be equal to the variance of the highpass subbands.

Example 7.4   Decompose the signal in Example 7.3 using a 4-level filter bank. In this example, use periodic convolution in the analysis and synthesis filters and a 4-element Daubechies filter. Examine the two highest resolution highpass subbands. These subbands will reside in the last $N/4$ to N samples. Set all values in these segments that are below a given threshold value to zero. Use the net variance of the subbands as the threshold.

```
% Example 7.4 and Figure 7.9
% Application of DWT to nonlinear filtering
% Construct the waveform in Example 7.3.
% Decompose the waveform in 4 levels, plot each level, then
%   reconstruct.
% Use Daubechies 4-element filter and periodic convolution.
%   Evaluate the two highest resolution highpass subbands and
%     zero out those samples below some threshold value.
%
close all; clear all;
fs = 1000;                       % Sample frequency
N = 1024;                        % Number of points in
                                 %   waveform
%
freqsin = [.63 1.1 2.7 5.6];     % Sinusoid frequencies
ampl = [1.2 1 1.2 .75 ];         % Amplitude of sinusoids
[x t] = signal(freqsin,ampl,N);  % Construct signal
x = x + (.25 * randn(1,N));      %   and add noise
h0 = daub(4);
figure(fig1);
```

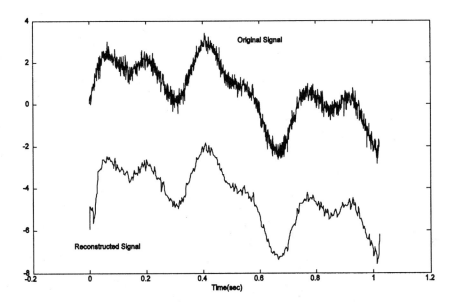

FIGURE 7.9 Application of the dyadic wavelet transform to nonlinear filtering. After subband decomposition using an analysis filter bank, a threshold process is applied to the two highest resolution highpass subbands before reconstruction using a synthesis filter bank. Periodic convolution was used so that there is no phase shift between the input and output signals.

```
an = analyze1(x,h0,4);              % Decompose signal, analytic
                                    %   filter bank of level 4
% Set the threshold times to equal the variance of the two higher
%   resolution highpass subbands.
threshold = var(an(N/4:N));
for i = (N/4:N)                     % Examine the two highest
                                    %   resolution highpass
                                    %   subbands

    if an(i) < threshold
      an(i) = 0;
    end
end
sy = synthesize1(an,h0,4);          % Reconstruct original
                                    %   signal

figure(fig2);
    plot(t,x,'k',t,sy-5,'k');       % Plot signals
    axis([-.2 1.2-8 4]);  xlabel('Time(sec)')
```

The routines for the analysis and synthesis filter banks differ slightly from those used in Example 7.3 in that they use circular convolution. In the analysis filter bank routine (analysis1), the data are first extended using the periodic or wraparound approach: the initial points are added to the end of the original data sequence (see Figure 2.10B). This extension is the same length as the filter. After convolution, these added points and the extra points generated by convolution are removed in a symmetrical fashion: a number of points equal to the filter length are removed from the initial portion of the output and the remaining extra points are taken off the end. Only the code that is different from that shown in Example 7.3 is shown below. In this code, symmetric elimination of the additional points and downsampling are done in the same instruction.

```
function an = analyze1(x,h0,L)..........
. . . . . . . . . . .
for i = 1:L
  a_ext = [an an(1:1f)];      % Extend data for "periodic
                              %   convolution"
  lpf = conv(a_ext,h0);       % Lowpass FIR filter
  hpf = conv(a_ext,h1);       % Highpass FIR filter
  lpfd = lpf(1f:2:1f+lx-1);   % Remove extra points. Shift to
  hpfd = hpf(1f:2:1f+lx-1);   %   obtain circular segment; then
                              %   downsample
  an(1:lx) = [lpfd hpfd];     % Lowpass output at beginning of
                              %   array, but now occupies only
                              %   half the data points as last
                              %   pass
  lx = lx/2; ....................
```

The synthesis filter bank routine is modified in a similar fashion except that the initial portion of the data is extended, also in wraparound fashion (by adding the end points to the beginning). The extended segments are then upsampled, convolved with the filters, and added together. The extra points are then removed in the same manner used in the analysis routine. Again, only the modified code is shown below.

```
function y = synthesize1(an,h0,L) ......................
. . . . . . . . . . . .
for i = 1:L
  lpx = y(1:lseg);                    % Get lowpass segment
  hpx = y(lseg+1:2*lseg);             % Get highpass outputs
  lpx = [lpx(lseg-1f/2+1:lseg) lpx];  % Circular extension:
                                      %   lowpass comp.
  hpx = [hpx(lseg-1f/2+1:lseg) hpx];  % and highpass component
  l_ext = length(lpx);
```

```
up_lpx = zeros(1,2*l_ext);          % Initialize vector for
                                    %  upsampling
up_lpx(1:2:2*l_ext) = lpx;          % Up sample lowpass (every
                                    %  odd point)
up_hpx = zeros(1,2*l_ext);          % Repeat for highpass
up_hpx(1:2:2*l_ext) = hpx;
syn = conv(up_lpx,g0) + conv(up_hpx,g1);  % Filter and
                                          %  combine
y(1:2*lseg) = syn(lf+1:(2*lseg)+lf);  % Remove extra
                                      %  points
lseg = lseg * 2;                    % Double segment lengths
                                    %  for next pass
end
    . . . . . . . . . . . . . . . . . . . . . . .
```

The original and reconstructed waveforms are shown in Figure 7.9. The filtering produced by thresholding the highpass subbands is evident. Also there is no phase shift between the original and reconstructed signal due to the use of periodic convolution, although a small artifact is seen at the beginning and end of the data set. This is because the data set was not really periodic.

Discontinuity Detection

Wavelet analysis based on filter bank decomposition is particularly useful for detecting small discontinuities in a waveform. This feature is also useful in image processing. Example 7.5 shows the sensitivity of this method for detecting small changes, even when they are in the higher derivatives.

Example 7.5 Construct a waveform consisting of 2 sinusoids, then add a small (approximately 1% of the amplitude) offset to this waveform. Create a new waveform by double integrating the waveform so that the offset is in the second derivative of this new signal. Apply a three-level analysis filter bank. Examine the high frequency subband for evidence of the discontinuity.

```
% Example 7.5 and Figures 7.10 and 7.11. Discontinuity detection
% Construct a waveform of 2 sinusoids with a discontinuity
%  in the second derivative
% Decompose the waveform into 3 levels to detect the
%  discontinuity.
% Use Daubechies 4-element filter
%
close all; clear all;
fig1 = figure('Units','inches','Position',[0 2.5 3 3.5]);
fig2 = figure('Units', 'inches','Position',[3 2.5 5 5]);
fs = 1000;                          % Sample frequency
```

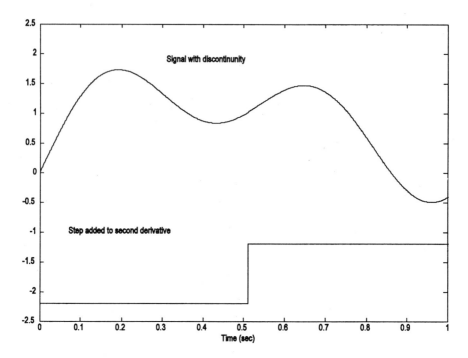

FIGURE 7.10 Waveform composed of two sine waves with an offset discontinuity in its second derivative at 0.5 sec. Note that the discontinuity is not apparent in the waveform.

```
N = 1024;                           % Number of points in
                                    %  waveform
freqsin = [.23 .8 1.8];             % Sinusoidal frequencies
ampl = [1.2 1 .7];                  % Amplitude of sinusoid
incr = .01;                         % Size of second derivative
                                    %  discontinuity
offset = [zeros(1,N/2) ones(1,N/2)];
h0 = daub(4)                        % Daubechies 4
%
[x1 t] = signal(freqsin,ampl,N);    % Construct signal
x1 = x1 + offset*incr;              % Add discontinuity at
                                    %  midpoint
x = integrate(integrate(x1));       % Double integrate
figure(fig1);
  plot(t,x,'k',t,offset-2.2,'k');   % Plot new signal
  axis([0 1-2.5 2.5]);
  xlabel('Time (sec)');
```

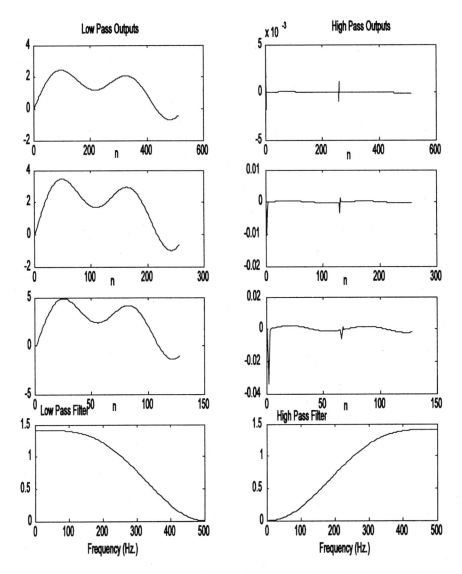

FIGURE 7.11 Analysis filter bank output of the signal shown in Figure 7.10. Although the discontinuity is not visible in the original signal, its presence and location are clearly identified as a spike in the highpass subbands.

```
figure(fig2);
a = analyze(x,h0,3);           % Decompose signal, analytic
                               %  filter bank of level 3
```

Figure 7.10 shows the waveform with a discontinuity in its second derivative at 0.5 sec. The lower trace indicates the position of the discontinuity. Note that the discontinuity is not visible in the waveform.

The output of the three-level analysis filter bank using the Daubechies 4-element filter is shown in Figure 7.11. The position of the discontinuity is clearly visible as a spike in the highpass subbands.

Feature Detection: Wavelet Packets

The DWT can also be used to construct useful descriptors of a waveform. Since the DWT is a bilateral transform, all of the information in the original waveform must be contained in the subband signals. These subband signals, or some aspect of the subband signals such as their energy over a given time period, could provide a succinct description of some important aspect of the original signal.

In the decompositions described above, only the lowpass filter subband signals were sent on for further decomposition, giving rise to the filter bank structure shown in the upper half of Figure 7.12. This decomposition structure is also known as a *logarithmic tree*. However, other decomposition structures are valid, including the *complete* or *balanced tree* structure shown in the lower half of Figure 7.12. In this decomposition scheme, both highpass and lowpass subbands are further decomposed into highpass and lowpass subbands up till the terminal signals. Other, more general, tree structures are possible where a decision on further decomposition (whether or not to split a subband signal) depends on the activity of a given subband. The scaling functions and wavelets associated with such general tree structures are known as *wavelet packets*.

Example 7.6 Apply *balanced tree* decomposition to the waveform consisting of a mixture of three equal amplitude sinusoids of 1 10 and 100 Hz. The main routine in this example is similar to that used in Examples 7.3 and 7.4 except that it calls the balanced tree decomposition routine, `w_packet`, and plots out the terminal waveforms. The `w_packet` routine is shown below and is used in this example to implement a 3-level decomposition, as illustrated in the lower half of Figure 7.12. This will lead to 8 output segments that are stored sequentially in the output vector, a.

```
% Example 7.5 and Figure 7.13
% Example of "Balanced Tree Decomposition"
% Construct a waveform of 4 sinusoids plus noise
% Decompose the waveform in 3 levels, plot outputs at the terminal
%  level
```

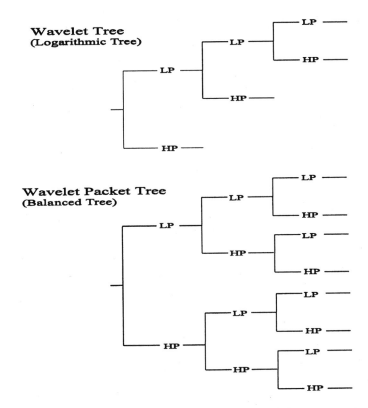

FIGURE 7.12 Structure of the analysis filter bank (wavelet tree) used in the DWT in which only the lowpass subbands are further decomposed and a more general structure in which all nonterminal signals are decomposed into highpass and lowpass subbands.

```
% Use a Daubechies 10 element filter
%
clear all; close all;
fig1 = figure('Units','inches','Position',[0 2.5 3 3.5]);
fig2 = figure('Units', 'inches','Position',[3 2.5 5 4]);
fs = 1000;                      % Sample frequency
N = 1024;                       % Number of points in
                                %  waveform
levels = 3                      % Number of decomposition
                                %  levels
nu_seg = 2^levels;              % Number of decomposed
                                %  segments
freqsin = [1 10 100];           % Sinusoid frequencies
```

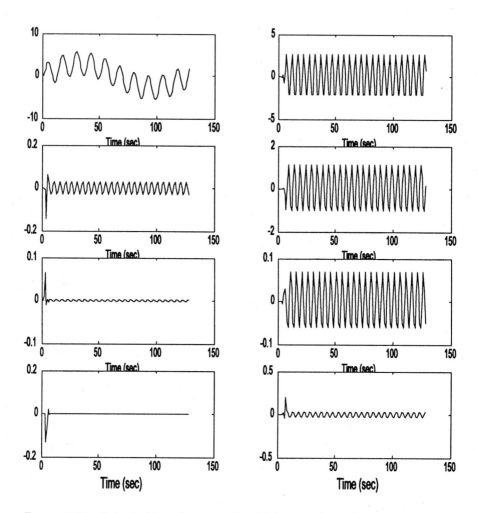

FIGURE 7.13 Balanced tree decomposition of the waveform shown in Figure 7.8. The signal from the upper left plot has been lowpass filtered 3 times and represents the lowest terminal signal in Figure 7.11. The upper right has been lowpass filtered twice then highpass filtered, and represents the second from the lowest terminal signal in Figure 7.11. The rest of the plots follow sequentially.

```
ampl = [1 1 1];                    % Amplitude of sinusoid
h0 = daub(10);                     % Get filter coefficients:
                                   %  Daubechies 10
%
[x t] = signal(freqsin,ampl,N);    % Construct signal
a = w_packet(x,h0,levels);         % Decompose signal, Balanced
                                   %  Tree
for i = 1:nu_seg
  i_s = 1 + (N/nu_seg) * (i-1);    % Location for this segment
  a_p = a(i_s:i_s+(N/nu_seg)-1);
  subplot(nu_seg/2,2,i);           % Plot decompositions
    plot((1:N/nu_seg),a_p,'k');
    xlabel('Time (sec)');
end
```

The balanced tree decomposition routine, w_packet, operates similarly to the DWT analysis filter banks, except for the filter structure. At each level, signals from the previous level are isolated, filtered (using standard convolution), downsampled, and both the high- and lowpass signals overwrite the single signal from the previous level. At the first level, the input waveform is replaced by the filtered, downsampled high- and lowpass signals. At the second level, the two high- and lowpass signals are each replaced by filtered, downsampled high- and lowpass signals. After the second level there are now four sequential signals in the original data array, and after the third level there be will be eight.

```
% Function to generate a "balanced tree" filter bank
% All arguments are the same as in routine 'analyze'
% an = w_packet(x,h,L)
% where
%  x = input waveform (must be longer than 2^L + L and power of
%       two)
%  h0 = filter coefficients (low pass)
%  L = decomposition level (number of High pass filter in bank)
%
function an = w_packet(x,h0,L)

lf = length(h0);                   % Filter length
lx = length(x);                    % Data length
an = x;                            % Initialize output
% Calculate High pass coefficients from low pass coefficients
for i = 0:(lf-1)
  h1(i+1) = (-1)^i * h0(lf-i);     % Uses Eq. (18)
end
% Calculate filter outputs for all levels
for i = 1:L
```

```
nu_low = 2^(i-1);                  % Number of lowpass filters
                                   %   at this level
l_seg = 1x/2^(i-1);                % Length of each data seg. at
                                   %   this level
for j = 1:nu_low;
  i_start = 1 + l_seg * (j-1);     % Location for current
                                   %   segment
  a_seg = an(i_start:i_start+l_seg-1);
  lpf = conv(a_seg,h0);            % Lowpass filter
  hpf = conv(a_seg,h1);            % Highpass filter
  lpf = lpf(1:2:l_seg);            % Downsample
  hpf = hpf(1:2:l_seg);
  an(i_start:i_start+l_seg-1) = [lpf hpf];
  end
end
```

The output produced by this decomposition is shown in Figure 7.13. The filter bank outputs emphasize various components of the three-sine mixture. Another example is given in Problem 7 using a chirp signal.

One of the most popular applications of the dyadic wavelet transform is in data compression, particularly of images. However, since this application is not so often used in biomedical engineering (although there are some applications regrading the transmission of radiographic images), it will not be covered here.

PROBLEMS

1. (A) Plot the frequency characteristics (magnitude and phase) of the Mexican hat and Morlet wavelets.

(B) The plot of the phase characteristics will be incorrect due to phase wrapping. Phase wrapping is due to the fact that the arctan function can never be greater that $\pm 2\pi$; hence, once the phase shift exceeds $\pm 2\pi$ (usually minus), it *warps around* and appears as positive. Replot the phase after correcting for this wrap-around effect. (*Hint*: Check for discontinuities above a certain amount, and when that amount is exceeded, subtract 2π from the rest of the data array. This is a simple algorithm that is generally satisfactory in linear systems analysis.)

2. Apply the continuous wavelet analysis used in Example 7.1 to analyze a chirp signal running between 2 and 30 Hz over a 2 sec period. Assume a sample rate of 500 Hz as in Example 7.1. Use the Mexican hat wavelet. Show both contour and 3-D plot.

3. Plot the frequency characteristics (magnitude and phase) of the Haar and Daubechies 4-and 10-element filters. Assume a sample frequency of 100 Hz.

4. Generate a Daubechies 10-element filter and plot the magnitude spectrum as in Problem 3. Construct the highpass filter using the alternating flip algorithm (Eq. (20)) and plot its magnitude spectrum. Generate the lowpass and highpass synthesis filter coefficients using the order flip algorithm (Eqs. (23) and (24)) and plot their respective frequency characteristics. Assume a sampling frequency of 100 Hz.

5. Construct a waveform of a chirp signal as in Problem 2 plus noise. Make the variance of the noise equal to the variance of the chirp. Decompose the waveform in 5 levels, operate on the lowest level (i.e., the high resolution highpass signal), then reconstruct. The operation should zero all elements below a given threshold. Find the best threshold. Plot the signal before and after reconstruction. Use Daubechies 6-element filter.

6. Discontinuity detection. Load the waveform **x** in file **Prob7_6_data** which consists of a waveform of 2 sinusoids the same as in Figure 7.9, but with a series of diminishing discontinuities in the second derivative. The discontinuities in the second derivative begin at approximately 0.5% of the sinusoidal amplitude and decrease by a factor of 2 for each pair of discontinuities. (The offset array can be obtained in the variable **offset**.) Decompose the waveform into three levels and examine and plot only the highest resolution highpass filter output to detect the discontinuity. *Hint*: The highest resolution output will be located in $N/2$ to N of the **analysis** output array. Use a Harr and a Daubechies 10-element filter and compare the difference in detectability. (Note that the Haar is a very weak filter so that some of the low frequency components will still be found in its output.)

7. Apply the balanced tree decomposition to a chirp signal similar to that used in Problem 5 except that the chirp frequency should range between 2 and 100 Hz. Decompose the waveform into 3 levels and plot the outputs at the terminal level as in Example 7.5. Use a Daubechies 4-element filter. Note that each output filter responds to different portions of the chirp signal.

8

Advanced Signal Processing Techniques: Optimal and Adaptive Filters

OPTIMAL SIGNAL PROCESSING: WIENER FILTERS

The FIR and IIR filters described in Chapter 4 provide considerable flexibility in altering the frequency content of a signal. Coupled with MATLAB filter design tools, these filters can provide almost any desired frequency characteristic to nearly any degree of accuracy. The actual frequency characteristics attained by the various design routines can be verified through Fourier transform analysis. However, these design routines do not tell the user what frequency characteristics are best; i.e., what type of filtering will most effectively separate out signal from noise. That decision is often made based on the user's knowledge of signal or source properties, or by trial and error. Optimal filter theory was developed to provide structure to the process of selecting the most appropriate frequency characteristics.

A wide range of different approaches can be used to develop an optimal filter, depending on the nature of the problem: specifically, what, and how much, is known about signal and noise features. If a representation of the desired signal is available, then a well-developed and popular class of filters known as *Wiener filters* can be applied. The basic concept behind Wiener filter theory is to minimize the difference between the filtered output and some desired output. This minimization is based on the least mean square approach, which adjusts the filter coefficients to reduce the square of the difference between the desired and actual waveform after filtering. This approach requires

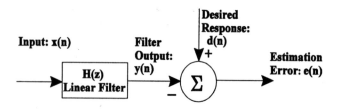

FIGURE 8.1 Basic arrangement of signals and processes in a Wiener filter.

an estimate of the desired signal which must somehow be constructed, and this estimation is usually the most challenging aspect of the problem.*

The Wiener filter approach is outlined in Figure 8.1. The input waveform containing both signal and noise is operated on by a linear process, $H(z)$. In practice, the process could be either an FIR or IIR filter; however, FIR filters are more popular as they are inherently stable,† and our discussion will be limited to the use of FIR filters. FIR filters have only numerator terms in the transfer function (i.e., only zeros) and can be implemented using convolution first presented in Chapter 2 (Eq. (15)), and later used with FIR filters in Chapter 4 (Eq. (8)). Again, the convolution equation is:

$$y(n) = \sum_{k=1}^{L} b(k) \, x(n - k) \tag{1}$$

where $h(k)$ is the impulse response of the linear filter. The output of the filter, $y(n)$, can be thought of as an estimate of the desired signal, $d(n)$. The difference between the estimate and desired signal, $e(n)$, can be determined by simple subtraction: $e(n) = d(n) - y(n)$.

As mentioned above, the least mean square algorithm is used to minimize the error signal: $e(n) = d(n) - y(n)$. Note that $y(n)$ is the output of the linear filter, $H(z)$. Since we are limiting our analysis to FIR filters, $h(k) \equiv b(k)$, and $e(n)$ can be written as:

$$e(n) = d(n) - y(n) = d(n) - \sum_{k=0}^{L-1} h(k) \, x(n - k) \tag{2}$$

where L is the length of the FIR filter. In fact, it is the sum of $e(n)^2$ which is minimized, specifically:

---

*As shown below, only the crosscorrelation between the unfiltered and the desired output is necessary for the application of these filters.

†IIR filters contain internal feedback paths and can oscillate with certain parameter combinations.

$$\varepsilon = \sum_{n=1}^{N} e^2(n) = \sum_{n=1}^{N} \left[d(n) - \sum_{k=1}^{L} b(k) \, x(n-k) \right]^2 \tag{3}$$

After squaring the term in brackets, the sum of error squared becomes a quadratic function of the FIR filter coefficients, b(k), in which two of the terms can be identified as the autocorrelation and cross correlation:

$$\varepsilon = \sum_{n=1}^{N} d(n) - 2 \sum_{k=1}^{L} b(k) r_{dx}(k) + \sum_{k=1}^{L} \sum_{\ell=1}^{L} b(k) \, b(\ell) r_{xx}(k-\ell) \tag{4}$$

where, from the original definition of cross- and autocorrelation (Eq. (3), Chapter 2):

$$r_{dx}(k) = \sum_{\ell=1}^{L} d(\ell) \, x(\ell + k)$$

$$r_{xx}(k) = \sum_{\ell=1}^{L} x(\ell) \, x(\ell + k)$$

Since we desire to minimize the error function with respect to the FIR filter coefficients, we take derivatives with respect to $b(k)$ and set them to zero:

$$\frac{\partial \varepsilon}{\partial b(k)} = 0; \qquad \text{which leads to:}$$

$$\sum_{k=1}^{L} b(k) \, r_{xx}(k-m) = r_{dx}(m), \qquad \text{for } 1 \le m \le L \tag{5}$$

Equation (5) shows that the optimal filter can be derived knowing only the autocorrelation function of the input and the crosscorrelation function between the input and desired waveform. In principle, the actual functions are not necessary, only the auto- and crosscorrelations; however, in most practical situations the auto- and crosscorrelations are derived from the actual signals, in which case some representation of the desired signal is required.

To solve for the FIR coefficients in Eq. (5), we note that this equation actually represents a series of L equations that must be solved simultaneously. The matrix expression for these simultaneous equations is:

$$\begin{bmatrix} r_{xx}(0) & r_{xx}(1) & \cdots & r_{xx}(L) \\ r_{xx}(1) & r_{xx}(0) & \cdots & r_{xx}(L-1) \\ \vdots & \vdots & \ddots & \vdots \\ r_{xx}(L) & r_{xx}(L-1) & \cdots & r_{xx}(0) \end{bmatrix} \begin{bmatrix} b(0) \\ b(1) \\ \vdots \\ b(L) \end{bmatrix} = \begin{bmatrix} r_{dx}(0) \\ r_{dx}(1) \\ \vdots \\ r_{dx}(L) \end{bmatrix} \tag{6}$$

Equation (6) is commonly known as the *Wiener-Hopf* equation and is a basic component of Wiener filter theory. Note that the matrix in the equation is

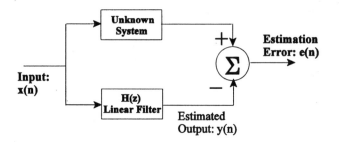

FIGURE 8.2   Configuration for using optimal filter theory for systems identification.

the correlation matrix mentioned in Chapter 2 (Eq. (21)) and has a symmetrical structure termed a Toeplitz structure.* The equation can be written more succinctly using standard matrix notation, and the FIR coefficients can be obtained by solving the equation through matrix inversion:

$$\mathbf{RB} = \mathbf{r}_{dx} \quad \text{and the solution is:} \quad \mathbf{b} = \mathbf{R}^{-1}\mathbf{r}_{dx} \tag{7}$$

The application and solution of this equation are given for two different examples in the following section on MATLAB implementation.

The Wiener-Hopf approach has a number of other applications in addition to standard filtering including systems identification, interference canceling, and inverse modeling or deconvolution. For system identification, the filter is placed in parallel with the unknown system as shown in Figure 8.2. In this application, the desired output is the output of the unknown system, and the filter coefficients are adjusted so that the filter's output best matches that of the unknown system. An example of this application is given in a subsequent section on *adaptive signal processing* where the *least mean squared* (LMS) algorithm is used to implement the optimal filter. Problem 2 also demonstrates this approach. In interference canceling, the desired signal contains both signal and noise while the filter input is a reference signal that contains only noise or a signal correlated with the noise. This application is also explored under the section on adaptive signal processing since it is more commonly implemented in this context.

MATLAB Implementation

The Wiener-Hopf equation (Eqs. (5) and (6), can be solved using MATLAB's matrix inversion operator ('\') as shown in the examples below. Alternatively,

---

*Due to this matrix's symmetry, it can be uniquely defined by only a single row or column.

since the matrix has the Toeplitz structure, matrix inversion can also be done using a faster algorithm known as the Levinson-Durbin recursion.

The MATLAB `toeplitz` function is useful in setting up the correlation matrix. The function call is:

```
Rxx = toeplitz(rxx);
```

where `rxx` is the input row vector. This constructs a symmetrical matrix from a single row vector and can be used to generate the correlation matrix in Eq. (6) from the autocorrelation function r_{xx}. (The function can also create an asymmetrical Toeplitz matrix if two input arguments are given.)

In order for the matrix to be inverted, it must be nonsingular; that is, the rows and columns must be independent. Because of the structure of the correlation matrix in Eq. (6) (termed *positive- definite*), it cannot be singular. However, it can be near singular: some rows or columns may be only slightly independent. Such an *ill-conditioned* matrix will lead to large errors when it is inverted. The MATLAB '\' matrix inversion operator provides an error message if the matrix is not well-conditioned, but this can be more effectively evaluated using the MATLAB `cond` function:

```
c = cond(X)
```

where `x` is the matrix under test and `c` is the ratio of the largest to smallest singular values. A very well-conditioned matrix would have singular values in the same general range, so the output variable, `c`, would be close to one. Very large values of `c` indicate an ill-conditioned matrix. Values greater than 10^4 have been suggested by Sterns and David (1996) as too large to produce reliable results in the Wiener-Hopf equation. When this occurs, the condition of the matrix can usually be improved by reducing its dimension, that is, reducing the range, L, of the autocorrelation function in Eq (6). This will also reduce the number of filter coefficients in the solution.

Example 8.1   Given a sinusoidal signal in noise (SNR = -8 db), design an optimal filter using the Wiener-Hopf equation. Assume that you have a copy of the actual signal available, in other words, a version of the signal without the added noise. In general, this would not be the case: if you had the desired signal, you would not need the filter! In practical situations you would have to estimate the desired signal or the crosscorrelation between the estimated and desired signals.

Solution The program below uses the routine `wiener_hopf` (also shown below) to determine the optimal filter coefficients. These are then applied to the noisy waveform using the `filter` routine introduced in Chapter 4 although correlation could also have been used.

```
% Example 8.1 and Figure 8.3 Wiener Filter Theory
% Use an adaptive filter to eliminate broadband noise from a
%   narrowband signal
% Implemented using Wiener-Hopf equations
%
close all; clear all;
fs = 1000;                              % Sampling frequency
```

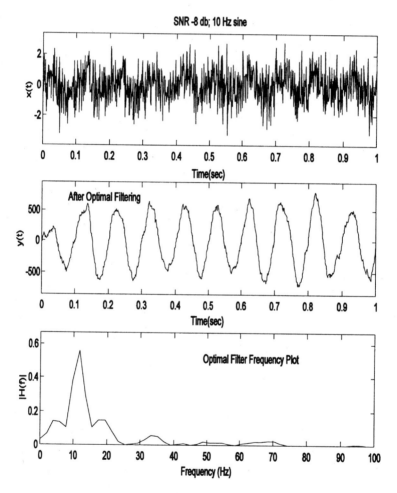

FIGURE 8.3 Application of the Wiener-Hopf equation to produce an optimal FIR filter to filter broadband noise (SNR = -8 db) from a single sinusoid (10 Hz.) The frequency characteristics (bottom plot) show that the filter coefficients were adjusted to approximate a bandpass filter with a small bandwidth and a peak at 10 Hz.

```
N = 1024;                          % Number of points
L = 256;                           % Optimal filter order
%
% Generate signal and noise data: 10 Hz sin in 8 db noise (SNR =
%  -8 db)
[xn, t, x] = sig_noise(10,-8,N);   % xn is signal + noise and
                                   %  x is noise free (i.e.,
                                   %  desired) signal
subplot(3,1,1); plot(t, xn,'k');   % Plot unfiltered data
  .........labels, table, axis.........
%
% Determine the optimal FIR filter coefficients and apply
b = wiener_hopf(xn,x,L);           % Apply Wiener-Hopf
                                   %  equations
y = filter(b,1,xn);                % Filter data using optimum
                                   %  filter weights
%
% Plot filtered data and filter spectrum
subplot(3,1,2); plot(t,y,'k');     % Plot filtered data
  .........labels, table, axis.........
%
subplot(3,1,3);
f = (1:N) * fs/N;      % Construct freq. vector for plotting
h = abs(fft(b,256)).^2             % Calculate filter power
plot(f,h,'k');                     %  spectrum and plot
  .........labels, table, axis.........
```

The function `Wiener_hopf` solves the Wiener-Hopf equations:

```
function b = wiener_hopf(x,y,maxlags)
% Function to compute LMS algol using Wiener-Hopf equations
% Inputs:       x = input
%               y = desired signal
%               Maxlags = filter length
% Outputs:      b = FIR filter coefficients
%
rxx = xcorr(x,maxlags,'coeff');    % Compute the autocorrela-
                                   %  tion vector
rxx = rxx(maxlags+1:end)';         % Use only positive half of
                                   %  symm. vector
rxy = xcorr(x,y,maxlags);          % Compute the crosscorrela-
                                   %  tion vector
rxy = rxy(maxlags+1:end)';         % Use only positive half
%
rxx_matrix = toeplitz(rxx);        % Construct correlation
                                   %  matrix
```

```
b = rxx_matrix\rxy;          % Calculate FIR coefficients
                             %  using matrix inversion,
                             %  Levinson could be used
                             %  here
```

Example 8.1 generates Figure 8.3 above. Note that the optimal filter approach, when applied to a single sinusoid buried in noise, produces a bandpass filter with a peak at the sinusoidal frequency. An equivalent—or even more effective—filter could have been designed using the tools presented in Chapter 4. Indeed, such a statement could also be made about any of the adaptive filters described below. However, this requires precise *a priori* knowledge of the signal and noise frequency characteristics, which may not be available. Moreover, a fixed filter will not be able to optimally filter signal and noise that changes over time.

Example 8.2   Apply the LMS algorithm to a systems identification task. The "unknown" system will be an all-zero linear process with a digital transfer function of:

$$H(z) = 0.5 + 0.75z^{-1} + 1.2z^{-2}$$

Confirm the match by plotting the magnitude of the transfer function for both the unknown and matching systems. Since this approach uses an FIR filter as the matching system, which is also an all-zero process, the match should be quite good. In Problem 2, this approach is repeated, but for an unknown system that has both poles and zeros. In this case, the FIR (all-zero) filter will need many more coefficients than the unknown pole-zero process to produce a reasonable match.

Solution   The program below inputs random noise into the unknown process using convolution and into the matching filter. Since the FIR matching filter cannot easily accommodate for a pure time delay, care must be taken to compensate for possible time shift due to the convolution operation. The matching filter coefficients are adjusted using the Wiener-Hopf equation described previously. Frequency characteristics of both unknown and matching system are determined by applying the FFT to the coefficients of both processes and the resultant spectra are plotted.

```
% Example 8.2 and Figure 8.4 Adaptive Filters System
%  Identification
%
% Uses optimal filtering implemented with the Wiener-Hopf
%  algorithm to identify an unknown system
%
% Initialize parameters
```

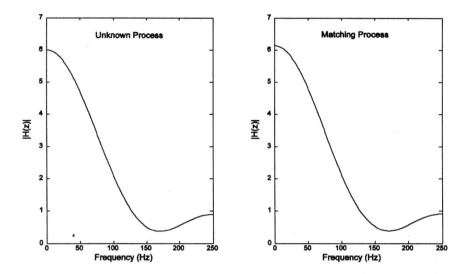

FIGURE 8.4 Frequency characteristics of an "unknown" process having coefficients of 0.5, 0.75, and 1.2 (an all-zero process). The matching process uses system identification implemented with the Wiener-Hopf adaptive filtering approach. This matching process generates a linear system with a similar spectrum to the unknown process. Since the unknown process is also an all-zero system, the transfer function coefficients also match.

```
close all; clear all;
fs = 500;                      % Sampling frequency
N = 1024;                      % Number of points
L = 8;                         % Optimal filter order
%
% Generate unknown system and noise input
b_unknown = [.5 .75 1.2];      % Define unknown process
xn = randn(1,N);
xd = conv(b_unknown,xn);       % Generate unknown system output
xd = xd(3:N+2);                % Truncate extra points.
%                                Ensure proper phase
% Apply Weiner filter
b = wiener_hopf(xn,xd,L);      % Compute matching filter
                               %  coefficients
b = b/N;                       % Scale filter coefficients
%
% Calculate frequency characteristics using the FFT
ps_match = (abs(fft(b,N))).^2;
ps_unknown = (abs(fft(b_unknown,N))).^2;
```

```
%
% Plot frequency characteristics of unknown and identified
%   process
f = (1:N) * fs/N;              % Construct freq. vector for
                               %   plotting
subplot(1,2,1);                % Plot unknown system freq. char.
   plot(f(1:N/2),ps_unknown(1:N/2),'k');
   ..........labels, table, axis.........
subplot(1,2,2);
                               % Plot matching system freq. char.
   plot(f(1:N/2),ps_match(1:N/2),'k');
   ..........labels, table, axis.........
```

The output plots from this example are shown in Figure 8.4. Note the close match in spectral characteristics between the "unknown" process and the matching output produced by the Wiener-Hopf algorithm. The transfer functions also closely match as seen by the similarity in impulse response coefficients:

$$h(n)_{\text{unknown}} = [0.5\ 0.75\ 1.2]; \qquad h(n)_{\text{match}} = [0.503\ 0.757\ 1.216].$$

ADAPTIVE SIGNAL PROCESSING

The area of adaptive signal processing is relatively new yet already has a rich history. As with optimal filtering, only a brief example of the usefulness and broad applicability of adaptive filtering can be covered here. The FIR and IIR filters described in Chapter 4 were based on an *a priori* design criteria and were fixed throughout their application. Although the Wiener filter described above does not require prior knowledge of the input signal (only the desired outcome), it too is fixed for a given application. As with classical spectral analysis methods, these filters cannot respond to changes that might occur during the course of the signal. Adaptive filters have the capability of modifying their properties based on selected features of signal being analyzed.

A typical adaptive filter paradigm is shown in Figure 8.5. In this case, the filter coefficients are modified by a feedback process designed to make the filter's output, $y(n)$, as close to some desired response, $d(n)$, as possible, by reducing the error, $e(n)$, to a minimum. As with optimal filtering, the nature of the desired response will depend on the specific problem involved and its formulation may be the most difficult part of the adaptive system specification (Stearns and David, 1996).

The inherent stability of FIR filters makes them attractive in adaptive applications as well as in optimal filtering (Ingle and Proakis, 2000). Accordingly, the adaptive filter, $H(z)$, can again be represented by a set of FIR filter coefficients,

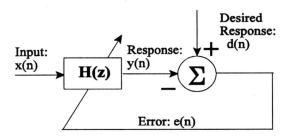

FIGURE 8.5 Elements of a typical adaptive filter.

$b(k)$. The FIR filter equation (i.e., convolution) is repeated here, but the filter coefficients are indicated as $b_n(k)$ to indicate that they vary with time (i.e., n).

$$y(n) = \sum_{k=1}^{L} b_n(k)\, x(n - k) \tag{8}$$

The adaptive filter operates by modifying the filter coefficients, $b_n(k)$, based on some signal property. The general adaptive filter problem has similarities to the Wiener filter theory problem discussed above in that an error is minimized, usually between the input and some desired response. As with optimal filtering, it is the squared error that is minimized, and, again, it is necessary to somehow construct a desired signal. In the Wiener approach, the analysis is applied to the entire waveform and the resultant optimal filter coefficients were similarly applied to the entire waveform (a so-called *block approach*). In adaptive filtering, the filter coefficients are adjusted and applied in an ongoing basis.

While the Wiener-Hopf equations (Eqs. (6) and (7)) can be, and have been, adapted for use in an adaptive environment, a simpler and more popular approach is based on gradient optimization. This approach is usually called the LMS recursive algorithm. As in Wiener filter theory, this algorithm also determines the optimal filter coefficients, and it is also based on minimizing the squared error, but it does not require computation of the correlation functions, r_{xx} and r_{xy}. Instead the LMS algorithm uses a recursive gradient method known as the *steepest-descent* method for finding the filter coefficients that produce the minimum sum of squared error.

Examination of Eq. (3) shows that the sum of squared errors is a quadratic function of the FIR filter coefficients, $b(k)$; hence, this function will have a single minimum. The goal of the LMS algorithm is to adjust the coefficients so that the sum of squared error moves toward this minimum. The technique used by the LMS algorithm is to adjust the filter coefficients based on the method of steepest descent. In this approach, the filter coefficients are modified based on an estimate of the negative gradient of the error function with respect to a given $b(k)$. This estimate is given by the partial derivative of the squared error, ε, with respect to the coefficients, $b_n(k)$:

$$\nabla_n = \frac{\partial \varepsilon_n^2}{\partial b_n(k)} = 2e(n) \frac{\partial(d(n) - y(n))}{\partial b_n(k)} \tag{9}$$

Since $d(n)$ is independent of the coefficients, $b_n(k)$, its partial derivative with respect to $b_n(k)$ is zero. As $y(n)$ is a function of the input times $b_n(k)$ (Eq. (8)), then its partial derivative with respect to $b_n(k)$ is just $x(n-k)$, and Eq. (9) can be rewritten in terms of the instantaneous product of error and the input:

$$\nabla_n = 2e(n)\, x(n - k) \tag{10}$$

Initially, the filter coefficients are set arbitrarily to some $b_0(k)$, usually zero. With each new input sample a new error signal, $e(n)$, can be computed (Figure 8.5). Based on this new error signal, the new gradient is determined (Eq. (10)), and the filter coefficients are updated:

$$b_n(k) = b_{n-1}(k) + \Delta e(n)\, x(n - k) \tag{11}$$

where Δ is a constant that controls the descent and, hence, the rate of convergence. This parameter must be chosen with some care. A large value of Δ will lead to large modifications of the filter coefficients which will hasten convergence, but can also lead to instability and oscillations. Conversely, a small value will result in slow convergence of the filter coefficients to their optimal values. A common rule is to select the convergence parameter, Δ, such that it lies in the range:

$$0 < \Delta < \frac{1}{10 L P_x} \tag{12}$$

where L is the length of the FIR filter and P_x is the power in the input signal. P_X can be approximated by:

$$P_x \approx \frac{1}{N - 1} \sum_{n=1}^{N} x^2(n) \tag{13}$$

Note that for a waveform of zero mean, P_x equals the variance of x. The LMS algorithm given in Eq. (11) can easily be implemented in MATLAB, as shown in the next section.

Adaptive filtering has a number of applications in biosignal processing. It can be used to suppress a narrowband noise source such as 60 Hz that is corrupting a broadband signal. It can also be used in the reverse situation, removing broadband noise from a narrowband signal, a process known as *adaptive line*

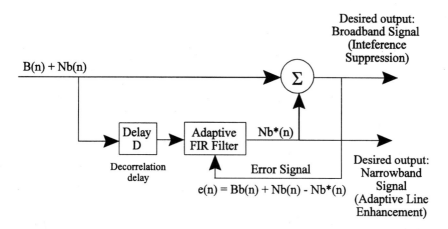

FIGURE 8.6 Configuration for Adaptive Line Enhancement (ALE) or Adaptive Interference Suppression. The Delay, D, decorrelates the narrowband component allowing the adaptive filter to use only this component. In ALE the narrowband component is the signal while in Interference suppression it is the noise.

enhancement (ALE).* It can also be used for some of the same applications as the Wiener filter such as system identification, inverse modeling, and, especially important in biosignal processing, adaptive noise cancellation. This last application requires a suitable reference source that is correlated with the noise, but not the signal. Many of these applications are explored in the next section on MATLAB implementation and/or in the problems.

The configuration for ALE and adaptive interference suppression is shown in Figure 8.6. When this configuration is used in adaptive interference suppression, the input consists of a broadband signal, $Bb(n)$, in narrowband noise, $Nb(n)$, such as 60 Hz. Since the noise is narrowband compared to the relatively broadband signal, the noise portion of sequential samples will remain correlated while the broadband signal components will be decorrelated after a few samples.† If the combined signal and noise is delayed by D samples, the broadband (signal) component of the delayed waveform will no longer be correlated with the broadband component in the original waveform. Hence, when the filter's output is subtracted from the input waveform, only the narrowband component

---

*The adaptive line enhancer is so termed because the objective of this filter is to enhance a narrowband signal, one with a spectrum composed of a single "line."

†Recall that the width of the autocorrelation function is a measure of the range of samples for which the samples are correlated, and this width is inversely related to the signal bandwidth. Hence, broadband signals remain correlated for only a few samples and vice versa.

can have an influence on the result. The adaptive filter will try to adjust its output to minimize this result, but since its output component, $Nb*(n)$, only correlates with the narrowband component of the waveform, $Nb(n)$, it is only the narrowband component that is minimized. In adaptive interference suppression, the narrowband component is the noise and this is the component that is minimized in the subtracted signal. The subtracted signal, now containing less noise, constitutes the output in adaptive interference suppression (upper output, Figure 8.6).

In adaptive line enhancement, the configuration is the same except the roles of signal and noise are reversed: the narrowband component is the signal and the broadband component is the noise. In this case, the output is taken from the filter output (Figure 8.6, lower output). Recall that this filter output is optimized for the narrowband component of the waveform.

As with the Wiener filter approach, a filter of equal or better performance could be constructed with the same number of filter coefficients using the traditional methods described in Chapter 4. However, the exact frequency or frequencies of the signal would have to be known in advance and these spectral features would have to be fixed throughout the signal, a situation that is often violated in biological signals. The ALE can be regarded as a *self-tuning narrowband filter* which will track changes in signal frequency. An application of ALE is provided in Example 8.3 and an example of adaptive interference suppression is given in the problems.

Adaptive Noise Cancellation

Adaptive noise cancellation can be thought of as an outgrowth of the interference suppression described above, except that a separate channel is used to supply the estimated noise or interference signal. One of the earliest applications of adaptive noise cancellation was to eliminate 60 Hz noise from an ECG signal (Widrow, 1964). It has also been used to improve measurements of the fetal ECG by reducing interference from the mother's EEG. In this approach, a reference channel carries a signal that is correlated with the interference, but not with the signal of interest. The adaptive noise canceller consists of an adaptive filter that operates on the reference signal, $N'(n)$, to produce an estimate of the interference, $N(n)$ (Figure 8.7). This estimated noise is then subtracted from the signal channel to produce the output. As with ALE and interference cancellation, the difference signal is used to adjust the filter coefficients. Again, the strategy is to minimize the difference signal, which in this case is also the output, since minimum output signal power corresponds to minimum interference, or noise. This is because the only way the filter can reduce the output power is to reduce the noise component since this is the only signal component available to the filter.

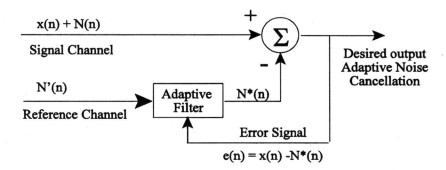

$e(n) = x(n) - N^*(n)$

FIGURE 8.7 Configuration for adaptive noise cancellation. The reference channel carries a signal, $N'(n)$, that is correlated with the noise, $N(n)$, but not with the signal of interest, $x(n)$. The adaptive filter produces an estimate of the noise, $N^*(n)$, that is in the signal. In some applications, multiple reference channels are used to provide a more accurate representation of the background noise.

MATLAB Implementation

The implementation of the LMS recursive algorithm (Eq. (11)) in MATLAB is straightforward and is given below. Its application is illustrated through several examples below.

The LMS algorithm is implemented in the function lms.

```
function [b,y,e] = lms(x,d,delta,L)
%
% Inputs:          x = input
%                  d = desired signal
%                  delta = the convergence gain
%                  L is the length (order) of the FIR filter
% Outputs:         b = FIR filter coefficients
%                  y = ALE output
%                  e = residual error
% Simple function to adjust filter coefficients using the LSM
%  algorithm
% Adjusts filter coefficients, b, to provide the best match
%  between the input, x(n), and a desired waveform, d(n),
% Both waveforms must be the same length
% Uses a standard FIR filter
%
M = length(x);
b = zeros(1,L); y = zeros(1,M);   % Initialize outputs
for n = L:M
```

```
x1 = x(n:-1:n-L+1);           % Select input for convolu-
                              %  tion
y(n) = b * x1';               % Convolve (multiply)
                              %  weights with input
e(n) = d(n)-y(n);             % Calculate error
b = b + delta*e(n)*x1;        % Adjust weights
end
```

Note that this function operates on the data as block, but could easily be modified to operate on-line, that is, as the data are being acquired. The routine begins by applying the filter with the current coefficients to the first L points (L is the filter length), calculates the error between the filter output and the desired output, then adjusts the filter coefficients accordingly. This process is repeated for another data segment L-points long, beginning with the second point, and continues through the input waveform.

Example 8.3   Optimal filtering using the LMS algorithm. Given the same sinusoidal signal in noise as used in Example 8.1, design an adaptive filter to remove the noise. Just as in Example 8.1, assume that you have a copy of the desired signal.

Solution   The program below sets up the problem as in Example 8.1, but uses the LMS algorithm in the routine lms instead of the Wiener-Hopf equation.

```
% Example 8.3 and Figure 8.8 Adaptive Filters
%  Use an adaptive filter to eliminate broadband noise from a
%    narrowband signal
%  Use LSM algorithm applied to the same data as Example 8.1
%
close all; clear all;
fs = 1000;*IH26*             % Sampling frequency
N = 1024;                    % Number of points
L = 256;                     % Optimal filter order
a = .25;                     % Convergence gain
%
% Same initial lines as in Example 8.1 .....
%% Calculate convergence parameter
PX = (1/(N+1))* sum(xn.^2); % Calculate approx. power in xn
delta = a * (1/(10*L*PX));   % Calculate Δ
b = lms(xn,x,delta,L);       % Apply LMS algorithm (see below)
%
% Plotting identical to Example 8.1. ...
```

Example 8.3 produces the data in Figure 8.8. As with the Wiener filter, the adaptive process adjusts the FIR filter coefficients to produce a narrowband filter centered about the sinusoidal frequency. The convergence factor, a, was

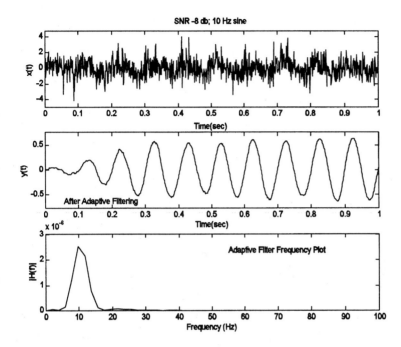

FIGURE 8.8 Application of an adaptive filter using the LSM recursive algorithm to data containing a single sinusoid (10 Hz) in noise (SNR = -8 db). Note that the filter requires the first 0.4 to 0.5 sec to adapt (400–500 points), and that the frequency characteristics of the coefficients produced after adaptation are those of a bandpass filter with a single peak at 10 Hz. Comparing this figure with Figure 8.3 suggests that the adaptive approach is somewhat more effective than the Wiener filter for the same number of filter weights.

empirically set to give rapid, yet stable convergence. (In fact, close inspection of Figure 8.8 shows a small oscillation in the output amplitude suggesting marginal stability.)

Example 8.4   The application of the LMS algorithm to a stationary signal was given in Example 8.3. Example 8.4 explores the adaptive characteristics of algorithm in the context of an adaptive line enhancement problem. Specifically, a single sinusoid that is buried in noise (SNR = -6 db) abruptly changes frequency. The ALE-type filter must readjust its coefficients to adapt to the new frequency.

The signal consists of two sequential sinusoids of 10 and 20 Hz, each lasting 0.6 sec. An FIR filter with 256 coefficients will be used. Delay and convergence gain will be set for best results. (As in many problems some adjustments must be made on a trial and error basis.)

Solution   Use the LSM recursive algorithm to implement the ALE filter.

```
% Example 8.4 and Figure 8.9 Adaptive Line Enhancement (ALE)
% Uses adaptive filter to eliminate broadband noise from a
%   narrowband signal
%.
% Generate signal and noise
close all; clear all;
fs = 1000;                          % Sampling frequency
```

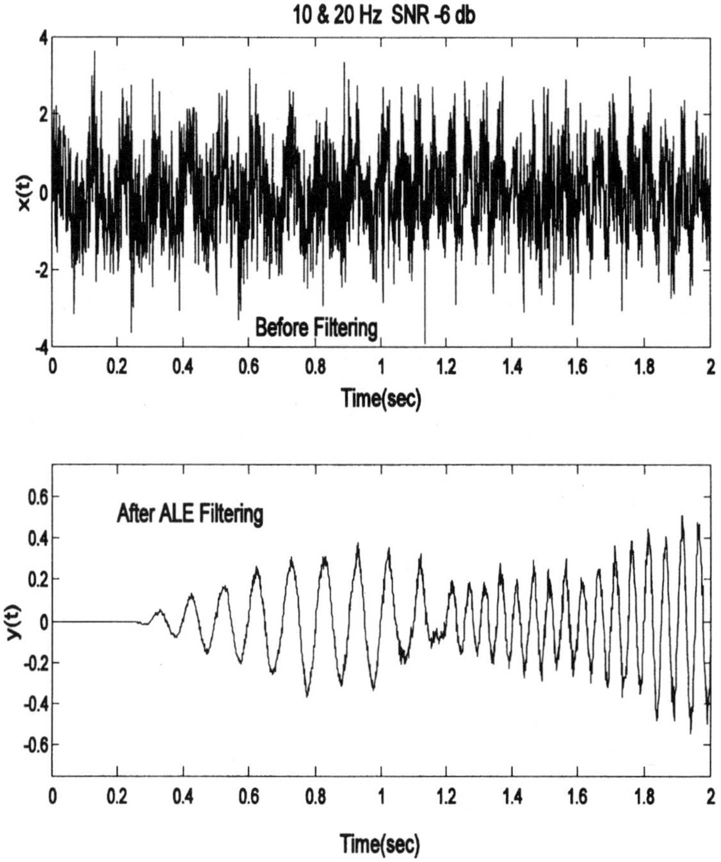

FIGURE 8.9   Adaptive line enhancer applied to a signal consisting of two sequential sinusoids having different frequencies (10 and 20 Hz). The delay of 5 samples and the convergence gain of 0.075 were determined by trial and error to give the best results with the specified FIR filter length.

```
L = 256;                        % Filter order
N = 2000;                       % Number of points
delay = 5;                      % Decorrelation delay
a = .075;                       % Convergence gain
t = (1:N)/fs;                   % Time vector for plotting
%
% Generate data: two sequential sinusoids, 10 & 20 Hz in noise
%  (SNR = -6)
x = [sig_noise(10,-6,N/2) sig_noise(20,-6,N/2)];
%
subplot(2,1,1);                 % Plot unfiltered data
  plot(t, x,'k');
  ........axis, title............

PX = (1/(N+1))* sum(x.^2);      % Calculate waveform
                                %  power for delta
delta = (1/(10*L*PX)) * a;      % Use 10% of the max.
                                %  range of delta
xd = [x(delay:N) zeros(1,delay-1)];  % Delay signal to decor-
                                %  relate broadband noise
[b,y] = lms(xd,x,delta,L);      % Apply LMS algorithm
subplot(2,1,2);                 % Plot filtered data
  plot(t,y,'k');
  ........axis, title............
```

The results of this code are shown in Figure 8.9. Several values of delay were evaluated and the delay chosen, 5 samples, showed marginally better results than other delays. The convergence gain of 0.075 (7.5% maximum) was also determined empirically. The influence of delay on ALE performance is explored in Problem 4 at the end of this chapter.

Example 8.5 The application of the LMS algorithm to adaptive noise cancellation is given in this example. Here a single sinusoid is considered as noise and the approach reduces the noise produced the sinusoidal interference signal. We assume that we have a scaled, but otherwise identical, copy of the interference signal. In practice, the reference signal would be correlated with, but not necessarily identical to, the interference signal. An example of this more practical situation is given in Problem 5.

```
% Example 8.5 and Figure 8.10 Adaptive Noise Cancellation
% Use an adaptive filter to eliminate sinusoidal noise from a
%  narrowband signal
%
% Generate signal and noise
close all; clear all;
```

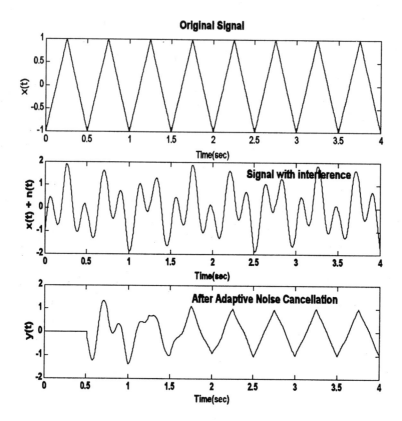

FIGURE 8.10 Example of adaptive noise cancellation. In this example the reference signal was simply a scaled copy of the sinusoidal interference, while in a more practical situation the reference signal would be correlated with, but not identical to, the interference. Note the near perfect cancellation of the interference.

```
fs = 500;                    % Sampling frequency
L = 256;                     % Filter order
N = 2000;                    % Number of points
t = (1:N)/fs;                % Time vector for plotting
a = 0.5;                     % Convergence gain (50%
                             %   maximum)
%
% Generate triangle (i.e., sawtooth) waveform and plot
w = (1:N) * 4 * pi/fs;       % Data frequency vector
x = sawtooth(w,.5);          % Signal is a triangle
%   (sawtooth)
```

```
subplot(3,1,1); plot(t,x,'k');     % Plot signal without noise
........axis, title.............

% Add interference signal: a sinusoid
intefer = sin(w*2.33);             % Interfer freq. = 2.33
                                   %  times signal freq.
x = x + intefer;                   % Construct signal plus
                                   %  interference
ref = .45 * intefer;               % Reference is simply a
                                   %  scaled copy of the
                                   %  interference signal
%
subplot(3,1,2); plot(t, x,'k');    % Plot unfiltered data

........axis, title.............
%
% Apply adaptive filter and plot
Px = (1/(N+1))* sum(x./\2);        % Calculate waveform power
                                   %  for delta
delta = (1/(10*L*Px)) * a;         % Convergence factor
[b,y,out] = lms(ref,x,delta,L);    % Apply LMS algorithm
subplot(3,1,3); plot(t,out,'k');   % Plot filtered data
........axis, title.............
```

Results in Figure 8.10 show very good cancellation of the sinusoidal interference signal. Note that the adaptation requires approximately 2.0 sec or 1000 samples.

PHASE SENSITIVE DETECTION

Phase sensitive detection, also known as *synchronous detection*, is a technique for demodulating *amplitude modulated* (AM) signals that is also very effective in reducing noise. From a frequency domain point of view, the effect of amplitude modulation is to shift the signal frequencies to another portion of the spectrum; specifically, to a range on either side of the modulating, or "carrier," frequency. Amplitude modulation can be very effective in reducing noise because it can shift signal frequencies to spectral regions where noise is minimal. The application of a narrowband filter centered about the new frequency range (i.e., the carrier frequency) can then be used to remove the noise outside the bandwidth of the effective bandpass filter, including noise that may have been present in the original frequency range.*

Phase sensitive detection is most commonly implemented using analog

---

*Many biological signals contain frequencies around 60 Hz, a major noise frequency.

hardware. Prepackaged phase sensitive detectors that incorporate a wide variety of optional features are commercially available, and are sold under the term *lock-in* amplifiers. While lock-in amplifiers tend to be costly, less sophisticated analog phase sensitive detectors can be constructed quite inexpensively. The reason phase sensitive detection is commonly carried out in the analog domain has to do with the limitations on digital storage and analog-to-digital conversion. AM signals consist of a *carrier* signal (usually a sinusoid) which has an amplitude that is varied by the signal of interest. For this to work without loss of information, the frequency of the carrier signal must be much higher than the highest frequency in the signal of interest. (As with sampling, the greater the spread between the highest signal frequency and the carrier frequency, the easier it is to separate the two after demodulation.) Since sampling theory dictates that the sampling frequency be at least twice the highest frequency in the *input signal*, the sampling frequency of an AM signal must be more than twice the carrier frequency. Thus, the sampling frequency will need to be much higher than the highest frequency of interest, much higher than if the AM signal were demodulated before sampling. Hence, digitizing an AM signal before demodulation places a higher burden on memory storage requirements and analog-to-digital conversion rates. However, with the reduction in cost of both memory and highspeed ADC's, it is becoming more and more practical to decode AM signals using the software equivalent of phase sensitive detection. The following analysis applies to both hardware and software PSD's.

AM Modulation

In an AM signal, the amplitude of a sinusoidal carrier signal varies in proportion to changes in the signal of interest. AM signals commonly arise in bioinstrumentation systems when transducer based on variation in electrical properties is excited by a sinusoidal voltage (i.e., the current through the transducer is sinusoidal). The strain gage is an example of this type of transducer where resistance varies in proportion to small changes in length. Assume that two strain gages are differential configured and connected in a bridge circuit, as shown in Figure 1.3. One arm of the bridge circuit contains the transducers, $R + \Delta R$ and $R - \Delta R$, while the other arm contains resistors having a fixed value of R, the nominal resistance value of the strain gages. In this example, ΔR will be a function of time, specifically a sinusoidal function of time, although in the general case it would be a time varying signal containing a range of sinusoid frequencies. If the bridge is balanced, and $\Delta R \ll R$, then it is easy to show using basic circuit analysis that the bridge output is:

$$V_{in} = \Delta R V / 2R \tag{14}$$

where V is source voltage of the bridge. If this voltage is sinusoidal, $V = V_s$ cos $(\omega_c t)$, then $V_{in}(t)$ becomes:

$$V_{in}(t) = (V_s \Delta R / 2R) \cos (\omega_c t) \tag{15}$$

If the input to the strain gages is sinusoidal, then $\Delta R = k \cos(\omega_s t)$; where ω_s is the signal frequency and is assumed to be $<< \omega_c$ and k is the strain gage sensitivity. Still assuming $\Delta R << R$, the equation for $V_{in}(t)$ becomes:

$$V_{in}(t) = V_s k / 2R \ [\cos(\omega_s t) \cos(\omega_c t)] \tag{16}$$

Now applying the trigonometric identity for the product of two cosines:

$$\cos(x) \cos(y) = \frac{1}{2} \cos(x + y) + \frac{1}{2} \cos(x - y) \tag{17}$$

the equation for $V_{in}(t)$ becomes:

$$V_{in}(t) = V_s k / 4R \ [\cos(\omega_c + \omega_s)t + \cos(\omega_c - \omega_s)t] \tag{18}$$

This signal would have the magnitude spectrum given in Figure 8.11. This signal is termed a *double side band suppressed-carrier modulation* since the carrier frequency, ω_c, is missing as seen in Figure 8.11.

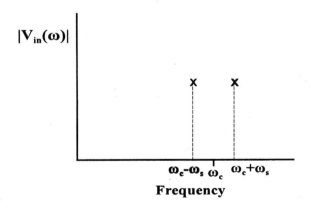

FIGURE 8.11 Frequency spectrum of the signal created by sinusoidally exciting a variable resistance transducer with a carrier frequency ω_c. This type of modulation is termed *double sideband suppressed-carrier modulation* since the carrier frequency is absent.

Note that using the identity:

$$\cos(x) + \cos(y) = 2 \, \cos\left(\frac{x + y}{2}\right) \cos\left(\frac{x - y}{2}\right) \tag{19}$$

then $V_{in}(t)$ can be written as:

$$V_{in}(t) = V_s k/2R \, (\cos(\omega_c t) \cos(\omega_s t)) = A(t) \cos(\omega_c t) \tag{20}$$

where

$$A(t) = V_s k/2R \, (\cos(\omega_{cs} t)) \tag{21}$$

Phase Sensitive Detectors

The basic configuration of a phase sensitive detector is shown in Figure 8.12 below. The first step in phase sensitive detection is multiplication by a phase shifted carrier.

Using the identity given in Eq. (18) the output of the multiplier, $V'(t)$, in Figure 8.12 becomes:

$$V'(t) = V_{in}(t) \, \cos(\omega_c t + \theta) = A(t) \, \cos(\omega_c t) \cos(\omega_c t + \theta)$$
$$= A(t)/2 \, [\cos(2\omega_c t + \theta) + \cos \theta] \tag{22}$$

To get the full spectrum, before filtering, substitute Eq. (21) for $A(t)$ into Eq. (22):

$$V'(t) = V_s k/4R \, [\cos(2\omega_c t + \theta) \cos(\omega_s t) + \cos(\omega_s t) \cos \theta)] \tag{23}$$

again applying the identity in Eq. (17):

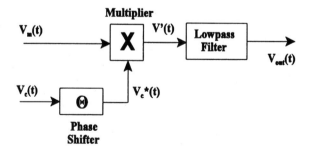

FIGURE 8.12 Basic elements and configuration of a phase sensitive detector used to demodulate AM signals.

$$V'(t) = V_s k/4R \, [\cos(2\omega_c t + \theta + \omega_s t) + \cos(2\omega_c t + \theta - \omega_s t)$$
$$+ \cos(\omega_s t + \theta) + \cos(\omega_s t - \theta)] \tag{24}$$

The spectrum of $V'(t)$ is shown in Figure 8.13. Note that the phase angle, θ, would have an influence on the magnitude of the signal, but not its frequency.

After lowpass digital filtering the higher frequency terms, $\omega_c t \pm \omega_s$ will be reduced to near zero, so the output, $V_{out}(t)$, becomes:

$$V_{out}(t) = A(t) \cos\theta = (V_s k/2R) \cos \theta \tag{25}$$

Since $\cos \theta$ is a constant, the output of the phase sensitive detector is the demodulated signal, $A(t)$, multiplied by this constant. The term *phase sensitive* is derived from the fact that the constant is a function of the phase difference, θ, between $V_c(t)$ and $V_{in}(t)$. Note that while θ is generally constant, any shift in phase between the two signals will induce a change in the output signal level, so this approach could also be used to detect phase changes between signals of constant amplitude.

The multiplier operation is similar to the sampling process in that it generates additional frequency components. This will reduce the influence of low frequency noise since it will be shifted up to near the carrier frequency. For example, consider the effect of the multiplier on 60 Hz noise (or almost any noise that is not near to the carrier frequency). Using the principle of superposition, only the noise component needs to be considered. For a noise component at frequency, ω_n ($V_{in}(t)_{NOISE} = V_n \cos (\omega_n t)$). After multiplication the contribution at $V'(t)$ will be:

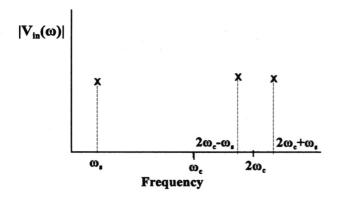

FIGURE 8.13 Frequency spectrum of the signal created by multiplying the $V_{in}(t)$ by the carrier frequency. After lowpass filtering, only the original low frequency signal at ω_s will remain.

$$V_{in}(t)_{\text{NOISE}} = V_n \left[\cos(\omega_c t + \omega_n t) + \cos(\omega_c t + \omega_s t) \right] \tag{26}$$

and the new, complete spectrum for $V'(t)$ is shown in Figure 8.14.

The only frequencies that will not be attenuated in the input signal, $V_{in}(t)$, are those around the carrier frequency that also fall within the bandwidth of the lowpass filter. Another way to analyze the noise attenuation characteristics of phase sensitive detection is to view the *effect* of the multiplier as shifting the lowpass filter's spectrum to be symmetrical about the carrier frequency, giving it the form of a narrow bandpass filter (Figure 8.15). Not only can extremely narrowband bandpass filters be created this way (simply by having a low cutoff frequency in the lowpass filter), but more importantly the center frequency of the effective bandpass filter *tracks* any changes in the carrier frequency. It is these two features, narrowband filtering and tracking, that give phase sensitive detection its signal processing power.

MATLAB Implementation

Phase sensitive detection is implemented in MATLAB using simple multiplication and filtering. The application of a phase sensitive detector is given in Exam-

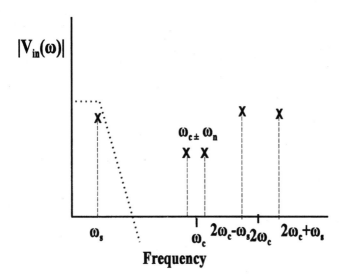

FIGURE 8.14 Frequency spectrum of the signal created by multiplying $V_{in}(t)$ including low frequency noise by the carrier frequency. The low frequency noise is shifted up to $\pm$ the carrier frequency. After lowpass filtering, both the noise and higher frequency signal are greatly attenuated, again leaving only the original low frequency signal at ω_s remaining.

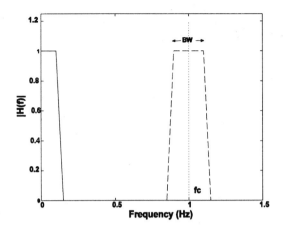

FIGURE 8.15 Frequency characteristics of a phase sensitive detector. The frequency response of the lowpass filter (solid line) is effectively "reflected" about the carrier frequency, fc, producing the effect of a narrowband bandpass filter (dashed line). In a phase sensitive detector the center frequency of this virtual bandpass filter tracks the carrier frequency.

ple 8.6 below. A carrier sinusoid of 250 Hz is modulated with a sawtooth wave with a frequency of 5 Hz. The AM signal is buried in noise that is 3.16 times the signal (i.e., SNR = -10 db).

Example 8.6 Phase Sensitive Detector. This example uses a phase sensitive detection to demodulate the AM signal and recover the signal from noise. The filter is chosen as a second-order Butterworth lowpass filter with a cutoff frequency set for best noise rejection while still providing reasonable fidelity to the sawtooth waveform. The example uses a sampling frequency of 2 kHz.

```
% Example 8.6 and Figure 8.16 Phase Sensitive Detection
%
% Set constants
close all; clear all;
fs = 2000;                        % Sampling frequency
f = 5;                            % Signal frequency
fc = 250;                         % Carrier frequency
N = 2000;                         % Use 1 sec of data
t = (1:N)/fs;                     % Time axis for plotting
wn = .02;                         % PSD lowpass filter cut-
                                  %  off frequency

[b,a] = butter(2,wn);            % Design lowpass filter
%
```

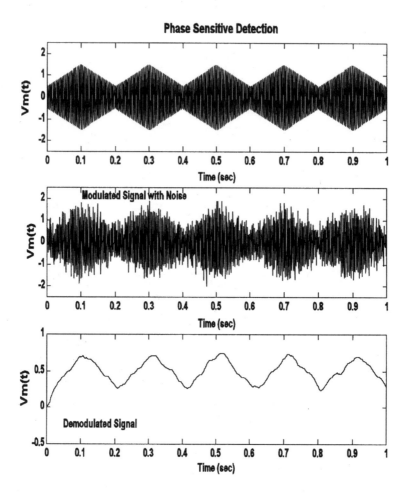

FIGURE 8.16 Application of phase sensitive detection to an amplitude-modulated signal. The AM signal consisted of a 250 Hz carrier modulated by a 5 Hz sawtooth (upper graph). The AM signal is mixed with white noise (SNR = −10db, middle graph). The recovered signal shows a reduction in the noise (lower graph).

```
% Generate AM signal
w = (1:N) * 2*pi*fc/fs;              % Carrier frequency =
                                     %   250 Hz
w1 = (1:N)*2*pi*f/fs;                % Signal frequency = 5 Hz
vc = sin(w);                         % Define carrier
vsig = sawtooth(w1,.5);              % Define signal
vm = (1 + .5 * vsig) .* vc;          % Create modulated signal
```

```
                                    %  with a Modulation
                                    %  constant = 0.5
subplot(3,1,1);
  plot(t,vm,'k');                   % Plot AM Signal
  .......axis, label,title.......
%
% Add noise with 3.16 times power (10 db) of signal for SNR of
%  -10 db
noise = randn(1,N);
scale = (var(vsig)/var(noise)) * 3.16;
vm = vm + noise * scale;            % Add noise to modulated
                                    %  signal
subplot(3,1,2);
  plot(t,vm,'k');                   % Plot AM signal
  .......axis, label,title.......

% Phase sensitive detection
ishift = fix(.125 * fs/fc);         % Shift carrier by 1/4
vc = [vc(ishift:N) vc(1:ishift-1)]; %  period (45 deg) using
                                    %  periodic shift
v1 = vc .* vm;                      % Multiplier
vout = filter(b,a,v1);              % Apply lowpass filter
subplot(3,1,3);
  plot(t,vout,'k');                 % Plot AM Signal
  .......axis, label,title.......
```

The lowpass filter was set to a cutoff frequency of 20 Hz (0.02 * f_s/2) as a compromise between good noise reduction and fidelity. (The fidelity can be roughly assessed by the sharpness of the peaks of the recovered sawtooth wave.) A major limitation in this process were the characteristics of the lowpass filter: digital filters do not perform well at low frequencies. The results are shown in Figure 8.16 and show reasonable recovery of the demodulated signal from the noise.

Even better performance can be obtained if the interference signal is narrowband such as 60 Hz interference. An example of using phase sensitive detection in the presence of a strong 60 Hz signal is given in Problem 6 below.

PROBLEMS

1.   Apply the Wiener-Hopf approach to a signal plus noise waveform similar to that used in Example 8.1, except use two sinusoids at 10 and 20 Hz in 8 db noise. Recall, the function **sig_noise** provides the noiseless signal as the third output to be used as the desired signal. Apply this optimal filter for filter lengths of 256 and 512.

2. Use the LMS adaptive filter approach to determine the FIR equivalent to the linear process described by the digital transfer function:

$$H(z) = \frac{0.2 + 0.5z^{-1}}{1 - 0.2z^{-1} + 0.8z^{-2}}$$

As with Example 8.2, plot the magnitude digital transfer function of the "unknown" system, $H(z)$, and of the FIR "matching" system. Find the transfer function of the IIR process by taking the square of the magnitude of `fft(b,n)./fft(a,n)` (or use `freqz`). Use the MATLAB function `filtfilt` to produce the output of the IIR process. This routine produces no time delay between the input and filtered output. Determine the approximate minimum number of filter coefficients required to accurately represent the function above by limiting the coefficients to different lengths.

3. Generate a 20 Hz *interference signal* in noise with and SNR + 8 db; that is, the interference signal is 8 db stronger that the noise. (Use `sig_noise` with an SNR of +8.) In this problem the noise will be considered as the desired signal. Design an adaptive interference filter to remove the 20 Hz "noise." Use an FIR filter with 128 coefficients.

4. Apply the ALE filter described in Example 8.3 to a signal consisting of two sinusoids of 10 and 20 Hz that are present simultaneously, rather that sequentially as in Example 8.3. Use a FIR filter lengths of 128 and 256 points. Evaluate the influence of modifying the delay between 4 and 18 samples.

5. Modify the code in Example 8.5 so that the reference signal is correlated with, but not the same as, the interference data. This should be done by convolving the reference signal with a lowpass filter consisting of 3 equal weights; i.e:

   $b = [0.333\ 0.333\ 0.333]$.

   For this more realistic scenario, note the degradation in performance as compared to Example 8.5 where the reference signal was identical to the noise.

6. Redo the phase sensitive detector in Example 8.6, but replace the white noise with a 60 Hz interference signal. The 60 Hz interference signal should have an amplitude that is 10 times that of the AM signal.

9

Multivariate Analyses:
Principal Component Analysis
and Independent Component Analysis

INTRODUCTION

Principal component analysis and *independent component analysis* fall within a branch of statistics known as multivariate analysis. As the name implies, multivariate analysis is concerned with the analysis of multiple variables (or measurements), but treats them as a single entity (for example, variables from multiple measurements made on the same process or system). In multivariate analysis, these multiple variables are often represented as a single vector variable that includes the different variables:

$$\mathbf{x} = [x_1(t), x_2(t) \ldots x_m(t)]^T \qquad \text{For } 1 \leq m \leq M \qquad (1)$$

The 'T' stands for transposed and represents the matrix operation of switching rows and columns.* In this case, $\mathbf{x}$ is composed of M variables, each containing N ($t = 1, \ldots, N$) observations. In signal processing, the observations are time samples, while in image processing they are pixels. Multivariate data, as represented by $\mathbf{x}$ above can also be considered to reside in M-dimensional space, where each spatial dimension contains one signal (or image).

In general, multivariate analysis seeks to produce results that take into

---

*Normally, all vectors including these multivariate variables are taken as column vectors, but to save space in this text, they are often written as row vectors with the transpose symbol to indicate that they are actually column vectors.

account the relationship between the multiple variables as well as within the variables, and uses tools that operate on all of the data. For example, the covariance matrix described in Chapter 2 (Eq. (19), Chapter 2, and repeated in Eq. (4) below) is an example of a multivariate analysis technique as it includes information about the relationship between variables (their covariance) and information about the individual variables (their variance). Because the covariance matrix contains information on both the variance within the variables and the covariance between the variables, it is occasionally referred to as the *variance–covariance* matrix.

A major concern of multivariate analysis is to find transformations of the multivariate data that make the data set smaller or easier to understand. For example, is it possible that the relevant information contained in a multidimensional variable could be expressed using fewer dimensions (i.e., variables) and might the reduced set of variables be more meaningful than the original data set? If the latter were true, we would say that the more meaningful variables were hidden, or *latent*, in the original data; perhaps the new variables better represent the underlying processes that produced the original data set. A biomedical example is found in EEG analysis where a large number of signals are acquired above the region of the cortex, yet these multiple signals are the result of a smaller number of neural sources. It is the signals generated by the neural sources—not the EEG signals per se—that are of interest.

In transformations that reduce the dimensionality of a multi-variable data set, the idea is to transform one set of variables into a new set where some of the new variables have values that are quite small compared to the others. Since the values of these variables are relatively small, they must not contribute very much information to the overall data set and, hence, can be eliminated.* With the appropriate transformation, it is sometimes possible to eliminate a large number of variables that contribute only marginally to the total information.

The data transformation used to produce the new set of variables is often a linear function since linear transformations are easier to compute and their results are easier to interpret. A linear transformation can be represent mathematically as:

$$y_i(t) = \sum_{j=1}^{M} w_{ij} x_j(t) \qquad i = 1, \ldots N \tag{2}$$

where w_{ij} is a constant coefficient that defines the transformation.

---

*Evaluating the significant of a variable by the range of its values assumes that all the original variables have approximately the same range. If not, some form of normalization should be applied to the original data set.

Since this transformation is a series of equations, it can be equivalently expressed using the notation of linear algebra:

$$
\begin{bmatrix} y_1(t) \\ y_2(t) \\ \vdots \\ y_M(t) \end{bmatrix} = \mathbf{W} \begin{bmatrix} x_1(t) \\ x_2(t) \\ \vdots \\ x_M(t) \end{bmatrix}
\tag{3}
$$

As a linear transformation, this operation can be interpreted as a rotation and possibly scaling of the original data set in M-dimensional space. An example of how a rotation of a data set can produce a new data set with fewer major variables is shown in Figure 9.1 for a simple two-dimensional (i.e., two variable) data set. The original data set is shown as a plot of one variable against the other, a so-called *scatter plot*, in Figure 9.1A. The variance of variable x_1 is 0.34 and the variance of x_2 is 0.20. After rotation the two new variables, y_1 and y_2 have variances of 0.53 and 0.005, respectively. This suggests that one variable, y_1, contains most of the information in the original two-variable set. The

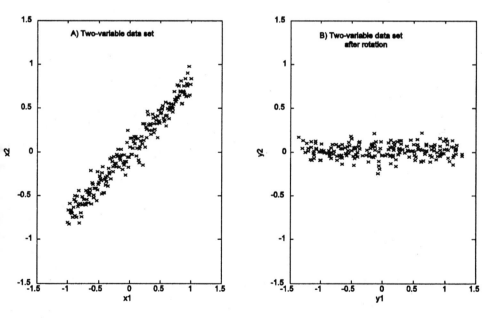

FIGURE 9.1 A data set consisting of two variables before (left graph) and after (right graph) linear rotation. The rotated data set still has two variables, but the variance on one of the variables is quite small compared to the other.

goal of this approach to data reduction is to find a matrix **W** that will produce such a transformation.

The two multivariate techniques discussed below, principal component analysis and independent component analysis, differ in their goals and in the criteria applied to the transformation. In principal component analysis, the object is to transform the data set so as to produce a new set of variables (termed principal components) that are uncorrelated. The goal is to reduce the dimensionality of the data, not necessarily to produce more meaningful variables. We will see that this can be done simply by rotating the data in M-dimensional space. In independent component analysis, the goal is a bit more ambitious: to find new variables (components) that are both statistically independent and nongaussian.

PRINCIPAL COMPONENT ANALYSIS

Principal component analysis (PCA) is often referred to as a technique for reducing the number of variables in a data set without loss of information, and as a possible process for identifying new variables with greater meaning. Unfortunately, while PCA can be, and is, used to transform one set of variables into another smaller set, the newly created variables are not usually easy to interpret. PCA has been most successful in applications such as image compression where data reduction—and not interpretation—is of primary importance. In many applications, PCA is used only to provide information on the true dimensionality of a data set. That is, if a data set includes M variables, do we really need all M variables to represent the information, or can the variables be recombined into a smaller number that still contain most of the essential information (Johnson, 1983)? If so, what is the most appropriate dimension of the new data set?

PCA operates by transforming a set of correlated variables into a new set of uncorrelated variables that are called the *principal components*. Note that if the variables in a data set are already uncorrelated, PCA is of no value. In addition to being uncorrelated, the principal components are orthogonal and are ordered in terms of the variability they represent. That is, the first principle component represents, for a single dimension (i.e., variable), the greatest amount of variability in the original data set. Each succeeding orthogonal component accounts for as much of the remaining variability as possible.

The operation performed by PCA can be described in a number of ways, but a geometrical interpretation is the most straightforward. While PCA is applicable to data sets containing any number of variables, it is easier to describe using only two variables since this leads to readily visualized graphs. Figure 9.2A shows two waveforms: a two-variable data set where each variable is a different mixture of the same two sinusoids added with different scaling factors. A small amount of noise was also added to each waveform (see Example 9.1).

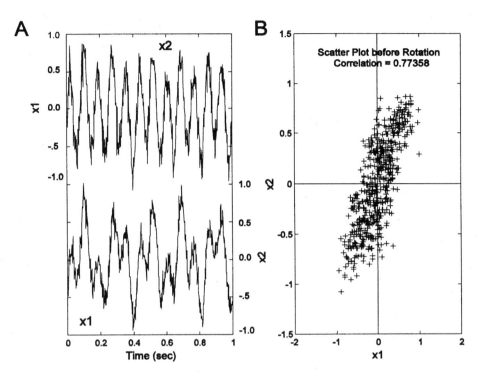

FIGURE 9.2 (A) Two waveforms made by mixing two sinusoids having different frequencies and amplitudes, then adding noise to the two mixtures. The resultant waveforms can be considered related variables since they both contain information from the same two sources. (B) The scatter plot of the two variables (or waveforms) was obtained by plotting one variable against the other for each point in time (i.e., each data sample). The correlation between the two samples ($r = 0.77$) can be seen in the diagonal clustering of points.

Since the data set was created using two separate sinusoidal sources, it should require two spatial dimensions. However, since each variable is composed of mixtures of the two sources, the variables have a considerable amount of covariance, or correlation.* Figure 9.2B is a scatter plot of the two variables, a plot of x_1 against x_2 for each point in time, and shows the correlation between the variables as a diagonal spread of the data points. (The correlation between the two variables is 0.77.) Thus, knowledge of the x value gives information on the

---

*Recall that covariance and correlation differ only in scaling. Definitions of these terms are given in Chapter 2 and are repeated for covariance below.

range of possible *y* values and vice versa. Note that the *x* value does not uniquely determine the *y* value as the correlation between the two variables is less than one. If the data were uncorrelated, the *x* value would provide no information on possible *y* values and vice versa. A scatter plot produced for such uncorrelated data would be roughly symmetrical with respect to both the horizontal and vertical axes.

For PCA to decorrelate the two variables, it simply needs to rotate the two-variable data set until the data points are distributed symmetrically about the mean. Figure 9.3B shows the results of such a rotation, while Figure 9.3A plots the time response of the transformed (i.e., rotated) variables. In the decorrelated condition, the variance is maximally distributed along the two orthogonal axes. In general, it may be also necessary to *center* the data by removing the means before rotation. The original variables plotted in Figure 9.2 had zero means so this step was not necessary.

While it is common in everyday language to take the word *uncorrelated* as meaning *unrelated* (and hence *independent*), this is not the case in statistical analysis, particularly if the variables are nonlinear. In the statistical sense, if two

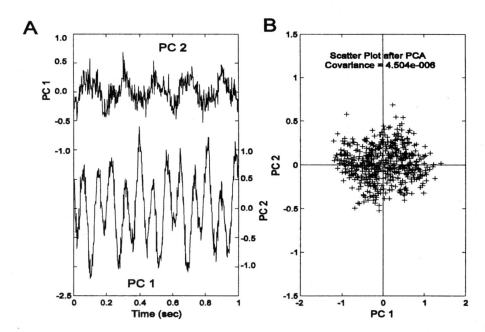

FIGURE 9.3 (A) Principal components of the two variables shown in Figure 9.2. These were produced by an orthogonal rotation of the two variables. (B) The scatter plot of the rotated principal components. The symmetrical shape of the data indicates that the two new components are uncorrelated.

(or more) variables are independent they will also be uncorrelated, but the reverse is not generally true. For example, the two variables plotted as a scatter plot in Figure 9.4 are uncorrelated, but they are highly related and not independent. They are both generated by a single equation, the equation for a circle with noise added. Many other nonlinear relationships (such as the quadratic function) can generate related (i.e., not independent) variables that are uncorrelated. Conversely, if the variables have a Gaussian distribution (as in the case of most noise), then when they are uncorrelated they are also independent. Note that most signals do not have a Gaussian distribution and therefore are not likely to be independent after they have been decorrelated using PCA. This is one of the reasons why the principal components are not usually meaningful variables: they are still mixtures of the underlying sources. This inability to make two signals independent through decorrelation provides the motivation for the methodology known as *independent component analysis* described later in this chapter.

If only two variables are involved, the rotation performed between Figure 9.2 and Figure 9.3 could be done by trial and error: simply rotate the data until

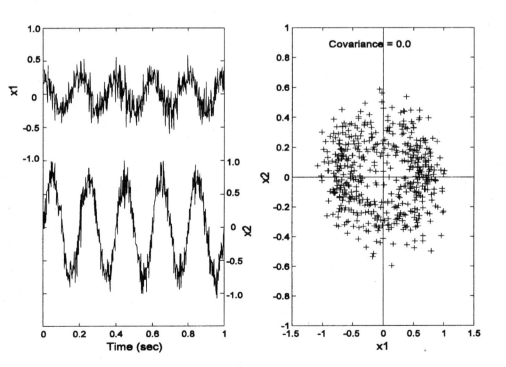

FIGURE 9.4   Time and scatter plots of two variables that are uncorrelated, but not independent. In fact, the two variables were generated by a single equation for a circle with added noise.

the covariance (or correlation) goes to zero. An example of this approach is given as an exercise in the problems. A better way to achieve zero correlation is to use a technique from linear algebra that generates a rotation matrix that reduces the covariance to zero. A well-known technique exists to reduce a matrix that is positive-definite (as is the covariance matrix) into a diagonal matrix by pre- and post-multiplication with an orthonormal matrix (Jackson, 1991):

$$\mathbf{U'SU} = \mathbf{D} \tag{4}$$

where $\mathbf{S}$ is the m-by-m covariance matrix, $\mathbf{D}$ is a diagonal matrix, and $\mathbf{U}$ is an orthonormal matrix that does the transformation. Recall that a diagonal matrix has zeros for the off-diagonal elements, and it is the off-diagonal elements that correspond to *covariance* in the covariance matrix (Eq. (19) in Chapter 2 and repeated as Eq. (5) below). The covariance matrix is defined by:

$$S = \begin{bmatrix} \sigma_{1,1} & \sigma_{1,2} & \cdots & \sigma_{1,N} \\ \sigma_{2,1} & \sigma_{2,2} & \cdots & \sigma_{2,N} \\ \vdots & \vdots & \ddots & \vdots \\ \sigma_{N,1} & \sigma_{N,2} & \cdots & \sigma_{N,N} \end{bmatrix} \tag{5}$$

Hence, the rotation implied by $\mathbf{U}$ will produce a new covariance matrix, $\mathbf{D}$, that has zero covariance. The diagonal elements of $\mathbf{D}$ are the variances of the new data, more generally known as the characteristic roots, or eigenvalues, of $\mathbf{S}$: $\lambda_1, \lambda_2, \ldots \lambda_n$. The columns of $\mathbf{U}$ are the characteristic vectors, or eigenvectors $\mathbf{u}_1, \mathbf{u}_2, \ldots \mathbf{u}_n$. Again, the eigenvalues of the new covariance matrix, $\mathbf{D}$, correspond to the variances of the rotated variables (now called the principle components). Accordingly, these eigenvalues (variances) can be used to determine what percentage of the total variance (which is equal to the sum of all eigenvalues) a given principal component represents. As shown below, this is a measure of the associated principal component's importance, at least with regard to how much of the total information it represents.

The eigenvalues or roots can be solved by the following determinant equation:

$$\det |\mathbf{S} - \lambda \mathbf{I}| = 0 \tag{6}$$

where $\mathbf{I}$ is the identity matrix. After solving for λ, the eigenvectors can be solved using the equation:

$$\det |\mathbf{S} - \lambda \mathbf{I}| \mathbf{b}_i = 0 \tag{7}$$

where the eigenvectors are obtained from $\mathbf{b}_i$ by the equation

$$u_i = b_i / \sqrt{b_i' b_i} \tag{8}$$

This approach can be carried out by hand for two or three variables, but is very tedious for more variables or long data sets. It is much easier to use singular value composition which has the advantage of working directly from the data matrix and can be done in one step. Moreover, singular value decomposition can be easily implemented with a single function call in MATLAB. Singular value decomposition solves an equation similar to Eq. (4), specifically:

$$X = U * D^{1/2}U' \tag{9}$$

In the case of PCA, X is the data matrix that is decomposed into (1) D, the diagonal matrix that contains, in this case, the square root of the eigenvalues; and (2) U, the principle components matrix. An example of this approach is given in the next section on MATLAB Implementation.

Order Selection

The eigenvalues describe how much of the variance is accounted for by the associated principal component, and when singular value decomposition is used, these eigenvalues are ordered by size; that is: $\lambda_1 > \lambda_2 > \lambda_3 \ldots > \lambda_M$. They can be very helpful in determining how many of the components are really significant and how much the data set can be reduced. Specifically, if several eigenvalues are zero or close to zero, then the associated principal components contribute little to the data and can be eliminated. Of course, if the eigenvalues are identically zero, then the associated principal component should clearly be eliminated, but where do you make the cut when the eigenvalues are small, but nonzero? There are two popular methods for determining eigenvalue thresholds. (1) Take the sum of all eigenvectors (which must account for all the variance), then delete those eigenvalues that fall below some percentage of that sum. For example, if you want the remaining variables to account for 90% of the variance, then chose a cutoff eigenvalue where the sum of all lower eigenvalues is less than 10% of the total eigenvalue sum. (2) Plot the eigenvalues against the order number, and look for breakpoints in the slope of this curve. Eigenvalues representing noise should not change much in value and, hence, will plot as a flatter slope when plotted against eigenvalue number (recall the eigenvalues are in order of large to small). Such a curve was introduced in Chapter 5 and is known as the *scree plot* (see Figure 5.6 D) These approaches are explored in the first example of the following section on MATLAB Implementation.

MATLAB Implementation

Data Rotation

Many multivariate techniques rotate the data set as part of their operation. Imaging also uses data rotation to change the orientation of an object or image.

From basic trigonometry, it is easy to show that, in two dimensions, rotation of a data point $(x1, y1)$ can be achieved by multiplying the data points by the sines and cosines of the rotation angle:

$$y_2 = y_1 \cos(\theta) + x_1 \sin(\theta) \tag{10}$$

$$x_2 = y_1 (-\sin(\theta)) + x_1 \cos(\theta) \tag{11}$$

where θ is the angle through which the data set is rotated in radians. Using matrix notation, this operation can be done by multiplying the data matrix by a *rotation* matrix:

$$R = \begin{bmatrix} \cos(\theta) & \sin(\theta) \\ -\sin(\theta) & \cos(\theta) \end{bmatrix} \tag{12}$$

This is the strategy used by the routine `rotation` given in Example 9.1 below. The generalization of this approach to three or more dimensions is straightforward. In PCA, the rotation is done by the algorithm as described below so explicit rotation is not required. (Nonetheless, it is required for one of the problems at the end of this chapter, and later in image processing.) An example of the application of rotation in two dimensions is given in the example.

Example 9.1 This example generate two cycles of a sine wave and rotate the wave by 45 deg.

Solution: The routine below uses the function `rotation` to perform the rotation. This function operates only on two-dimensional data. In addition to multiplying the data set by the matrix in Eq. (12), the function `rotation` checks the input matrix and ensures that it is in the right orientation for rotation with the variables as columns of the data matrix. (It assumes two-dimensional data, so the number of columns, i.e., number of variables, should be less than the number of rows.)

```
% Example 9.1 and Figure 9.5
% Example of data rotation
% Create a two variable data set of y = sin (x)
%   then rotate the data set by an angle of 45 deg
%
clear all; close all;
N = 100;                          % Variable length
x(1,:) = (1:N)/10;                % Create a two variable data
x(2,:) = sin(x(1,:)*4*pi/10);     %   set: x1 linear; x2 =
                                  %   sin(x1)—two periods
plot(x(1,:),x(2,:),'*k');         % Plot data set
  xlabel('x1'); ylabel('x2');
phi = 45*(2*pi/360);              % Rotation angle equals 45 deg
```

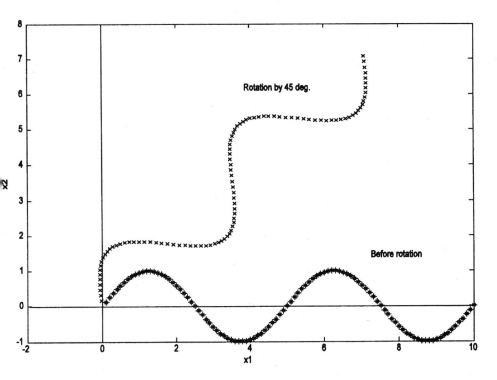

FIGURE 9.5 A two-cycle sine wave is rotated 45 deg. using the function `rotation` that implements Eq. (12).

```
y = rotation(x,phi);              % Rotate
hold on;
plot(y(1,:),y(2,:),'xk');         % Plot rotated data
```

The rotation is performed by the function `rotation` following Eq. (12).

```
% Function rotation
% Rotates the first argument by an angle phi given in the second
% argument function out = rotate(input,phi)
% Input variables
%   input            A matrix of the data to be rotated
    phi              The rotation angle in radians
% Output variables
%   out              The rotated data
%
[r c] = size(input);
if r < c                          % Check input format and
```

```
input = input';              % transpose if necessary
transpose_flag = 'y';
end
% Set up rotation matrix
R = [cos(phi) sin(phi); -sin(phi) cos(phi)];
out = input * R;             % Rotate input
if transpose_flag == 'y'     % Restore original input format
  out = out';
end
```

Principal Component Analysis Evaluation

PCA can be implemented using singular value decomposition. In addition, the MATLAB Statistics Toolbox has a special program, princomp, but this just implements the singular value decomposition algorithm. Singular value decomposition of a data array, X, uses:

```
[V,D,U] = svd(X);
```

where D is a diagonal matrix containing the eigenvalues and V contains the principal components in columns. The eigenvalues can be obtained from D using the diag command:

```
eigen = diag(D);
```

Referring to Eq. (9), these values will actually be the square root of the eigenvalues, λ_i. If the eigenvalues are used to measure the variance in the rotated principal components, they also need to be scaled by the number of points.

It is common to normalize the principal components by the eigenvalues so that different components can be compared. While a number of different normalizing schemes exist, in the examples here, we multiply the eigenvector by the square root of the associated eigenvalue since this gives rise to principal components that have the same value as a rotated data array (See Problem 1).

Example 9.2 Generate a data set with five variables, but from only two sources and noise. Compute the principal components and associated eigenvalues using singular value decomposition. Compute the eigenvalue ratios and generate the scree plot. Plot the significant principal components.

```
% Example 9.2 and Figures 9.6, 9.7, and 9.8
% Example of PCA
% Create five variable waveforms from only two signals and noise
% Use this in PCA Analysis
%
% Assign constants
```

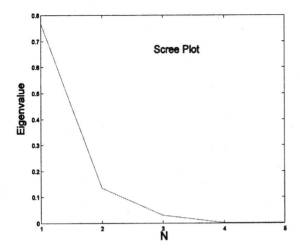

FIGURE 9.6 Plot of eigenvalue against component number, the scree plot. Since the eigenvalue represents the variance of a given component, it can be used as a measure of the amount of information the associated component represents. A break is seen at 2, suggesting that only the first two principal components are necessary to describe most of the information in the data.

```
clear all; close all;
N = 1000;                        % Number points (4 sec of
                                 %  data)
fs = 500;                        % Sample frequency
w = (1:N) * 2*pi/fs;             % Normalized frequency
                                 %  vector
t = (1:N);*IH26*                 % Time vector for plotting
%
% Generate data
x = .75 *sin(w*5);               % One component a sine
y = sawtooth(w*7,.5);            % One component a sawtooth
%
% Combine data in different proportions
D(1,:) = .5*y + .5*x + .1*rand(1,N);
D(2,:) = .2*y + .7*x + .1*rand(1,N);
D(3,:) = .7*y + .2*x + .1*rand(1,N);
D(4,:) = -.6*y + -.24*x + .2*rand(1,N);
D(5,:) = .6* rand(1,N);          % Noise only
%
% Center data subtract mean
for i = 1:5
    D(i,:) = D(i,:)-mean(D(i,:)); % There is a more efficient
```

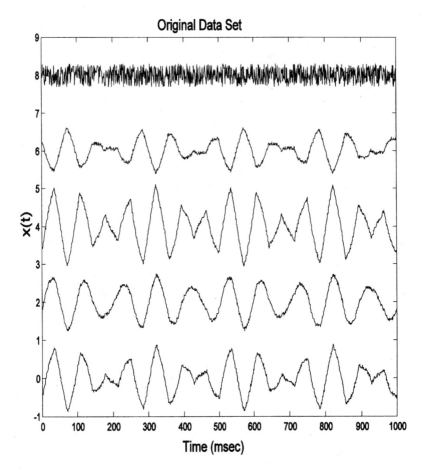

FIGURE 9.7 Plot of the five variables used in Example 9.2. They were all produced from only two sources (see Figure 9.8B) and/or noise. (*Note*: one of the variables is pure noise.)

```
                                        % way to do this
    end
    %
    % Find Principal Components
    [U,S,pc]= svd(D,0);                 % Singular value decompo-
                                        % sition

    eigen = diag(S).^2;                 % Calculate eigenvalues
```

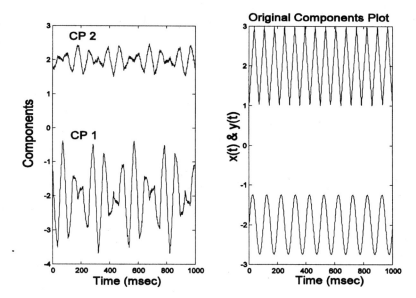

FIGURE 9.8 Plot of the first two principal components and the original two sources. Note that the components are not the same as the original sources. Even thought they are uncorrelated (see covariance matrix on the next page), they cannot be independent since they are still mixtures of the two sources.

```
pc = pc(:,1:5);                    % Reduce size of principal
                                   %   comp. matrix
for i = 1:5                        % Scale principal components
  pc(:,i) = pc(:,i) * sqrt(eigen(i));
end
eigen = eigen/N                    % Eigenvalues now equal
                                   %   variances
plot(eigen);                       % Plot scree plot
.......labels and title....................
%
% Calculate Eigenvalue ratio
total_eigen = sum(eigen);
for i = 1:5
  pct(i) = sum(eigen(i:5))/total_eigen;
end
disp(pct*100)                      % Display eigenvalue ratios
                                   %   in percent
%
% Print Scaled Eigenvalues and Covariance Matrix of Principal
```

```
%  Components
S = cov(pc)
%
% Plot Principal Components and Original Data
figure;
subplot(1,2,1);          % Plot first two principal components
   plot(t,pc(:,1)-2,t,pc(:,2)+2); % Displaced for clarity
   ......labels and title....................

subplot(1,2,2);            % Plot Original components
   plot(t,x-2,'k',t,y+2,'k');     % Displaced for clarity
   ......labels and title....................
```

The five variables are plotted below in Figure 9.7. Note that the strong dependence between the variables (they are the product of only two different sources plus noise) is not entirely obvious from the time plots. The new covariance matrix taken from the principal components shows that all five components are uncorrelated, and also gives the variance of the five principal components

$$
\begin{array}{ccccc}
0.5708 & -0.0000 & 0.0000 & -0.0000 & 0.0000 \\
-0.0000 & 0.0438 & 0.0000 & -0.0000 & 0.0000 \\
0.0000 & 0.0000 & 0.0297 & -0.0000 & 0.0000 \\
-0.0000 & -0.0000 & -0.0000 & 0.0008 & 0.0000 \\
0.0000 & 0.0000 & 0.0000 & 0.0000 & 0.0008
\end{array}
$$

The percentage of variance accounted by the sums of the various eigenvalues is given by the program as:

CP 1-5	CP 2-5	CP 3-5	CP 4-5	CP 5
100%	11.63%	4.84%	0.25%	0.12%

Note that the last three components account for only 4.84% of the variance of the data. This suggests that the actual dimension of the data is closer to two than to five. The scree plot, the plot of eigenvalue versus component number, provides another method for checking data dimensionality. As shown in Figure 9.6, there is a break in the slope at 2, again suggesting that the actual dimension of the data set is two (which we already know since it was created using only two independent sources).

The first two principal components are shown in Figure 9.8, along with the waveforms of the original sources. While the principal components are uncorrelated, as shown by the covariance matrix above, they do not reflect the two independent data sources. Since they are still mixtures of the two sources they can not be independent even though they are uncorrelated. This occurs because the variables do not have a gaussian distribution, so that decorrelation does not imply independence. Another technique described in the next section can be used to make the variables independent, in which case the original sources can be recovered.

INDEPENDENT COMPONENT ANALYSIS

The application of principal component analysis described in Example 9.1 shows that decorrelating the data is not sufficient to produce independence between the variables, at least when the variables have nongaussian distributions. Independent component analysis seeks to transform the original data set into number of *independent* variables. The motivation for this transformation is primarily to uncover more meaningful variables, not to reduce the dimensions of the data set. When data set reduction is also desired it is usually accomplished by preprocessing the data set using PCA.

One of the more dramatic applications of independent component analysis (ICA) is found in the *cocktail party problem*. In this situation, multiple people are speaking simultaneously within the same room. Assume that their voices are recorded from a number of microphones placed around the room, where the number of microphones is greater than, or equal to, the number of speakers. Figure 9.9 shows this situation for two microphones and two speakers. Each microphone will pick up some mixture of all of the speakers in the room. Since presumably the speakers are generating signals that are independent (as would be the case in a real cocktail party), the successful application of independent component analysis to a data set consisting of microphone signals should recover the signals produced by the different speakers. Indeed, ICA has been quite successful in this problem. In this case, the goal is not to reduce the number of signals, but to produce signals that are more meaningful; specifically, the speech of the individual speakers. This problem is similar to the analysis of EEG signals where many signals are recorded from electrodes placed around the head, and these signals represent combinations of underlying neural sources.

The most significant computational difference between ICA and PCA is that PCA uses only second-order statistics (such as the variance which is a function of the data squared) while ICA uses higher-order statistics (such as functions of the data raised to the fourth power). Variables with a Gaussian distribution have zero statistical moments above second-order, but most *signals* do not have a Gaussian distribution and do have higher-order moments. These higher-order statistical properties are put to good use in ICA.

The basis of most ICA approaches is a generative model; that is, a model that describes how the measured signals are produced. The model assumes that

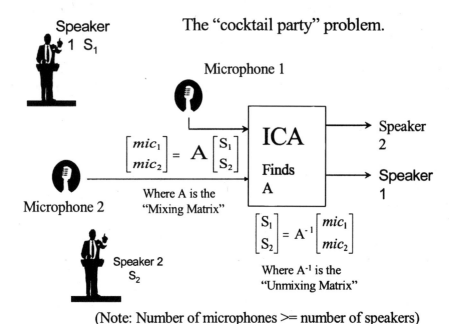

(Note: Number of microphones >= number of speakers)

FIGURE 9.9 A schematic of the *cocktail party problem* where two speakers are talking simultaneously and their voices are recorded by two microphones. Each microphone detects the output of both speakers. The problem is to unscramble, or unmix, the two signals from the combinations in the microphone signals. No information is known about the content of the speeches nor the placement of the microphones and speakers.

the measured signals are the product of instantaneous linear combinations of the independent sources. Such a model can be stated mathematically as:

$$x_i(t) = a_{i1}\, s_1(t) + a_{i2}\, s_2(t) + \cdots + a_{iN}\, s_N(t) \qquad \text{for } i = 1, \ldots, N \qquad (13)$$

Note that this is a series of equations for the N different signal variables, $x_i(t)$. In discussions of the ICA model equation, it is common to drop the time function. Indeed, most ICA approaches do not take into account the ordering of variable elements; hence, the fact that s and x are time functions is irrelevant.

In matrix form, Eq. (13) becomes similar to Eq. (3):

$$\begin{bmatrix} x_1(t) \\ x_2(t) \\ \vdots \\ x_n(t) \end{bmatrix} = A \begin{bmatrix} s_1(t) \\ s_2(t) \\ \vdots \\ s_n(t) \end{bmatrix} \qquad (14)$$

which can be written succinctly as:

$$\mathbf{x} = \mathbf{As} \tag{15}$$

where $\mathbf{s}$ is a vector composed of all the source signals,* $\mathbf{A}$ is the mixing matrix composed of the constant elements $a_{i,j}$, and $\mathbf{x}$ is a vector of the measured signals. The model described by Eqs. (13) and (14) is also known as a *latent variables* model since the source variables, $\mathbf{s}$, cannot be observed directly: they are hidden, or *latent*, in $\mathbf{x}$. Of course the principle components in PCA are also latent variables; however, since they are not independent they are usually difficult to interpret. Note that noise is not explicitly stated in the model, although ICA methods will usually work in the presence of moderate noise (see Example 9.3). ICA techniques are used to solve for the mixing matrix, $\mathbf{A}$, from which the independent components, $\mathbf{s}$, can be obtained through simple matrix inversion:

$$\mathbf{s} = \mathbf{A}^{-1}\mathbf{x} \tag{16}$$

If the mixing matrix is known or can be determined, then the underlying sources can be found simply by solving Eq. (16). However, ICA is used in the more general situation where the mixing matrix is not known. The basic idea is that if the measured signals, $\mathbf{x}$, are related to the underlying source signals, $\mathbf{s}$, by a linear transformation (i.e., a rotation and scaling operation) as indicated by Eqs. (14) and (15), then some inverse transformation (rotation/scaling) can be found that recovers the original signals. To estimate the mixing matrix, ICA needs to make only two assumptions: that the source variables, $\mathbf{s}$, are truly independent;† and that they are non-Gaussian. Both conditions are usually met when the sources are real signals. A third restriction is that the mixing matrix must be square; in other words, the number of sources should equal the number of measured signals. This is not really a restriction since PCA can be always be applied to reduce the dimension of the data set, $\mathbf{x}$, to equal that of the source data set, $\mathbf{s}$.

The requirement that the underlying signals be non-Gaussian stems from the fact that ICA relies on higher-order statistics to separate the variables. Higher-order statistics (i.e., moments and related measures) of Gaussian signals are zero. ICA does not require that the distribution of the source variables be known, only that they not be Gaussian. Note that if the measured variables are already independent, ICA has nothing to contribute, just as PCA is of no use if the variables are already uncorrelated.

The only information ICA has available is the measured variables; it has no information on either the mixing matrix, $\mathbf{A}$, or the underlying source vari-

---

*Note that the source signals themselves are also vectors. In this notation, the individual signals are considered as components of the single source vector, $\mathbf{s}$.

†In fact, the requirement for strict independence can be relaxed somewhat in many situations.

ables, **s**. Hence, there are some limits to what ICA can do: there are some unresolvable ambiguities in the components estimated by ICA. Specifically, ICA cannot determine the variances, hence the energies or amplitudes, of the actual sources. This is understandable if one considers the cocktail party problem. The sounds from a loudmouth at the party could be offset by the positions and gains of the various microphones, making it impossible to identify definitively his excessive volume. Similarly a soft-spoken party-goer could be closer to a number of the microphones and appear unduly loud in the recorded signals. Unless something is known about the mixing matrix (in this case the position and gains of the microphones with respect to the various speakers), this ambiguity cannot be resolved. Since the amplitude of the signals cannot be resolved, it is usual to fix the amplitudes so that a signal's variance is one. It is also impossible, for the same reasons, to determine the sign of the source signal, although this is not usually of much concern in most applications.

A second restriction is that, unlike PCA, the order of the components cannot be established. This follows from the arguments above: to establish the order of a given signal would require some information about the mixing matrix which, by definition, is unknown. Again, in most applications this is not a serious shortcoming.

The determination of the independent components begins by removing the mean values of the variables, also termed *centering* the data, as in PCA. The next step is to *whiten* the data, also know as *sphering* the data. Data that have been whitened are uncorrelated (as are the principal components), but, in addition, all of the variables have variances of one. PCA can be used for both these operations since it decorrelates the data and provides information on the variance of the decorrelated data in the form of the eigenvectors. Figure 9.10 shows the scatter plot of the data used in Figure 9.1 before and after whitening using PCA to decorrelate the data then scaling the components to have unit variances.

The independent components are determined by applying a linear transformation to the whitened data. Since the observations are a linear transformation of the underlying signals, **s**, (Eq. (15)) one should be able to be reconstruct them from a (inverse) linear transformation to the observed signals, **x**. That is, a given component could be obtained by the transformation:

$$ic_i = \mathbf{b}_i^T \mathbf{x} \tag{17}$$

where *ic*, the independent component, is an estimate of the original signal, and **b** is the appropriate vector to reconstruct that independent component. There are quite a number of different approaches for estimating **b**, but they all make use of an objective function that relates to variable independence. This function is maximized (or minimized) by an optimization algorithm. The various approaches differ in the specific *objective function* that is optimized and the *optimization* method that is used.

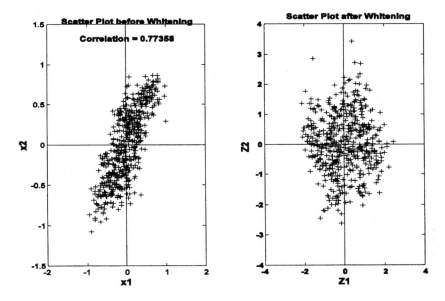

FIGURE 9.10 Two-variable multivariate data before (left) and after (right) whitening. Whitened data has been decorrelated and the resultant variables scaled so that their variance is one. Note that the whitened data has a generally circular shape. A whitened three-variable data set would have a spherical shape, hence the term *sphering* the data.

One of the most intuitive approaches uses an objective function that is related to the non-gaussianity of the data set. This approach takes advantage of the fact that mixtures tend to be more gaussian than the distribution of independent sources. This is a direct result of the central limit theorem which states that the sum of k independent, identically distributed random variables converges to a Gaussian distribution as k becomes large, regardless of the distribution of the individual variables. Hence, mixtures of non-Gaussian sources will be more Gaussian than the unmixed sources. This was demonstrated in Figure 2.1 using averages of uniformly distributed random data. Here we demonstrate the action of the central limit theorem using a deterministic function. In Figure 9.11A, a Gaussian distribution is estimated using the histogram of a 10,000-point sequence of Gaussian noise as produced by the MATLAB function `randn`. A distribution that is closely alined with an actual gaussian distribution (dotted line) is seen. A similarly estimated distribution of a single sine wave is shown in Figure 9.11B along with the Gaussian distribution. The sine wave distribution (solid line) is quite different from Gaussian (dashed line). However, a mixture of only two independent sinusoids (having different frequencies) is seen to be

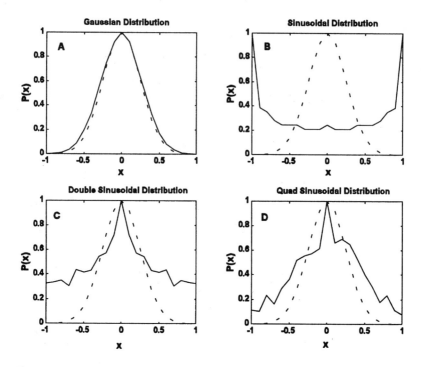

FIGURE 9.11 Approximate distributions for four variables determined from histograms of 10,0000-point waveforms. (A) Gaussian noise (from the MATLAB `randn` function). (B) Single sinusoid at 100 Hz. (C) Two sinusoids mixed together (100 and 30 Hz). (D) Four sinusoids mixed together (100, 70, 30, and 25 Hz). Note that larger mixtures produce distributions that look more like Gaussian distributions.

much closer to the Gaussian distribution (Figure 9.11C). The similarity improves as more independent sinusoids are mixed together, as seen in Figure 9.11D which shows the distribution obtained when four sinusoids (not harmonically related) are added together.

To take advantage of the relationship between non-gaussianity and component independence requires a method to measure gaussianity (or lack thereof). With such a measure, it would be possible to find **b** in Eq. (14) by adjusting **b** until the measured non-gaussianity of the transformed data set, ic_i, is maximum. One approach to quantifying non-gaussianity is to use kurtosis, the fourth-order cumulant of a variable, that is zero for Gaussian data and nonzero otherwise. Other approaches use an information-theoretic measure termed *negentropy*. Yet another set of approaches uses mutual information as the objective function to be minimized. An excellent treatment of the various approaches, their strengths and weaknesses, can be found in Hyvärinen et al. (2001), as well as Cichicki et al. (2002).

MATLAB Implementation

Development of an ICA algorithm is not a trivial task; however, a number of excellent algorithms can be downloaded from the Internet in the form of MATLAB m-files. Two particularly useful algorithms are the *FastICA* algorithm developed by the ICA Group at Helsinki University:

http://www.cis.hut.fi/projects/ica/fastica/fp.html

and the *Jade* algorithm for real-valued signals developed by J.-F. Cardoso:

http://sig.enst.fr/~cardoso/stuff.html.

The Jade algorithm is used in the example below, although the FastICA algorithm allows greater flexibility, including an interactive mode.

Example 9.3 Construct a data set consisting of five observed signals that are linear combinations of three different waveforms. Apply PCA and plot the scree plot to determine the actual dimension of the data set. Apply the Jade ICA algorithm given the proper dimensions to recover the individual components.

```
% Example 9.3 and Figure 9.12, 9.13, 9.14, and 9.15
% Example of ICA
% Create a mixture using three different signals mixed five ways
%   plus noise
% Use this in PCA and ICA analysis
%
clear all; close all;
% Assign constants
N = 1000;                    % Number points (4 sec of data)
fs = 500;                    % Sample frequency
w = (1:N) * 2*pi/fs;         % Normalized frequency vector
t = (1:N);
%
% Generate the three signals plus noise
s1 = .75 *sin(w*12) + .1*randn(1,N);  % Double sin, a sawtooth
s2 = sawtooth(w*5,.5) + .1*randn(1,N); % and a periodic
                                      %   function
s3 = pulstran((0:999),(0:5)'*180,kaiser(100,3)) +
    .07*randn(1,N);
%
% Plot original signals displaced for viewing
```

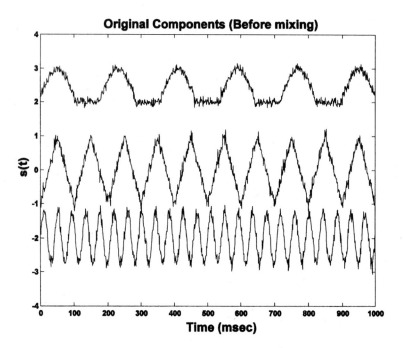

FIGURE 9.12 The three original source signals used to create the mixture seen in Figure 9.14 and used in Example 9.3.

```
plot(t,s1-2,'k',t,s2,'k',t,s3+2,'k');
  xlabel('Time (sec)');  ylabel('s(t)');
  title('Original Components (Before mixing)');
%
% Combine the 3 source signals 5 different ways. Define the mix-
% ing matrix
A = [.5 .5 .5; .2 .7 .7; .7 .4 .2; -.5      % Mixing matrix
  .2-.6; .7-.5-.4];
s = [s1; s2; s3];                          % Signal matrix
X = A * s;                        % Generate mixed signal output
figure;                           % Figure for mixed signals
%
% Center data and plot mixed signals
for i = 1:5
  X(i,:) = X(i,:)-mean(X(i,:));
  plot(t,X(i,:)+2*(i-1),'k');
  hold on;
end
......labels and title.........
```

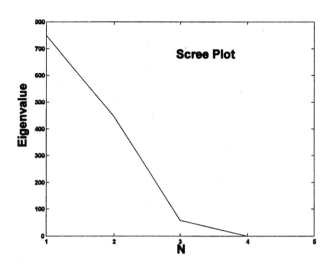

FIGURE 9.13   Scree plot of eigenvalues from the data set of Figure 9.12. Note the shape break at $N = 3$, indicating that there are only three independent variables in the data set of five waveforms. Hence, the ICA algorithm will be requested to search for only three components.

```
%
% Do PCA and plot Eigenvalues
figure;
[U,S,pc]= svd(X,0);              % Use single value decomposition
eigen = diag(S).^2;             % Get the eigenvalues
plot(eigen,'k');                % Scree plot
......labels and title..........
%
nu_ICA = input('Enter the number of independent components');
% Compute ICA
W = jadeR(X,nu_ICA);            % Determine the mixing matrix
ic = (W * X)';                  % Determine the IC's from the
                                %  mixing matrix
figure;                         % Plot independent components
plot(t,ic(:,1)-4,'k',t,ic(:,2),'k',t,ic(:,3)+4,'k');
......labels and title..........
```

The original source signals are shown in Figure 9.12. These are mixed together in different proportions to produce the five signals shown in Figure 9.14. The Scree plot of the eigenvalues obtained from the five-variable data set does show a marked break at 3 suggesting that there, in fact, only three separate components, Figure 9.13. Applying ICA to the five-variable mixture in Figure

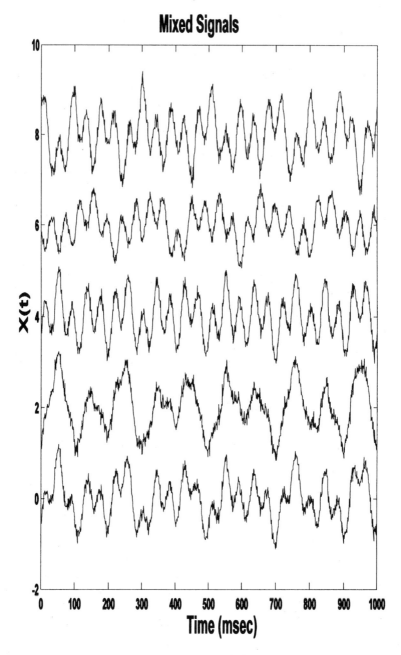

FIGURE 9.14 Five signals created by mixing three different waveforms and noise. ICA was applied to this data set to recover the original signals. The results of applying ICA to this data set are seen in Figure 9.15.

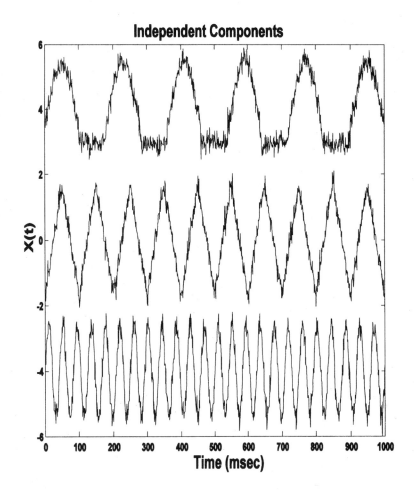

FIGURE 9.15 The three independent components found by ICA in Example 9.3. Note that these are nearly identical to the original, unmixed components. The presence of a small amount of noise does not appear to hinder the algorithm.

9.14 recovers the original source signals as shown in Figure 9.15. This figure dramatically demonstrates the ability of this approach to recover the original signals even in the presence of modest noise. ICA has been applied to biosignals to estimate the underlying sources in an multi-lead EEG signal, to improve the detection of active neural areas in functional magnetic resonance imaging, and to uncover the underlying neural control components in an eye movement motor control system. Given the power of the approach, many other applications are sure to follow.

PROBLEMS

1. Load the two-variable data set, X, contained in file `p1_data`. Assume for plotting that the sample frequency is 500 Hz. While you are not given the dimensions or orientation of the data set, you can assume the number of time samples is much greater than the number of measured signals.

(A) Rotate these data by an angle entered through the keyboard and output the covariance (from the covariance matrix) after each rotation. Use the function `rotate` to do the rotation. See comments in the function for details. Continue to rotate the data set *manually* until the covariances are very small (less than 10^{-4}). Plot the rotated and unrotated variables as a scatter plot and output their variances (also from covariance matrix). The variances will be the eigenvalues found by PCA and the rotated data the principal components.

(B) Now apply PCA using the approach given in Example 9.1 and compare the scatter plots with the manually rotated data. Compare the variances of the principal components from PCA (which can be obtained from the eigenvalues) with the variances obtained by manual rotation in (A) above.

2. Load the multi-variable data set, X, contained in file `p2_data`. Make the same assumptions with regard to sampling frequency and data set size as in Problem 1 above.

(A) Determine the actual dimension of the data using PCA and the scree plot.

(B) Perform an ICA analysis using either the Jade or FastICA algorithm limiting the number of components determined from the scree plot. Plot independent components.

10

Fundamentals of Image Processing: MATLAB Image Processing Toolbox

IMAGE PROCESSING BASICS: MATLAB IMAGE FORMATS

Images can be treated as two-dimensional data, and many of the signal processing approaches presented in the previous chapters are equally applicable to images: some can be directly applied to image data while others require some modification to account for the two (or more) data dimensions. For example, both PCA and ICA have been applied to image data treating the two-dimensional image as a single extended waveform. Other signal processing methods including Fourier transformation, convolution, and digital filtering are applied to images using two-dimensional extensions. Two-dimensional images are usually represented by two-dimensional data arrays, and MATLAB follows this tradition;* however, MATLAB offers a variety of data formats in addition to the standard format used by most MATLAB operations. Three-dimensional images can be constructed using multiple two-dimensional representations, but these multiple arrays are sometimes treated as a single volume image.

General Image Formats: Image Array Indexing

Irrespective of the image format or encoding scheme, an image is always represented in one, or more, two dimensional arrays, $I(m,n)$. Each element of the

---

*Actually, MATLAB considers image data arrays to be three-dimensional, as described later in this chapter.

variable, I, represents a single picture element, or *pixel*. (If the image is being treated as a volume, then the element, which now represents an elemental volume, is termed a *voxel*.) The most convenient indexing protocol follows the traditional matrix notation, with the horizontal pixel locations indexed left to right by the second integer, n, and the vertical locations indexed top to bottom by the first integer m (Figure 10.1). This indexing protocol is termed *pixel coordinates* by MATLAB. A possible source of confusion with this protocol is that the vertical axis positions increase from top to bottom and also that the second integer references the horizontal axis, the opposite of conventional graphs.

MATLAB also offers another indexing protocol that accepts non-integer indexes. In this protocol, termed *spatial coordinates*, the pixel is considered to be a square patch, the center of which has an integer value. In the default coordinate system, the *center* of the upper left-hand pixel still has a reference of (1,1), but the upper left-hand corner of this pixel has coordinates of (0.5,0.5) (see Figure 10.2). In this spatial coordinate system, the locations of image coordinates are positions on a (discrete) plane and are described by general variables *x* and *y*. The are two sources of potential confusion with this system. As with the pixel coordinate system, the vertical axis increases downward. In addition, the positions of the vertical and horizontal indexes (now better though of as coordinates) are switched: the horizontal index is first, followed by the vertical coordinate, as with conventional *x,y* coordinate references. In the default spatial coordinate system, integer coordinates correspond with their pixel coordinates, remembering the position swap, so that I(5,4) in pixel coordinates references the same pixel as I(4.0,5.0) in spatial coordinates. Most routines expect a specific pixel coordinate system and produce outputs in that system. Examples of spatial coordinates are found primarily in the spatial transformation routines described in the next chapter.

It is possible to change the baseline reference in the spatial coordinate

$$
\begin{array}{ccccc}
x(1,1) & x(1,2) & x(1,3) & \cdots & x(1,N) \\
x(2,1) & x(2,2) & x(2,3) & \cdots & x(2,N) \\
x(3,1) & x(3,2) & x(3,3) & \cdots & x(3,N) \\
\vdots & \vdots & \vdots & \ddots & \vdots \\
x(M,1) & x(M,2) & x(M,3) & \cdots & x(M,N)
\end{array}
$$

FIGURE 10.1 Indexing format for MATLAB images using the *pixel coordinate* system. This indexing protocol follows the standard matrix notation.

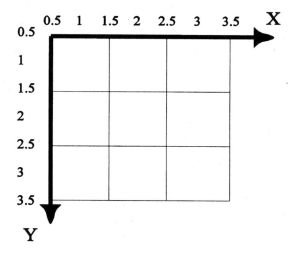

FIGURE 10.2   Indexing in the spatial coordinate system.

system as certain commands allow you to redefine the coordinates of the reference corner. This option is described in context with related commands.

Data Classes: Intensity Coding Schemes

There are four different data *classes*, or encoding schemes, used by MATLAB for image representation. Moreover, each of these data classes can store the data in a number of different formats. This variety reflects the variety in image types (color, grayscale, and black and white), and the desire to represent images as efficiently as possible in terms of memory storage. The efficient use of memory storage is motivated by the fact that images often require a large numbers of array locations: an image of 400 by 600 pixels will require 240,000 data points, each of which will need one or more bytes depending of the data format.

The four different image classes or encoding schemes are: *indexed* images, *RGB* images, *intensity* images, and *binary* images. The first two classes are used to store color images. In indexed images, the pixel values are, themselves, indexes to a table that *maps* the index value to a color value. While this is an efficient way to store color images, the data sets do not lend themselves to arithmetic operations (and, hence, most image processing operations) since the results do not always produce meaningful images. Indexed images also need an associated matrix variable that contains the *colormap*, and this map variable needs to accompany the image variable in many operations. Colormaps are N by 3 matrices that function as *lookup tables*. The indexed data variable points to a particular row in the map and the three columns associated with that row contain the intensity of the colors red, green, and blue. The values of the three columns range between 0 and 1 where 0 is the absence of the related color and 1 is the strongest intensity of that color. MATLAB convention suggests that indexed arrays use variable names beginning in `x..` (or simply `x`) and the suggested name for the colormap is `map`. While indexed variables are not very useful in image processing operations, they provide a compact method of storing color images, and can produce effective displays. They also provide a convenient and flexible method for colorizing grayscale data to produce a *pseudocolor* image.

The MATLAB Image Processing Toolbox provides a number of useful prepackaged colormaps. These colormaps can implemented with any number of rows, but the default is 64 rows. Hence, if any of these standard colormaps are used with the default value, the indexed data should be scaled to range between 0 and 64 to prevent saturation. An example of the application of a MATLAB colormap is given in Example 10.3. An extension of that example demonstrates methods for colorizing grayscale data using a colormap.

The other method for coding color image is the RGB coding scheme in which three different, but associated arrays are used to indicate the intensity of the three color components of the image: red, green, or blue. This coding scheme produces what is know as a *truecolor* image. As with the encoding used in indexed data, the larger the pixel value, the brighter the respective color. In this coding scheme, each of the color components can be operated on separately. Obviously, this color coding scheme will use more memory than indexed images, but this may be unavoidable if extensive processing is to be done on a color image. By MATLAB convention the variable name `RGB`, or something similar, is used for variables of this data class. Note that these variables are actually three-dimensional arrays having dimensions N by M by 3. While we have not used such three dimensional arrays thus far, they are fully supported by MATLAB. These arrays are indexed as `RGB(n,m,i)` where $i = 1,2,3$. In fact, all image variables are conceptualized in MATLAB as three-dimensional arrays, except that for non-RGB images the third dimension is simply 1.

Grayscale images are stored as intensity class images where the pixel value represents the brightness or *grayscale* value of the image at that point. MATLAB convention suggests variable names beginning with `I` for variables in class intensity. If an image is only black or white (not intermediate grays), then the binary coding scheme can be used where the representative array is a *logical* array containing either 0's or 1's. MATLAB convention is to use `BW` for variable names in the binary class. A common problem working with binary images is the failure to define the array as logical which would cause the image variable to be misinterpreted by the display routine. Binary class variables can be specified as logical (set the logical flag associated with the array) using the command `BW = logical(A)`, assuming `A` consists of only zeros and ones. A logical array can be converted to a standard array using the *unary plus* operator:

A = +BW. Since all binary images are of the form "logical," it is possible to check if a variable is logical using the routine: isa(I, 'logical'); which will return a1 if true and zero otherwise.

Data Formats

In an effort to further reduce image storage requirements, MATLAB provides three different data formats for most of the classes mentioned above. The *uint8* and *uint16* data formats provide 1 or 2 bytes, respectively, for each array element. Binary images do not support the uint16 format. The third data format, the double format, is the same as used in standard MATLAB operations and, hence, is the easiest to use. Image arrays that use the double format can be treated as regular MATLAB matrix variables subject to all the power of MATLAB and its many functions. The problem is that this format uses 8 bytes for each array element (i.e., pixel) which can lead to very large data storage requirements.

In all three data formats, a zero corresponds to the lowest intensity value, i.e., black. For the uint8 and uint16 formats, the brightest intensity value (i.e., white, or the brightest color) is taken as the largest possible number for that coding scheme: for uint8, 2^{8-1}, or 255; and for uint16, 2^{16}, or 65,535. For the double format, the brightest value corresponds to 1.0.

The isa routine can also be used to test the format of an image. The routine, isa(I, 'type') will return a 1 if I is encoded in the format type, and a zero otherwise. The variable type can be: unit8, unit16, or double. There are a number of other assessments that can be made with the isa routine that are described in the associated help file.

Multiple images can be grouped together as one variable by adding another dimension to the variable array. Since image arrays are already considered three-dimensional, the additional images are added to the fourth dimension. Multi-image variables are termed *multiframe* variables and each two-dimensional (or three-dimensional) image of a multiframe variable is termed a *frame*. Multiframe variables can be generated within MATLAB by incrementing along the fourth index as shown in Example 10.2, or by concatenating several images together using the cat function:

```
IMF = cat(4, I1, I2, I3,...);
```

The first argument, 4, indicates that the images are to concatenated along the fourth dimension, and the other arguments are the variable names of the images. All images in the list must be the same type and size.

Data Conversions

The variety of coding schemes and data formats complicates even the simplest of operations, but is necessary for efficient memory use. Certain operations require a given data format and/or class. For example, standard MATLAB operations require the data be in double format, and will not work correctly with Indexed images. Many MATLAB image processing functions also expect a specific format and/or coding scheme, and generate an output usually, but not always, in the same format as the input. Since there are so many combinations of coding and data type, there are a number of routines for converting between different types. For converting format types, the most straightforward procedure is to use the **im2xxx** routines given below:

```
I_uint8  = im2uint8(I);      % Convert to uint8 format
I_uint16 = im2uint16(I);     % Convert to uint16 format
I_double = im2double(I);     % Convert to double format
```

These routines accept any data class as input; however if the class is indexed, the input argument, **I**, must be followed by the term **indexed**. These routines also handle the necessary rescaling except for indexed images. When converting indexed images, variable range can be a concern: for example, to convert an indexed variable to uint8, the variable range must be between 0 and 255.

Converting between different image encoding schemes can sometimes be done by scaling. To convert a grayscale image in uint8, or uint16 format to an indexed image, select an appropriate grayscale colormap from the MATLAB's established colormaps, then scale the image variable so the values lie within the range of the colormap; i.e., the data range should lie between 0 and N, where N is the depth of the colormap (MATLAB's colormaps have a default depth of 64, but this can be modified). This approach is demonstrated in Example 10.3. However, an easier solution is simply to use MATLAB's **gray2ind** function listed below. This function, as with all the conversion functions, will scale the input data appropriately, and in the case of **gray2ind** will also supply an appropriate grayscale colormap (although alternate colormaps of the same depth can be substituted). The routines that convert to indexed data are:

```
[x, map] = gray2ind(I, N);   % Convert from grayscale to
                             %   indexed
% Convert from truecolor to indexed
[x, map] = rgb2ind(RGB, N or map);
```

Both these routines accept data in any format, including logical, and produce an output of type uint8 if the associated map length is less than or equal to 64, or uint16 if greater that 64. N specifies the colormap depth and must be less than 65,536. For **gray2ind** the colormap is **gray** with a depth of **N**, or the default value of 64 if N is omitted. For RGB conversion using **rgb2ind**, a colormap of **N** levels is generated to best match the RGB data. Alternatively, a colormap can be provided as the second argument, in which case `rgb2ind` will generate an output array, `x`, with values that best match the colors given in `map`. The `rgb2ind` function has a number of options that affect the image conversion, options that allow trade-offs between color accuracy and image resolution. (See the associated help file).

An alternative method for converting a grayscale image to indexed values is the routine `grayslice` which converts using thresholding:

```
x = grayslice(I, N or V);   % Convert grayscale to indexed using
                            %  thresholding
```

where any input format is acceptable. This function *slices* the image into N levels using a equal step thresholding process. Each slice is then assigned a specific level on whatever colormap is selected. This process allows some interesting color representations of grayscale images, as described in Example 10.4. If the second argument is a vector, `v`, then it contains the threshold levels (which can now be unequal) and the number of slices corresponds to the length of this vector. The output format is either `uint8` or `uint16` depending on the number of slices, similar to the two conversion routines above.

Two conversion routines convert from indexed images to other encoding schemes:

```
I = ind2gray(x, map);       % Convert to grayscale intensity
                            %  encoding
RGB = ind2rgb(x, map);      % Convert to RGB ("truecolor")
                            %  encoding
```

Both functions accept any format and, in the case of `ind2gray` produces outputs in the same format. Function `ind2rgb` produces outputs formatted as double. Function `ind2gray` removes the hue and saturation information while retaining the luminance, while function `ind2rgb` produces a truecolor RGB variable.

To convert an image to binary coding use:

```
BW = im2bw(I, Level);       % Convert to binary logical encoding
```

where `Level` specifies the threshold that will be used to determine if a pixel is white (1) or black (0). The input image, `I`, can be either intensity, RGB, or indexed,* and in any format (uint8, uint16, or double). While most functions output binary images in uint8 format, `im2bw` outputs the image in logical format.

---

*As with all conversion routines, and many other routines, when the input image is in indexed format it must be followed by the colormap variable.

In this format, the image values are either 0 or 1, but each element is the same size as the double format (8 bytes). This format can be used in standard MAT-LAB operations, but does use a great deal of memory. One of the applications of the dither function can also be used to generate binary images as described in the associated help file.

A final conversion routine does not really change the data class, but does scale the data and can be very useful. This routine converts general class double data to intensity data, scaled between 0 and 1:

```
I = mat2gray(A, [Anin Amax]);   % Scale matrix to intensity
                                %  encoding, double format.
```

where A is a matrix and the optional second term specifies the values of A to be scaled to zero, or black (Amin), or 1, or white (Amin). Since a matrix is already in double format, this routine provides only scaling. If the second argument is missing, the matrix is scaled so that its highest value is 1 and its lowest value is zero. Using the default scaling can be a problem if the image contains a few irrelevant pixels having large values. This can occur after certain image processing operations due to border (or edge) effects. In such cases, other scaling must be imposed, usually determined empirically, to achieve a suitable range of image intensities.

The various data classes, their conversion routines, and the data formats they support are summarized in Table 1 below. The output format of the various conversion routines is indicated by the superscript: (1) uint8 or unit 16 depending on the number of levels requested (N); (2) Double; (3) No format change (output format equals input format); and (4) Logical (size double).

Image Display

There are several options for displaying an image, but the most useful and easiest to use is the imshow function. The basic calling format of this routine is:

TABLE 10.1 Summary of Image Classes, Data Formats, and Conversion Routines

Class	Formats supported	Conversion routines
Indexed	All	gray2ind[1], grayslice[1], rgb2ind[1]
Intensity	All	ind2gray[2], mat2gray[2,3], rgb2gray[3]
RGB	All	ind2rgb[2]
Binary	uint8, double	im2bw[4], dither[1]

```
imshow(I,arg)
```

where I is the image array and **arg** is an argument, usually optional, that depends on the data format. For indexed data, the variable name must be followed by the colormap, **map**. This holds for all display functions when indexed data are involved. For intensity class image variables, **arg** can be a scalar, in which case it specifies the number of levels to use in rendering the image, or, if **arg** is a vector, [**low high**], **arg** specifies the values to be taken to readjust the range limits of a specific data format.* If the empty matrix, [ ], is given as **arg**, or it is simply missing, the maximum and minimum values in array I are taken as the **low** and **high** values. The **imshow** function has a number of other options that make it quite powerful. These options can be found with the help command. When I is an indexed variable, it should be followed by the **map** variable.

There are two functions designed to display multiframe variables. The function **montage (MFW)** displays the various images in a gird-like pattern as shown in Example 10.2. Alternatively, multiframe variables can be displayed as a movie using the **immovie** and **movie** commands:

```
mov = imovie(MFW);      % Generate movie variable
movie(mov);             % Display movie
```

Unfortunately the **movie** function cannot be displayed in a textbook, but is presented in one of the problems at the end of the chapter, and several amusing examples are presented in the problems at the end of the next chapter. The **immovie** function requires multiframe data to be in either Indexed or RGB format. Again, if **MFW** is an indexed variable, it must be followed by a colormap variable.

The basics features of the MATLAB Imaging Processing Toolbox are illustrated in the examples below.

Example 10.1 Generate an image of a *sinewave grating* having a *spatial frequency* of 2 cycles/inch. A sinewave grating is a pattern that is constant in the vertical direction, but varies sinusoidally in the horizontal direction. It is used as a visual stimulus in experiments dealing with visual perception. Assume the figure will be 4 inches square; hence, the overall pattern should contain 4 cycles. Assume the image will be placed in a 400-by-400 pixel array (i.e., 100 pixels per inch) using a uint16 format.

Solution Sinewave gratings usually consist of sines in the horizontal direction and constant intensity in the vertical direction. Since this will be a gray-

---

*Recall the default minimum and maximum values for the three non-indexed classes were: [0, 256] for uint8; [0, 65535] for uint16; and [0, 1] for double arrays.

scale image, we will use the intensity coding scheme. As most reproductions
have limited grayscale resolution, a uint8 data format will be used. However,
the sinewave will be generated in the double format, as this is MATLAB's
standard format. To save memory requirement, we first generate a 400-by-1
image line in double format, then convert it to uint8 format using the conversion
routine im2uint8. The uint8 image can then be extended vertically to 400 pixels.

```
% Example 10.1 and Figure 1.3
% Generate a sinewave grating 400 by 400 pixels
% The grating should vary horizontally with a spatial frequency
%   of 4 cycles per inch.
% Assume the horizontal and vertical dimensions are 4 inches
%
clear all; close all;
N = 400;                     % Vertical and horizontal size
Nu_cyc = 4;                  % Produce 4 cycle grating
x = (1:N)*Ny_cyc/N;          % Spatial (time equivalent) vector
%
```

Sinewave Grating

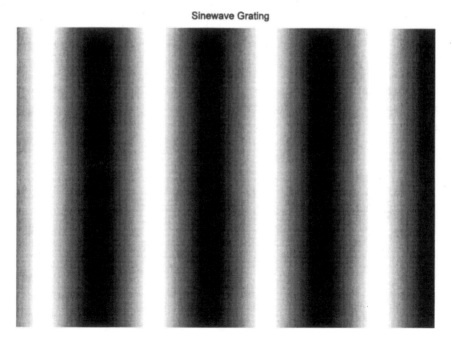

FIGURE 10.3 A *sinewave grating* generated by Example 10.1. Such images are
often used as stimuli in experiments on vision.

```
% Generate a single horizontal line of the image in a vector of
%  400 points
%
% Generate sin; scale between 0&1
I_sin(1,:) = .5 * sin(2*pi*x) + .5;
I_8 = im2uint8(I_sin);     % Convert to a uint8 vector
%
for i = 1:N                % Extend to N (400) vertical lines
   I(i,:) = I_8;
end
%
imshow(I);                 % Display image
   title('Sinewave Grating');
```

The output of this example is shown as Figure 10.3. As with all images shown in this text, there is a loss in both detail (resolution) and grayscale variation due to losses in reproduction. To get the best images, these figures, and all figures in this section can be reconstructed on screen using the code from the examples provided in the CD.

Example 10.2   Generate a multiframe variable consisting of a series of sinewave gratings having different phases. Display these images as a montage. Border the images with black for separation on the montage plot. Generate 12 frames, but reduce the image to 100 by 100 to save memory.

```
% Example 10.2 and Figure 10.4
% Generate a multiframe array consisting of sinewave gratings
%  that vary in phase from 0 to 2 * pi across 12 images
%
% The gratings should be the same as in Example 10.1 except with
%  fewer pixels (100 by 100) to conserve memory.
%
clear all; close all;
N = 100;                   % Vertical and horizontal points
Nu_cyc = 2;                % Produce 4 cycle grating
M = 12;                    % Produce 12 images
x = (1:N)*Nu_cyc/N;        % Generate spatial vector
%
for j = 1:M                % Generate M (12) images
  phase = 2*pi*(j-1)/M;    % Shift phase through 360 (2*pi)
                           %  degrees
                           % Generate sine; scale to be 0 & 1
  I_sin = .5 * sin(2*pi*x + phase) + .5'*;
                           % Add black at left and right borders
  I_sin = [zeros(1,10) I_sin(1,:) zeros(1,10)];
```

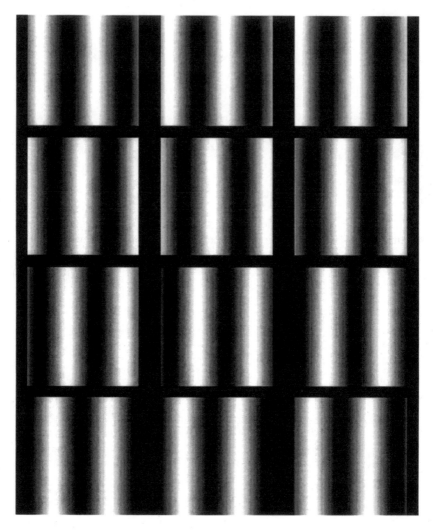

FIGURE 10.4 Montage of sinewave gratings created by Example 10.2.

```
    I_8 = im2uint8(I_sin);    % Convert to a uint8 vector
%
    for i = 1:N               % Extend to N (100) vertical lines
      if i < 10 | I > 90      % Insert black space at top and
                              %  bottom

        I(i,:,1:j) = 0;
      else
```

```
    I(i,:,1,j) = I_8;
      end
    end
  end
  montage(I);                    % Display image as montage
    title('Sinewave Grating');
```

The montage created by this example is shown in Figure 10.4 on the next page. The multiframe data set was constructed one frame at a time and the frame was placed in I using the frame index, the fourth index of I.* Zeros are inserted at the beginning and end of the sinewave and, in the image construction loop, for the first and last 9 points. This is to provide a dark band between the images. Finally the sinewave was phase shifted through 360 degrees over the 12 frames.

Example 10.3 Construct a multiframe variable with 12 sinewave grating images. Display these data as a movie. Since the immovie function requires the multiframe image variable to be in either RGB or indexed format, convert the uint16 data to indexed format. This can be done by the gray2ind(I,N) function. This function simply scales the data to be between 0 and N, where N is the depth of the colormap. If N is unspecified, gray2ind defaults to 64 levels. MATLAB colormaps can also be specified to be of any depth, but as with gray2ind the default level is 64.

```
% Example 10.3
% Generate a movie of a multiframe array consisting of sinewave
%   gratings that vary in phase from 0 to pi across 10 images
% Since function 'immovie' requires either RGB or indexed data
%   formats scale the data for use as Indexed with 64 gray levels.
% Use a standard MATLAB grayscale ('gray');
%
% The gratings should be the same as in Example 10.2.
%
clear all;
close all;
% Assign parameters
N = 100;                       % Vertical and horizontal points
Nu_cyc = 2;                    % Produce 2 cycle grating
M = 12;                        % Produce 12 images
%
x = (1:N)*Nu_cyc/N;            % Generate spatial vector
```

---

*Recall, the third index is reserved for referencing the color plane. For non-RGB variables, this index will always be 1. For images in RGB format the third index would vary between 1 and 3.

```
for j = 1:M                   % Generate M (100) images
   % Generate sine; scale between 0 and 1
   phase = 10*pi*j/M;         % Shift phase 180 (pi) over 12 images
   I_sin(1,:) = .5 * sin(2*pi*x + phase) + .5';
   for i = 1:N                % Extend to N (100) vertical lines
   for i = 1:N                % Extend to 100 vertical lines to
      Mf(i,:,1,j) = x1;       %   create 1 frame of the multiframe
                              %   image
   end
   end
%
%
[Mf, map] = gray2ind(Mf);    % Convert to indexed image
mov = immovie(Mf,map);       % Make movie, use default colormap
movie(mov,10);               % and show 10 times
```

To fully appreciate this example, the reader will need to run this program under MATLAB. The 12 frames are created as in Example 10.3, except the code that adds border was removed and the data scaling was added. The second argument in immovie, is the colormap matrix and this example uses the map generated by gray2ind. This map has the default level of 64, the same as all of the other MATLAB supplied colormaps. Other standard maps that are appropriate for grayscale images are 'bone' which has a slightly bluish tint, 'pink' which has a decidedly pinkish tint, and 'copper' which has a strong rust tint. Of course any colormap can be used, often producing interesting *pseudocolor* effects from grayscale data. For an interesting color alternative, try running Example 10.3 using the prepackaged colormap jet as the second argument of immovie. Finally, note that the size of the multiframe array, Mf, is $(100,100,1,12)$ or $1.2 \times 10^5 \times 2$ bytes. The variable mov generated by immovie is even larger!

Image Storage and Retrieval

Images may be stored on disk using the imwrite command:

```
imwrite(I, filename.ext, arg1, arg2, ...);
```

where I is the array to be written into file filename. There are a large variety of file formats for storing image data and MATLAB supports the most popular formats. The file format is indicated by the filename's extension, ext, which may be: .bmp (Microsoft bitmap), .gif (graphic interchange format), .jpeg (Joint photographic experts group), .pcs (Paintbrush), .png (portable network graphics), and .tif (tagged image file format). The arguments are optional and may be used to specify image compression or resolution, or other format dependent information.

The specifics can be found in the `imwrite` help file. The `imwrite` routine can be used to store any of the data formats or data classes mentioned above; however, if the data array, `I`, is an indexed array, then it must be followed by the colormap variable, `map`. Most image formats actually store uint8 formatted data, but the necessary conversions are done by the `imwrite`.

The `imread` function is used to retrieve images from disk. It has the calling structure:

```
[I map] = imread('filename.ext',fmt or frame);
```

where `filename` is the name of the image file and `.ext` is any of the extensions listed above. The optional second argument, `fmt`, only needs to be specified if the file format is not evident from the filename. The alternative optional argument `frame` is used to specify which frame of a multiframe image is to be read in `I`. An example that reads multiframe data is found in Example 10.4. As most file formats store images in uint8 format, `I` will often be in that format. File formats `.tif` and `.png` support uint16 format, so `imread` may generate data arrays in uint16 format for these file types. The output class depends on the manner in which the data is stored in the file. If the file contains a grayscale image data, then the output is encoded as an intensity image, if truecolor, then as RGB. For both these cases the variable `map` will be empty, which can be checked with the `isempty(map)` command (see Example 10.4). If the file contains indexed data, then both output, `I` and `map` will contain data.

The type of data format used by a file can also be obtained by *querying* a graphics file using the function `infinfo`.

```
information = infinfo('filename.ext')
```

where `information` will contain text providing the essential information about the file including the ColorType, FileSize, and BitDepth. Alternatively, the image data and map can be loaded using `imread` and the format image data determined from the MATLAB `whos` command. The `whos` command will also give the structure of the data variable (uint8, uint16, or double).

Basic Arithmetic Operations

If the image data are stored in the double format, then all MATLAB standard mathematical and operational procedures can be applied directly to the image variables. However, the double format requires 4 times as much memory as the uint16 format and 8 times as much memory as the uint8 format. To reduce the reliance on the double format, MATLAB has supplied functions to carry out some basic mathematics on uint8- and uint16-format arrays. These routines will work on either format; they actually carry out the operations in double precision on an element by element basis then convert back to the input format. This reduces roundoff and overflow errors. The basic arithmetic commands are:

```
I_diff = imabssdiff(I, J);        % Subtracts J from I on a pixel
                                  %  by pixel basis and returns
                                  %  the absolute difference
I_comp = imcomplement(I)          % Compliments image I
I_add = imadd(I, J);              % Adds image I and J (images and/
                                  %  or constants) to form image
                                  %  I_add
I_sub = imsubtract(I, J);         % Subtracts J from image I
I_divide = imdivide(I, J)         % Divides image I by J
I_multiply = immultiply(I, J)     % Multiply image I by J
```

For the last four routines, J can be either another image variable, or a constant. Several arithmetical operations can be combined using the imlincomb function. The function essentially calculates a weighted sum of images. For example to add 0.5 of image $I1$ to 0.3 of image $I2$, to 0.75 of Image $I3$, use:

```
% Linear combination of images
I_combined = imlincomb (.5, I1, .3, I2, .75, I3);
```

The arithmetic operations of multiplication and addition by constants are easy methods for increasing the contrast or brightness or an image. Some of these arithmetic operations are illustrated in Example 10.4.

Example 10.4   This example uses a number of the functions described previously. The program first loads a set of MRI (magnetic resonance imaging) images of the brain from the MATLAB Image Processing Toolbox's set of stock images. This image is actually a multiframe image consisting of 27 frames as can be determined from the command imifinfo. One of these frames is selected by the operator and this image is then manipulated in several ways: the contrast is increased; it is inverted; it is sliced into 5 levels (N_slice); it is modified horizontally and vertically by a Hanning window function, and it is thresholded and converted to a binary image.

```
% Example 10.4 and Figures 10.5 and 10.6
% Demonstration of various image functions.
% Load all frames of the MRI image in mri.tif from the the MATLAB
%  Image Processing Toolbox (in subdirectory imdemos).
% Select one frame based on a user input.
% Process that frame by: contrast enhancement of the image,
%  inverting the image, slicing the image, windowing, and
%  thresholding the image
```

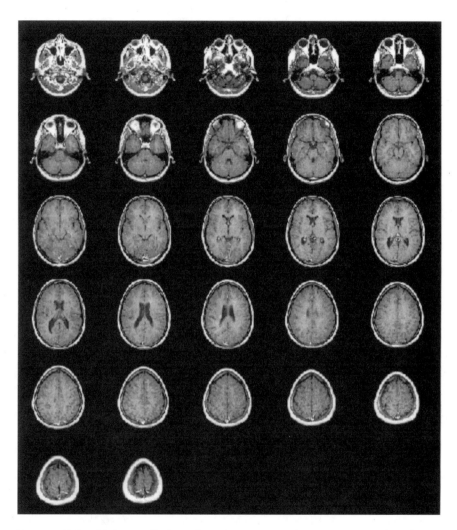

FIGURE 10.5 *Montage* display of 27 frames of magnetic resonance images of the brain plotted in Example 10.4. These multiframe images were obtained from MATLAB's `mri.tif` file in the images section of the Image Processing Toolbox. Used with permission from MATLAB, Inc. Copyright 1993–2003, The Math Works, Inc. Reprinted with permission.

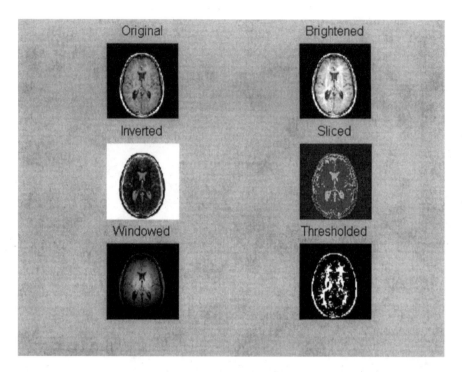

FIGURE 10.6 Figure showing various signal processing operations on frame 17 of the MRI images shown in Figure 10.5. Original from the MATLAB Image Processing Toolbox. Copyright 1993–2003, The Math Works, Inc. Reprinted with permission.

```
% Display original and all modifications on the same figure
%
clear all; close all;
N_slice = 5;                        % Number of sliced for
                                    %  sliced image
Level = .75;                        % Threshold for binary
                                    %  image
%
% Initialize an array to hold 27 frames of mri.tif
% Since this image is stored in tif format, it could be in either
%  unit8 or uint16.
% In fact, the specific input format will not matter, since it
%  will be converted to double format in this program.
mri = uint8(zeros(128,128,1,27));   % Initialize the image
                                    %  array for 27 frames
for frame = 1:27                    % Read all frames into
                                    %  variable mri
```

```
    [mri(:,:,:,frame), map ] = imread('mri.tif', frame);
end
montage(mri, map);                    % Display images as a
                                      %  montage
                                      % Include map in case
                                      %  Indexed
%
frame_select = input('Select frame for processing: ');
I = mri(:,:,:,frame_select);         % Select frame for
                                      %  processing
%
% Now check to see if image is Indexed (in fact 'whos' shows it
%  is).
if isempty(map) == 0                  % Check to see if
                                      %  indexed data
    I = ind2gray(I,map);             % If so, convert to
                                      %  intensity image
end
I1 = im2double(I);                    % Convert to double
                                      %  format
%
I_bright = immultiply(I1,1.2);        % Increase the contrast
I_invert = imcomplement(I1);          % Compliment image
x_slice = grayslice(I1,N_slice);      % Slice image in 5 equal
                                      %  levels
%
[r c] = size(I1);                     % Multiple
for i = 1:r                           %  horizontally by a
                                      %  Hamming window
    I_window(i,:) = I1(i,:) .* hamming(c)';
end
for i = 1:c                           % Multiply vertically
                                      %  by same window
    I_window(:,i) = I_window(:,i) .* hamming(r);
end
I_window = mat2gray(I_window);        % Scale windowed image
BW = im2bw(I1,Level);                 % Convert to binary
%
figure;
subplot(3,2,1);                       % Display all images in
                                      %  a single plot
    imshow(I1); title('Original');
subplot(3,2,2);
    imshow(I_bright), title('Brightened');
subplot(3,2,3);
```

```
   imshow(I_invert); title('Inverted');
subplot(3,2,4);
   I_slice = ind2rgb(x_slice, jet        % Convert to RGB (see
   (N_slice));                           %  text)
   imshow(I_slice); title('Sliced');     % Display color slices
subplot(3,2,5);
   imshow(I_window); title('Windowed');
subplot(3,2,6);
   imshow(BW); title('Thresholded');
```

Since the image file might be indexed (in fact it is), the `imread` function includes map as an output. If the image is not indexed, then map will be empty. Note that `imread` reads only one frame at a time, the frame specified as the second argument of `imread`. To read in all 27 frames, it is necessary to use a loop. All frames are then displayed in one figure (Figure 10.5) using the `montage` function. The user is asked to select one frame for further processing. Since montage can display any input class and format, it is not necessary to determine these data characteristics at this time.

After a particular frame is selected, the program checks if the map variable is empty (function `isempty`). If it is not (as is the case for these data), then the image data is converted to grayscale using function `ind2gray` which produces an intensity image in double format. If the image is not Indexed, the image variable is converted to double format. The program then performs the various signal processing operations. Brightening is done by multiplying the image by a constant greater that 1.0, in this case 1.2, Figure 10.6. Inversion is done using `imcomplement`, and the image is sliced into `N_slice` (5) levels using `grayslice`. Since `grayslice` produces an indexed image, it also generates a map variable. However, this `grayscale` map is not used, rather an alternative map is substituted to produce a color image, with the color being used to enhance certain features of the image.* The Hanning window is applied to the image in both the horizontal and vertical direction Figure 10.6. Since the image, `I1`, is in double format, the multiplication can be carried out directly on the image array; however, the resultant array, `I_window`, has to be rescaled using `mat2gray` to insure it has the correct range for `imshow`. Recall that if called without any arguments; `mat2gray` scales the array to take up the full intensity range (i.e., 0 to 1). To place all the images in the same figure, `subplot` is used just as with other graphs, Figure 10.6. One potential problem with this approach is that Indexed data may plot incorrectly due to limited display memory allocated to

---

*More accurately, the image should be termed a pseudocolor image since the original data was grayscale. Unfortunately the image printed in this text is in grayscale; however the example can be rerun by the reader to obtain the actual color image.

the map variables. (This problem actually occurred in this example when the sliced array was displayed as an Indexed variable.) The easiest solution to this potential problem is to convert the image to RGB before calling `imshow` as was done in this example.

Many images that are grayscale can benefit from some form of color coding. With the RGB format, it is easy to highlight specific features of a grayscale image by placing them in a specific color plane. The next example illustrates the use of color planes to enhance features of a grayscale image.

Example 10.5   In this example, brightness levels of a grayscale image that are 50% or less are coded into shades of blue, and those above are coded into shades of red. The grayscale image is first put in double format so that the maximum range is 0 to 1. Then each pixel is tested to be greater than 0.5. Pixel values less that 0.5 are placed into the blue image plane of an RGB image (i.e., the third plane). These pixel values are multiplied by two so they take up the full range of the blue plane. Pixel values above 0.5 are placed in the red plane (plane 1) after scaling to take up the full range of the red plane. This image is displayed in the usual way. While it is not reproduced in color here, a homework problem based on these same concepts will demonstrate pseudocolor.

```
% Example 10.5 and Figure 10.7 Example of the use of pseudocolor
% Load frame 17 of the MRI image (mri.tif)
%  from the Image Processing Toolbox in subdirectory 'imdemos'.
```

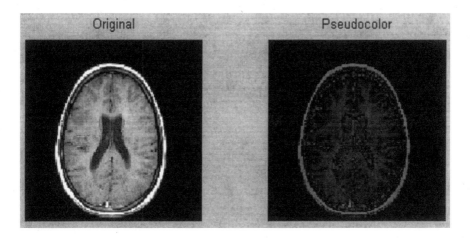

FIGURE 10.7   Frame 17 of the MRI image given in Figure 10.5 plotted directly and in pseudocolor using the code in Example 10.5. (Original image from MATLAB). Copyright 1993–2003, The Math Works, Inc. Reprinted with permission.

```
% Display a pseudocolor image in which all values less that 50%
%   maximum are in shades of blue and values above are in shades
%   of red.
%
clear all; close all;
frame = 17;
[I(:,:,1,1), map ] = imread('mri.tif', frame);
% Now check to see if image is Indexed (in fact 'whos' shows it is).
if isempty(map) == 0          % Check to see if Indexed data
  I = ind2gray(I,map);        % If so, convert to Intensity image
end
  I = im2double(I);           % Convert to double
[M N] = size(I);
RGB = zeros(M,N,3);           % Initialize RGB array
for i = 1:M
  for j = 1:N                 % Fill RGB planes
    if I(i,j) > .5
      RGB(i,j,1) = (I(i,j)-.5)*2;
    else
      RGB(i,j,3) = I(i,j)*2;
    end
  end
end
%
subplot(1,2,1);               % Display images in a single plot
  imshow(I); title('Original');
subplot(1,2,2);
  imshow(RGB) title('Pseudocolor');
```

The pseudocolor image produced by this code is shown in Figure 10.7. Again, it will be necessary to run the example to obtain the actual color image.

ADVANCED PROTOCOLS: BLOCK PROCESSING

Many of the signal processing techniques presented in previous chapters operated on small, localized groups of data. For example, both FIR and adaptive filters used data samples within the same general *neighborhood*. Many image processing techniques also operate on neighboring data elements, except the neighborhood now extends in two dimensions, both horizontally and vertically. Given this extension into two dimensions, many operations in image processing are quite similar to those in signal processing. In the next chapter, we examine both two-dimensional filtering using two-dimensional convolution and the two-dimensional Fourier transform. While many image processing operations are conceptually the same as those used on signal processing, the implementation is somewhat more involved due to the additional *bookkeeping* required to operate on data in two dimensions. The MATLAB Image Processing Toolbox simplifies much of the tedium of working in two dimensions by introducing functions that facilitate two-dimensional block, or neighborhood operations. These *block processing operations* fall into two categories: *sliding neighborhood* operations and *distinct block* operation. In sliding neighborhood operations, the block slides across the image as in convolution; however, the block must slide in both horizontal and vertical directions. Indeed, two-dimensional convolution described in the next chapter is an example of one very useful sliding neighborhood operation. In distinct block operations, the image area is divided into a number of fixed groups of pixels, although these groups may overlap. This is analogous to the overlapping segments used in the Welch approach to the Fourier transform described in Chapter 3. Both of these approaches to dealing with blocks of localized data in two dimensions are supported by MATLAB routines.

Sliding Neighborhood Operations

The sliding neighborhood operation alters one pixel at a time based on some operation performed on the surrounding pixels; specifically those pixels that lie within the neighborhood defined by the block. The block is placed as symmetrically as possible around the pixel being altered, termed the *center pixel* (Figure 10.8). The center pixel will only be in the center if the block is odd in both

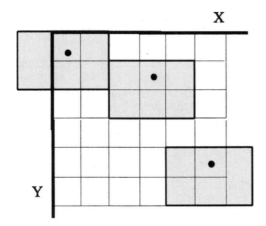

FIGURE 10.8 A 3-by-2 pixel *sliding neighborhood* block. The block (gray area), is shown in three different positions. Note that the block sometimes falls off the picture and padding (usually zero padding) is required. In actual use, the block slides, one element at a time, over the entire image. The dot indicates the center pixel.

dimensions, otherwise the center pixel position favors the left and upper sides of the block (Figure 10.8).* Just as in signal processing, there is a problem that occurs at the edge of the image when a portion of the block will extend beyond the image (Figure 10.8, upper left block). In this case, most MATLAB sliding block functions automatically perform zero padding for these pixels. (An exception, is the `imfilter` routine described in the next capter.)

The MATLAB routines `conv2` and `filter2` are both siding neighborhood operators that are directly analogous to the one dimensional convolution routine, `conv`, and filter routine, `filter`. These functions will be discussed in the next chapter on image filtering. Other two-dimensional functions that are directly analogous to their one-dimensional counterparts include: `mean2`, `std2`, `corr2`, and `fft2`. Here we describe a general sliding neighborhood routine that can be used to implement a wide variety of image processing operations. Since these operations can be—but are not necessarily—nonlinear, the function has the name `nlfilter`, presumably standing for nonlinear filter. The calling structure is:

```
I1 = nlfilter(I, [M N], func, P1, P2, ...);
```

where `I` is the input image array, `M` and `N` are the dimensions of the neighborhood block (horizontal and vertical), and `func` specifies the function that will operate over the block. The optional parameters `P1`, `P2`, ..., will be passed to the function if it requires input parameters. The function should take an *M* by *N* input and must produce a *single, scalar output* that will be used for the value of the center pixel. The input can be of any class or data format supported by the function, and the output image array, `I1`, will depend on the format provided by the routine's output.

The function may be specified in one of three ways: as a string containing the desired operation, as a *function handle* to an *M*-file, or as a function established by the routine `inline`. The first approach is straightforward: simply embed the function operation, which could be any appropriate MATLAB statment(s), within single quotes. For example:

```
I1 = nlfilter(I; [3 3], 'mean2');
```

This command will slide a 3 by 3 moving average across the image producing a lowpass filtered version of the original image (analogous to an FIR filter of [1/3 1/3 1/3]). Note that this could be more effectively implemented using the filter routines described in the next chapter, but more complicated, perhaps nonlinear, operations could be included within the quotes.

---

*In MATLAB notation, the center pixel of an *M* by *N* block is located at: `floor(([M N] + 1)/2)`.

The use of a function handle is shown in the code:

```
I1 = nlfilter(I, [3 3], @my_function);
```

where `my_function` is the name of an *M*-file function. The function handle `@my_function` contains all the information required by MATLAB to execute the function. Again, this file should produce a single, scalar output from an *M* by *N* input, and it has the possibility of containing input arguments in addition to the block matrix.

The `inline` routine has the ability to take string text and convert it into a function for use in `nlfilter` as in this example string:

```
F = inline('2*x(2,2) -sum( x(1:3,1))/3- sum(x(1:3,3))/3
      - x(1,2)-x(3,2)');
I1 = nlfilter(I, [3 3], F);
```

Function `inline` assumes that the input variable is x, but it also can find other variables based on the context and it allows for additional arguments, `P1`, `P2`, ... (see associated help file). The particular function shown above would take the difference between the center point and its 8 surrounding neighbors, performing a differentiator-like operation. There are better ways to perform spatial differentiation described in the next chapter, but this form will be demonstrated as one of the operations in Example 10.6 below.

Example 10.6 Load the image of blood cells in `blood.tiff` in MATLAB's image files. Convert the image to class intensity and double format. Perform the following sliding neighborhood operations: averaging over a 5 by 5 sliding block, differencing (spatial differentiation) using the function, `F`, above; and vertical boundary detection using a 2 by 3 vertical differencer. This differencer operator subtracts a vertical set of three left hand pixels from the three adjacent right hand pixels. The result will be a brightening of vertical boundaries that go from dark to light and a darkening of vertical boundaries that go from light to dark. Display all the images in the same figure including the original. Also include binary images of the vertical boundary image thresholded at two different levels to emphasize the left and right boundaries.

```
% Example 10.6 and Figure 10.9
% Demonstration of sliding neighborhood operations
% Load image of blood cells, blood.tiff from the Image Processing
%   Toolbox in subdirectory imdemos.
% Use a sliding 3 by 3 element block to perform several sliding
%   neighborhood operations including taking the average over the
%   block, implementing the function 'F' in the example
```

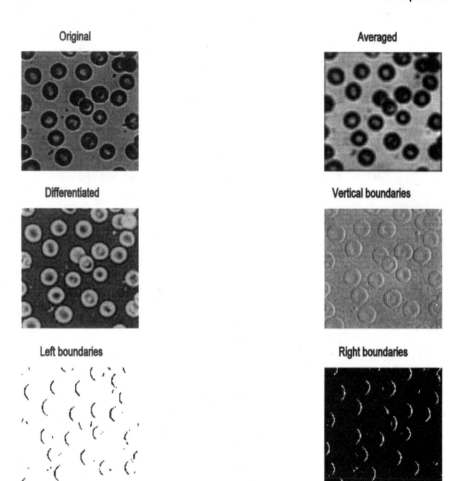

FIGURE 10.9 A variety of sliding neighborhood operations carried out on an image of blood cells. (Original reprinted with permission from The Image Processing Handbook, 2nd ed. Copyright CRC Press, Boca Raton, Florida.)

```
%  above, and implementing a function that enhances vertical
%  boundaries.
% Display the original and all modification on the same plot
%
clear all; close all;
[I map] = imread('blood1.tif');% Input image
% Since image is stored in tif format, it could be in either uint8
%  or uint16 format (although the 'whos' command shows it is in
%  uint8).
```

```
% The specific data format will not matter since the format will
%  be converted to double either by 'ind2gray,' if it is an In-
%  dexed image or by 'im2gray' if it is not.
%
if isempty(map) == 0            % Check to see if indexed data
   I = ind2gray(I,map);         % If so, convert to intensity
                                %  image
end
I = im2double(I);               % Convert to double and scale
                                % If not already
%
% Perform the various sliding neighborhood operations.
% Averaging
I_avg = nlfilter(I,[5 5], 'mean2');
%
% Differencing
F = inline('x(2,2)-sum(x(1:3,1))/3- sum(x(1:3,3))/3 - ...
   x(1,2)-x(3,2)');
I_diff = nlfilter(I, [3 3], F);
%
% Vertical boundary detection
F1 = inline ('sum(x(1:3,2))-sum(x(1:3,1))');
I_vertical = nlfilter(I,[3 2], F1);
%
% Rescale all arrays
I_avg = mat2gray(I_avg);
I_diff = mat2gray(I_diff);
I_vertical = mat2gray(I_vertical);
%
subplot(3,2,1);                 % Display all images in a single
                                %  plot
   imshow(I);
   title('Original');
subplot(3,2,2);
   imshow(I_avg);
   title('Averaged');
subplot(3,2,3);
   imshow(I_diff);
   title('Differentiated');
subplot(3,2,4);
   imshow(I_vertical);
   title('Vertical boundaries');
subplot(3,2,5);
   bw = im2bw(I_vertical,.6);   % Threshold data, low threshold
   imshow(bw);
```

```
    title('Left boundaries');
subplot(3,2,6);
    bw1 = im2bw(I_vertical,.8);   % Threshold data, high
                                  %  threshold
    imshow(bw1);
    title('Right boundaries');
```

The code in Example 10.6 produces the images in Figure 10.9. These operations are quite time consuming: Example 10.6 took about 4 minutes to run on a 500 MHz PC. Techniques for increasing the speed of Sliding Operations can be found in the help file for `colfilt`. The vertical boundaries produced by the 3 by 2 sliding block are not very apparent in the intensity image, but become quite evident in the thresholded binary images. The averaging has improved contrast, but the resolution is reduced so that edges are no longer distinct.

Distinct Block Operations

All of the sliding neighborhood options can also be implemented using configurations of fixed blocks (Figure 10.10). Since these blocks do not slide, but are

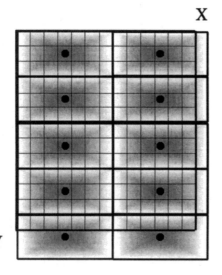

FIGURE 10.10 A 7-by-3 pixel *distinct block.* As with the sliding neighborhood block, these fixed blocks can fall off the picture and require padding (usually zero padding). The dot indicates the center pixel although this point usually has little significance in this approach.

fixed with respect to the image (although they may overlap), they will produce very different results. The MATLAB function for implementing *distinct block* operations is similar in format to the sliding neighborhood function:

```
I1 = blkproc(I, [M N], [Vo Ho], func);
```

where M and N specify the vertical and horizontal size of the block, Vo and Ho are optional arguments that specify the vertical and horizontal overlap of the block, func is the function that operates on the block, I is the input array, and I1 is the output array. As with nlfilter the data format of the output will depend on the output of the function. The function is specified in the same manner as described for nlfilter; however the function output will be different.

Function outputs for sliding neighborhood operations had to be single scalars that then became the value of the center pixel. In distinct block operations, the block does not move, so the function output will normally produce values for every pixel in the block. If the block produces a single output, then only the center pixel of each block will contain a meaningful value. If the function is an operation that normally produces a single value, the output of this routine can be expanded by multiplying it by an array of ones that is the same size as the block This will place that single output in every pixel in the block:

```
I1 = blkproc(I [4 5], 'std2 * ones(4,5)');
```

In this example the output of the MATLAB function std2 is placed into a 4 by 5 array and this becomes the output of the function, an array the same size as the block. It is also possible to use the inline function to describe the function:

```
F = inline('std2(x) * ones(size(x))');
I1 = blkproc(I, [4 5], F);
```

Of course, it is possible that certain operations could produce a different output for each pixel in the block. An example of block processing is given in Example 10.7.

Example 10.7   Load the blood cell image used in Example 10.6 and perform the following distinct block processing operations: 1) Display the average for a block size of 8 by 8; 2) For a 3 by 3 block, perform the differentiator operation used in Example 10.6; and 3) Apply the vertical boundary detector form Example 10.6 to a 3 by 3 block. Display all the images including the original in a single figure.

```
% Example 10.7 and Figure 10.11
% Demonstration of distinct block operations
% Load image of blood cells used in Example 10.6
% Use a 8 by 8 distinct block to get averages for the entire block
% Apply the 3 by 3 differentiator from Example 10.6 as a distinct
%   block operation.
% Apply a 3 by 3 vertical edge detector as a block operation
% Display the original and all modification on the same plot
%
..... Image load, same as in Example 10.6.......
%
```

Original

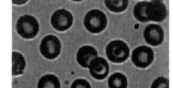

Averaged

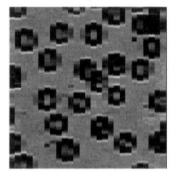

Differentiated

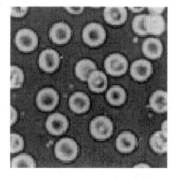

Vertical Edge

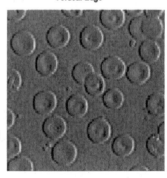

FIGURE 10.11   The blood cell image of Example 10.6 processed using three *Distinct block* operations: block averaging, block differentiation, and block vertical edge detection. (Original image reprinted from The Image Processing Handbook, 2nd edition. Copyright CRC Press, Boca Raton, Florida.)

```
% Perform the various distinct block operations.
% Average of the image
I_avg = blkproc(I,[10 10], 'mean2 * ones(10,10)');
%
% Deferentiator-place result in all blocks
F = inline('(x(2,2)-sum(x(1:3,1))/3- sum(x(1:3,3))/3 ...
      - x(1,2)-x(3,2)) * ones(size(x))');
I_diff = blkproc(I, [3 3], F);
%
% Vertical edge detector-place results in all blocks
F1 = inline('(sum(x(1:3,2))-sum(x(1:3,1))) ...
      * ones(size(x))');
I_vertical = blkproc(I, [3,2], F1);
........Rescale and plotting as in Example 10.6.......
```

Figure 10.11 shows the images produced by Example 10.7. The "differentiator" and edge detection operators look similar to those produced the Sliding Neighborhood operation because they operate on fairly small block sizes. The averaging operator shows images that appear to have large pixels since the neighborhood average is placed in block of 8 by 8 pixels.

The topics covered in this chapter provide a basic introduction to image processing and basic MATLAB formats and operations. In subsequent chapters we use this foundation to develop some useful image processing techniques such as filtering, Fourier and other transformations, and registration (alignment) of multiple images.

PROBLEMS

1. (A) Following the approach used in Example 10.1, generate an image that is a sinusoidal grating in both horizontal and vertical directions (it will look somewhat like a checkerboard). (*Hint*: This can be done with very few additional instructions.) (B) Combine this image with its inverse as a multiframe image and show it as a movie. Use multiple repetitions. The movie should look like a flickering checkerboard. Submit the two images.

2. Load the x-ray image of the spine (**spine.tif**) from the MATLAB Image Processing Toolbox. Slice the image into 4 different levels then plot in pseudocolor using yellow, red, green, and blue for each slice. The 0 level slice should be blue and the highest level slice should be yellow. Use **grayslice** and *construct you own colormap*. Plot original and sliced image in the same figure. (If the "original" image also displays in pseudocolor, it is because the computer display is using the same 3-level colormap for both images. In this case, you should convert the sliced image to RGB before displaying.)

3.   Load frame 20 from the MRI image (`mri.tif`) and code it in pseudocolor by coding the image into green and the inverse of the image into blue. Then take a threshold and plot pixels over 80% maximum as red.

4.   Load the image of a cancer cell (from rat prostate, courtesy of Alan W. Partin, M.D., Johns Hopkins University School of Medicine) `cell.tif` and apply a correction to the intensity values of the image (a *gamma correction* described in later chapters). Specifically, modify each pixel in the image by a function that is a quarter wave sine wave. That is, the corrected pixels are the output of the sine function of the input pixels: Out(m,n) = f(In(m,n)) (see plot below).

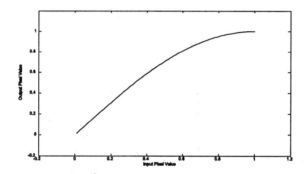

FIGURE PROB. 10.4   Correction function to be used in Problem 4. The input pixel values are on the horizontal axis, and the output pixels values are on the vertical axis.

5.   Load the blood cell image in `blood1.tif`. Write a sliding neighborhood function to enhance *horizontal* boundaries that go from dark to light. Write a second function that enhances boundaries that go from light to dark. Threshold both images so as to enhance the boundaries. Use a 3 by 2 sliding block. (*Hint*: This program may require several minutes to run. You do *not* need to rerun the program each time to adjust the threshold for the two binary images.)

6.   Load the blood cells in `blood.tif`. Apply a distinct block function that replaces all of the values within a block by the maximum value in that block. Use a 4 by 4 block size. Repeat the operation using a function that replaces all the values by the minimum value in the block.

11

Image Processing:
Filters, Transformations,
and Registration

SPECTRAL ANALYSIS: THE FOURIER TRANSFORM

The Fourier transform and the efficient algorithm for computing it, the fast Fourier transform, extend in a straightforward manner to two (or more) dimensions. The two-dimensional version of the Fourier transform can be applied to images providing a spectral analysis of the image content. Of course, the resulting spectrum will be in two dimensions, and usually it is more difficult to interpret than a one-dimensional spectrum. Nonetheless, it can be a very useful analysis tool, both for describing the contents of an image and as an aid in the construction of imaging filters as described in the next section. When applied to images, the spatial directions are equivalent to the time variable in the one-dimensional Fourier transform, and this analogous *spatial frequency* is given in terms of cycles/unit length (i.e., cycles/cm or cycles/inch) or normalized to cycles per sample. Many of the concerns raised with sampled time data apply to sampled spatial data. For example, undersampling an image will lead to aliasing. In such cases, the spatial frequency content of the original image is greater than $f_S/2$, where f_S now is 1/(pixel size). Figure 11.1 shows an example of aliasing in the frequency domain. The upper left-hand upper image contains a chirp signal increasing in spatial frequency from left to right. The high frequency elements on the right side of this image are adequately sampled in the left-hand image. The same pattern is shown in the upper right-hand image except that the sampling frequency has been reduced by a factor of 6. The right side of this image also contains sinusoidally varying intensities, but at additional frequencies as

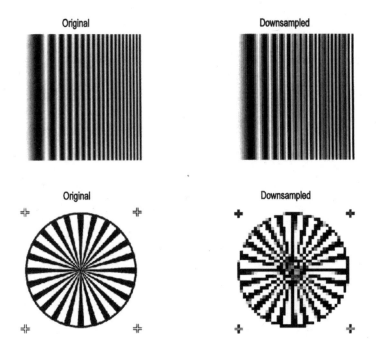

FIGURE 11.1 The influence of aliasing due to undersampling on two images with high spatial frequency. The aliased images show addition sinusoidal frequencies in the upper right image and jagged diagonals in the lower right image. (Lower original image from file 'testpostl.png' from the MATLAB Image Processing Toolbox. Copyright 1993–2003, The Math Works, Inc. Reprinted with permission.)

the aliasing folds other sinusoids on top of those in the original pattern. The lower figures show the influence of aliasing on a diagonal pattern. The jagged diagonals are characteristic of aliasing as are moire patterns seen in other images. The problem of determining an appropriate sampling size is even more acute in image acquisition since oversampling can quickly lead to excessive memory storage requirements.

The two-dimensional Fourier transform in continuous form is a direct extension of the equation given in Chapter 3:

$$F(\omega_1,\omega_2) = \int\limits_{m=-\infty}^{\infty} \int\limits_{n=-\infty}^{\infty} f(m,n)e^{-j\omega_1 m}e^{-j\omega_2 n}dm\ dn \tag{1}$$

The variables ω_1 and ω_2 are still frequency variables, although they define spatial frequencies and their units are in radians per sample. As with the time domain spectrum, $F(\omega_1,\omega_2)$ is a complex-valued function that is periodic in both ω_1 and ω_2. Usually only a single period of the spectral function is displayed, as was the case with the time domain analog.

The inverse two-dimensional Fourier transform is defined as:

$$f(m,n) = \frac{1}{4\pi^2} \int\limits_{\omega_1=-\pi}^{\pi} \int\limits_{\omega_2=-\pi}^{\pi} F(\omega_1,\omega_2)e^{-j\omega_1 m}e^{-j\omega_2 n}d\omega_1\, d\omega_2 \qquad (2)$$

As with the time domain equivalent, this statement is a reflection of the fact that any two-dimensional function can be represented by a series (possibly infinite) of sinusoids, but now the sinusoids extend over the two dimensions.

The discrete form of Eqs. (1) and (2) is again similar to their time domain analogs. For an image size of M by N, the discrete Fourier transform becomes:

$$F(p,q) = \sum_{m=0}^{M-1} \sum_{n=0}^{N-1} f(m,n)e^{-j(2\pi/M)p\, m}e^{-j(2\pi/N)q\, n} \qquad (3)$$

$$p = 0,1 \ldots, M-1; \qquad q = 0,1 \ldots, N-1$$

The values $F(p,q)$ are the Fourier Transform coefficients of $f(m,n)$. The discrete form of the inverse Fourier Transform becomes:

$$f(m,n) = \frac{1}{MN} \sum_{p=0}^{M-1} \sum_{q=0}^{N-1} F(p,q)e^{-j(2\pi/M)p\, m}e^{-j(2\pi/N)q\, n} \qquad (4)$$

$$m = 0,1 \ldots, M-1; \qquad n = 0,1 \ldots, N-1$$

MATLAB Implementation

Both the Fourier transform and inverse Fourier transform are supported in two (or more) dimensions by MATLAB functions. The two-dimensional Fourier transform is evoked as:

```
F = fft2(x,M,N);
```

where F is the output matrix and x is the input matrix. M and N are optional arguments that specify padding for the vertical and horizontal dimensions, respectively. In the time domain, the frequency spectrum of simple waveforms can usually be anticipated and the spectra of even relatively complicated waveforms can be readily understood. With two dimensions, it becomes more difficult to visualize the expected Fourier transform even of fairly simple images. In Example 11.1 a simple thin rectangular bar is constructed, and the Fourier transform of the object is constructed. The resultant spatial frequency function is plotted both as a three-dimensional function and as an intensity image.

Example 11.1 Determine and display the two-dimensional Fourier transform of a thin rectangular object. The object should be 2 by 10 pixels in size and solid white against a black background. Display the Fourier transform as both a function (i.e., as a mesh plot) and as an image plot.

```
% Example 11.1 Two-dimensional Fourier transform of a simple
%   object.
% Construct a simple 2 by 10 pixel rectangular object, or bar.
% Take the Fourier transform padded to 256 by 256 and plot the
%   result as a 3-dimensional function (using mesh) and as an
%   intensity image.
%
% Construct object
close all; clear all;
% Construct the rectangular object
f = zeros(22,30);        % Original figure can be small since it
f(10:12,10:20) = 1;      %  will be padded
  %
F = fft2(f,128,128);     % Take FT; pad to 128 by 128
F = abs(fftshift(F));,   % Shift center; get magnitude
%
imshow(f,'notruesize'); % Plot object
  .....labels..........
figure;
mesh(F);                 % Plot Fourier transform as function
  .......labels..........
figure;
F = log(F);              % Take log function
```

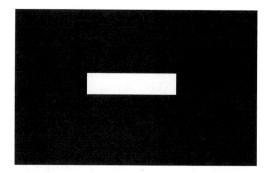

FIGURE 11.2A The rectangular object (2 pixels by 10 pixels used in Example 11.1. The Fourier transform of this image is shown in Figure 11.2B and C.

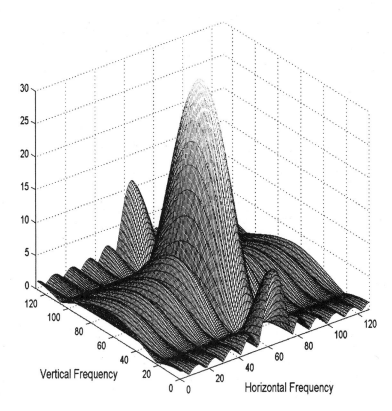

FIGURE 11.2B Fourier transform of the rectangular object in Figure 11.2A plotted as a function. More energy is seen, particularly at the higher frequencies, along the vertical axis because the object's vertical cross sections appear as a narrow pulse. The border horizontal cross sections produce frequency characteristics that fall off rapidly at higher frequencies.

```
I = mat2gray(F);        % Scale as intensity image
imshow(I);              % Plot Fourier transform as image
```

Note that in the above program the image size was kept small (22 by 30) since the image will be padded (with zeros, i.e., black) by 'fft2.' The fft2 routine places the DC component in the upper-left corner. The fftshift routine is used to shift this component to the center of the image for plotting purposes. The log of the function was taken before plotting as an image to improve the grayscale quality in the figure.

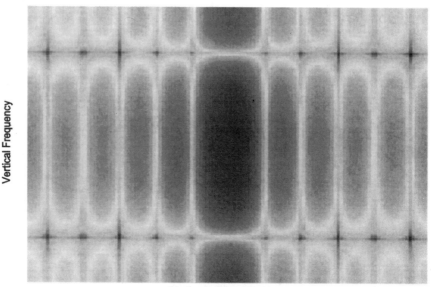

Vertical Frequency

Horizontal Frequency

FIGURE 11.2C   The Fourier transform of the rectangular object in Figure 11.2A plotted as an image. The log of the function was taken before plotting to improve the details. As in the function plot, more high frequency energy is seen in the vertical direction as indicated by the dark vertical band.

The horizontal chirp signal plotted in Figure 11.1 also produces a easily interpretable Fourier transform as shown in Figure 11.3. The fact that this image changes in only one direction, the horizontal direction, is reflected in the Fourier transform. The linear increase in spatial frequency in the horizontal direction produces an approximately constant spectral curve in that direction.

The two-dimensional Fourier transform is also useful in the construction and evaluation of linear filters as described in the following section.

LINEAR FILTERING

The techniques of linear filtering described in Chapter 4 can be directly extended to two dimensions and applied to images. In image processing, FIR filters are usually used because of their linear phase characteristics. Filtering an image is a local, or neighborhood, operation just as it was in signal filtering, although in this case the neighborhood extends in two directions around a given pixel. In image filtering, the value of a filtered pixel is determined from a linear combination of surrounding pixels. For the FIR filters described in Chapter 4,

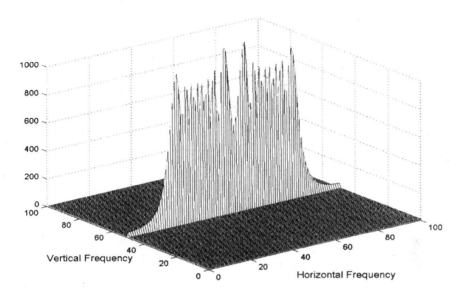

FIGURE 11.3 Fourier transform of the horizontal chirp signal shown in Figure 11.1. The spatial frequency characteristics of this image are zero in the vertical direction since the image is constant in this direction. The linear increase in spatial frequency in the horizontal direction is reflected in the more or less constant amplitude of the Fourier transform in this direction.

the linear combination for a given FIR filter was specified by the impulse response function, the filter coefficients, $b(n)$. In image filtering, the filter function exists in two dimensions, $h(m,n)$. These two-dimensional filter weights are applied to the image using convolution in an approach analogous to one-dimensional filtering.

The equation for two-dimensional convolution is a straightforward extension of the one-dimensional form (Eq. (15), Chapter 2):

$$y(m,n) = \sum_{k_1=-\infty}^{\infty} \sum_{k_2=-\infty}^{\infty} x(k_1, k_2) b(m - k_1, n - k_2) \tag{5}$$

While this equation would not be difficult to implement using MATLAB statements, MATLAB has a function that implements two-dimensional convolution directly.

Using convolution to perform image filtering parallels its use in signal imaging: the image array is convolved with a set of filter coefficients. However, in image analysis, the filter coefficients are defined in two dimensions, $h(m,n)$. A classic example of a digital image filter is the *Sobel* filter, a set of coefficients that perform a horizontal spatial derivative operation for enhancement of horizontal edges (or vertical edges if the coefficients are rotated using transposition):

$$h(m,n)_{\text{Sobel}} = \begin{bmatrix} 1 & 2 & 1 \\ 0 & 0 & 0 \\ -1 & -2 & -1 \end{bmatrix}.$$

These two-dimensional filter coefficients are sometimes referred to as the *convolution kernel*. An example of the application of a Sobel filter to an image is provided in Example 11.2.

When convolution is used to apply a series of weights to either image or signal data, the weights represent a two-dimensional impulse response, and, as with a one-dimensional impulse response, the weights are applied to the data in reverse order as indicated by the negative sign in the one- and two-dimensional convolution equations (Eq. (15) from Chapter 2 and Eq. (5).* This can become a source of confusion in two-dimensional applications. Image filtering is easier to conceptualize if the weights are applied directly to the image data in the same orientation. This is possible if digital filtering is implemented using *correlation* rather that convolution. Image filtering using correlation is a sliding neighborhood operation, where the value of the center pixel is just the weighted sum of neighboring pixels with the weighting given by the filter coefficients. When correlation is used, the set of weighting coefficients is termed the *correlation kernel* to distinguish it from the standard filter coefficients. In fact, the operations of correlation and convolution both involve weighted sums of neighboring pixels, and the only difference between correlation kernels and convolution kernels is a 180-degree rotation of the coefficient matrix. MATLAB filter routines use correlation kernels because their application is easier to conceptualize.

MATLAB Implementation

Two dimensional-convolution is implemented using the routine `conv2`:

```
I2 = conv2(I1, h, shape)
```

where `I1` and `h` are image and filter coefficients (or two images, or simply two matrices) to be convolved and **shape** is an optional argument that controls the size of the output image. If shape is `full`, the default, then the size of the output matrix follows the same rules as in one-dimensional convolution: each

---

*In one dimension, this is equivalent to applying the weights in reverse order. In two dimensions, this is equivalent to rotating the filter matrix by 180 degrees before multiplying corresponding pixels and coefficients.

dimension of the output is the sum of the two matrix lengths along that dimension minus one. Hence, if the two matrices have sizes I1(M1, N1) and h(M2, N2), the output size is: I2(M1 + M2 - 1, N2 + N2 - 1). If shape is 'valid', then any pixel evaluation that requires image padding is ignored and the size of the output image is: Ic(M1-M2 + 1, N1-N2 + 1). Finally, if **shape** is 'same' the size of the output matrix is the same size as I1; that is: I2(M1, N1). These options allow a great deal in flexibility and can simplify the use of two-dimensional convolution; for example, the 'same' option can eliminate the need for dealing with the additional points generated by convolution.

Two-dimensional correlation is implemented with the routine 'imfilter' that provides even greater flexibility and convenience in dealing with size and boundary effects. The calling structure of this routine is given in the next page.

```
I2 = imfilter(I1, h, options);
```

where again I1 and h are the input matrices and **options** can include up to three separate control options. One option controls the size of the output array using the same terms as in 'conv2' above: 'same' and 'full' ('valid' is not valid in this routine!). With 'imfilter' the default output size is 'same' (not 'full'), since this is the more likely option in image analysis. The second possible option controls how the edges are treated. If a constant is given, then the edges are padded with the value of that constant. The default is to use a constant of zero (i.e., standard zero padding). The boundary option 'symmetric' uses a mirror reflection of the end points as shown in Figure 2.10. Similarly the option 'circular' uses periodic extension also shown in Figure 2.10. The last boundary control option is 'replicate', which pads using the nearest edge pixel. When the image is large, the influence of the various border control options is subtle, as shown in Example 11.4. A final option specifies the use of convolution instead of correlation. If this option is activated by including the argument **conv**, imfilter is redundant with 'conv2' except for the options and defaults. The **imfilter** routine will accept all of the data format and types defined in the previous chapter and produces an output in the same format; however, filtering is not usually appropriate for indexed images. In the case of RGB images, **imfilter** operates on all three image planes.

Filter Design

The MATLAB Image Processing Toolbox provides considerable support for generating the filter coefficients.* A number of filters can be generated using MATLAB's **fspecial** routine:

---

*Since MATLAB's preferred implementation of image filters is through correlation, not convolution, MATLAB's filter design routines generate correlation kernels. We use the term "filter coefficient" for either kernel format.

```
h = fspecial(type, parameters);
```

where `type` specifies a specific filter and the optional parameters are related to the filter selected. Filter type options include: `'gaussian'`, `'disk'`, `'sobel'`, `'prewitt'`, `'laplacian'`, `'log'`, `'average'`, and `'unsharp'`. The `'gaussian'` option produces a Gaussian lowpass filter. The equation for a Gaussian filter is similar to the equation for the gaussian distribution:

$$h(m,n) = e^{-(d/\sigma)/2} \qquad \text{where} \quad d = \sqrt{(m^2 + n^2)}$$

This filter has particularly desirable properties when applied to an image: it provides an optimal compromise between smoothness and filter sharpness. The MATLAB routine for this filter accepts two parameters: the first specifies the filter size (the default is 3) and the second the value of sigma. The value of sigma will influence the cutoff frequency while the size of the filter determines the number of pixels over which the filter operates. In general, the size should be 3–5 times the value of sigma.

Both the `'sobel'` and `'prewitt'` options produce a 3 by 3 filter that enhances horizontal edges (or vertical if transposed). The `'unsharp'` filter produces a contrast enhancement filter. This filter is also termed *unsharp masking* because it actually suppresses low spatial frequencies where the low frequencies are presumed to be the unsharp frequencies. In fact, it is a special highpass filter. This filter has a parameter that specifies the shape of the highpass characteristic. The `'average'` filter simply produces a constant set of weights each of which equals $1/N$, where N = the number of elements in the filter (the default size of this filter is 3 by 3, in which case the weights are all $1/9 = 0.1111$). The filter coefficients for a 3 by 3 Gaussian lowpass filter (sigma = 0.5) and the unsharpe filter (alpha = 0.2) are shown below:

$$h_{\text{unsharp}} = \begin{bmatrix} -0.1667 & -0.6667 & -0.1667 \\ -0.6667 & 4.3333 & -0.6667 \\ -0.1667 & -0.6667 & -0.1667 \end{bmatrix}; \quad h_{\text{gaussian}} = \begin{bmatrix} 0.0113 & 0.0838 & 0.0113 \\ 0.0838 & 0.6193 & 0.0838 \\ 0.0113 & 0.0838 & 0.0113 \end{bmatrix}$$

The *Laplacian* filter is used to take the second derivative of an image: $\partial^2/\partial x$. The *log* filter is actually the *log of Gaussian* filter and is used to take the first derivative, $\partial/\partial x$, of an image.

MATLAB also provides a routine to transform one-dimensional FIR filters, such as those described in Chapter 4, into two-dimensional filters. This approach is termed the *frequency transform* method and preserves most of the characteristics of the one-dimensional filter including the transition bandwidth and ripple features. The frequency transformation method is implemented using:

```
h = ftrans2(b);
```

where **h** are the output filter coefficients (given in correlation kernel format), and **b** are the filter coefficients of a one-dimensional filter. The latter could be produced by any of the FIR routines described in Chapter 4 (i.e., **fir1**, **fir2**, or **remez**). The function **ftrans2** can take an optional second argument that specifies the transformation matrix, the matrix that converts the one-dimensional coefficients to two dimensions. The default transformation is the *McClellan transformation* that produces a nearly circular pattern of filter coefficients. This approach brings a great deal of power and flexibility to image filter design since it couples all of the FIR filter design approaches described in Chapter 4 to image filtering.

The two-dimensional Fourier transform described above can be used to evaluate the frequency characteristics of a given filter. In addition, MATLAB supplies a two-dimensional version of **freqz**, termed **freqz2**, that is slightly more convenient to use since it also handles the plotting. The basic call is:

```
[H fx fy]  =  freqz2(h, Ny, Nx);.
```

where **h** contains the two-dimensional filter coefficients and **Nx** and **Ny** specify the size of the desired frequency plot. The output argument, **H**, contains the two-dimensional frequency spectra and **fx** and **fy** are plotting vectors; however, if **freqz2** is called with no output arguments then it generates the frequency plot directly. The examples presented below do not take advantage of this function, but simply use the two-dimensional Fourier transform for filter evaluation.

Example 11.2   This is an example of linear filtering using two of the filters in **fspecial**. Load one frame of the MRI image set (**mri.tif**) and apply the sharpening filter, $h_{unsharp}$, described above. Apply a horizontal Sobel filter, h_{Sobel}, (also shown above), to detect horizontal edges. Then apply the Sobel filter to detect the vertical edges and combine the two edge detectors. Plot both the horizontal and combined edge detectors.

Solution   To generate the vertical Sobel edge detector, simply transpose the horizontal Sobel filter. While the two Sobel images could be added together using **imadd,** the program below first converts both images to binary then combines them using a logical or. This produces a more dramatic black and white image of the boundaries.

```
% Example 11.2 and Figure 11.4A and B
% Example of linear filtering using selected filters from the
%   MATLAB 'fspecial' function.
% Load one frame of the MRI image and apply the 3 by 3 "unshape"
%   contrast enhancement filter shown in the text. Also apply two
```

Original

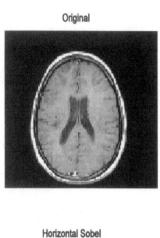

Unsharp

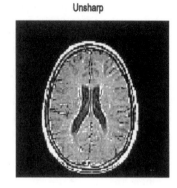

Horizontal Sobel

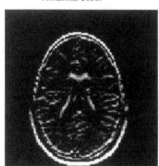

Combined Image

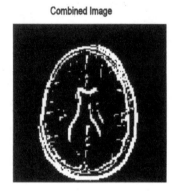

FIGURE 11.4A   MRI image of the brain before and after application of two filters from MATLAB's `fspecial` routine. Upper right: Image sharpening using the filter `unsharp`. Lower images: Edge detection using the `sobel` filter for horizontal edges (left) and for both horizontal and vertical edges (right). (Original image from MATLAB. Image Processing Toolbox. Copyright 1993–2003, The Math Works, Inc. Reprinted with permission.)

```
%   3 by 3 Sobel edge detector filters to enhance horizontal and
%   vertical edges.
% Combine the two edge detected images
%
clear all; close all;
%
frame = 17;                                    % Load MRI frame 17
[I(:,:,:,1), map ] = imread('mri.tif', frame);
```

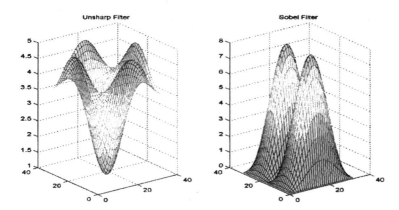

FIGURE 11.4B Frequency characteristics of the unsharp and Sobel filters used in Example 11.2.

```
if isempty(map) == 0              % Usual check and
    I = ind2gray(I,map);          %   conversion if
                                  %   necessary.
else
    I = im2double(I);
end
%
h_unsharp = fspecial('unsharp',.5);   % Generate 'unsharp'
I_unsharp = imfilter(I,h_unsharp);    %   filter coef. and
                                      %   apply
%
h_s = fspecial('Sobel');              % Generate basic Sobel
                                      %   filter.
I_sobel_horin = imfilter(I,h_s);      % Apply to enhance
I_sobel_vertical = imfilter(I,h_s');  %   horizontal and
                                      %   vertical edges
%
% Combine by converting to binary and or-ing together
I_sobel_combined = im2bw(I_sobel_horin) | ...
    im2bw(I_sobel_vertical);
%
subplot(2,2,1); imshow(I);            % Plot the images
    title('Original');
subplot(2,2,2); imshow(I_unsharp);
    title('Unsharp');
subplot(2,2,3); imshow(I_sobel_horin);
```

```
title('Horizontal Sobel');
subplot(2,2,4); imshow(I_sobel_combined);
  title('Combined Image'); figure;
%
% Now plot the unsharp and Sobel filter frequency
% characteristics
F= fftshift(abs(fft2(h_unsharp,32,32)));
subplot(1,2,1); mesh(1:32,1:32,F);
  title('Unsharp Filter'); view([-37,15]);
%
F = fftshift(abs(fft2(h_s,32,32)));
subplot(1,2,2); mesh(1:32,1:32,F);
  title('Sobel Filter'); view([-37,15]);
```

The images produced by this example program are shown below along with the frequency characteristics associated with the 'unsharp' and 'sobel' filter. Note that the 'unsharp' filter has the general frequency characteristics of a highpass filter, that is, a positive slope with increasing spatial frequencies (Figure 11.4B). The double peaks of the Sobel filter that produce edge enhancement are evident in Figure 11.4B. Since this is a magnitude plot, both peaks appear as positive.

In Example 11.3, routine ftrans2 is used to construct two-dimensional filters from one-dimensional FIR filters. Lowpass and highpass filters are constructed using the filter design routine fir1 from Chapter 4. This routine generates filter coefficients based on the ideal rectangular window approach described in that chapter. Example 11.3 also illustrates the use of an alternate padding technique to reduce the edge effects caused by zero padding. Specifically, the 'replicate' option of imfilter is used to pad by repetition of the last (i.e., image boundary) pixel value. This eliminates the dark border produced by zero padding, but the effect is subtle.

Example 11.3   Example of the application of standard one-dimensional FIR filters extended to two dimensions. The blood cell images (blood1.tif) are loaded and filtered using a 32 by 32 lowpass and highpass filter. The one-dimensional filter is based on the rectangular window filter (Eq. (10), Chapter 4), and is generated by fir. It is then extended to two dimensions using ftrans2.

```
% Example 11.3 and Figure 11.5A and B
% Linear filtering. Load the blood cell image
% Apply a 32nd order lowpass filter having a bandwidth of .125
%  fs/2, and a highpass filter having the same order and band-
%  width. Implement the lowpass filter using 'imfilter' with the
```

Original

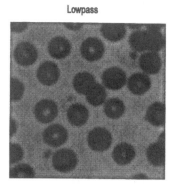

Lowpass

Replicated Boundary

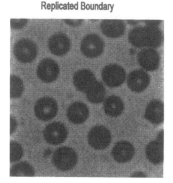

Highpass

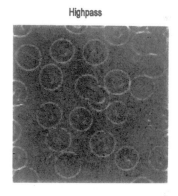

FIGURE 11.5A Image of blood cells before and after lowpass and highpass filtering. The upper lowpass image (upper right) was filtered using zero padding, which produces a slight black border around the image. Padding by extending the edge pixel eliminates this problem (lower left). (Original Image reprinted with permission from The Image Processing Handbook, 2nd edition. Copyright CRC Press, Boca Raton, Florida.)

```
%   zero padding (the default) and with replicated padding
%   (extending the final pixels).
% Plot the filter characteristics of the high and low pass filters
%
% Load the image and transform if necessary
clear all; close all;
N = 32;                          % Filter order
w_lp = .125;                     % Lowpass cutoff frequency
```

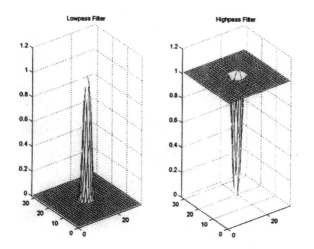

FIGURE 11.5B Frequency characteristics of the lowpass (left) and highpass (right) filters used in Figure 11.5A.

```
w_hp = .125;                    % Highpass cutoff frequency
.......load image blood1.tif and convert as in Example
    11.2 ......
%
b = fir1(N,w_lp);              % Generate the lowpass filter
h_lp = ftrans2(b);            % Convert to 2-dimensions
I_lowpass = imfilter(I,h_lp);   %  and apply with,
%  and without replication
I_lowpass_rep = imfilter (I,h_lp,'replicate');
b = fir1(N,w_hp,'high');      % Repeat for highpass
h_hp = ftrans2(b);
I_highpass = imfilter(I, h_hp);
I_highpass = mat2gray(I_highpass);
%
........plot the images and filter characteristics as in
    Example 11.2.......
```

The figures produced by this program are shown below (Figure 11.5A and B). Note that there is little difference between the image filtered using zero padding and the one that uses extended ('replicate') padding. The highpass filtered image shows a slight derivative-like characteristic that enhances edges. In the plots of frequency characteristics, Figure 11.5B, the lowpass and highpass filters appear to be circular, symmetrical, and near opposites.

The problem of aliasing due to downsampling was discussed above and demonstrated in Figure 11.1. Such problems could occur whenever an image is displayed in a smaller size that will require fewer pixels, for example when the size of an image is reduced during reshaping of a computer window. Lowpass filtering can be, and is, used to prevent aliasing when an image is downsized. In fact, MATLAB automatically performs lowpass filtering when downsizing an image. Example 11.4 demonstrates the ability of lowpass filtering to reduce aliasing when downsampling is performed.

Example 11.4 Use lowpass filtering to reduce aliasing due to downsampling. Load the radial pattern (`'testpat1.png'`) and downsample by a factor of six as was done in Figure 11.1. In addition, downsample that image by the same amount, but after it has been lowpass filtered. Plot the two downsampled images side-by-side. Use a 32 by 32 FIR rectangular window lowpass filter. Set the cutoff frequency to be as high as possible and still eliminate most of the aliasing.

```
% Example 11.4 and Figure 11.6
% Example of the ability of lowpass filtering to reduce aliasing.
% Downsample the radial pattern with and without prior lowpass
%   filtering.
% Use a cutoff frequency sufficient to reduce aliasing.
%
clear all; close all;
N = 32;                      % Filter order
w = .5;                      % Cutoff frequency (see text)
```

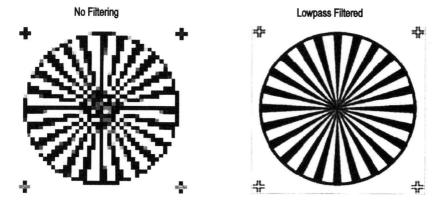

FIGURE 11.6 Two images of the radial pattern shown in Figure 11.1 after downsampling by a factor of 6. The right-hand image was filtered by a lowpass filter before downsampling.

```
dwn = 6;                          % Downsampling coefficient
b = fir1(N,w);                    % Generate the lowpass filter
h = ftrans2(b);                   % Convert to 2-dimensions
%
[Imap] = imread('testpat1.png'); % Load image
I_lowpass = imfilter(I,h);       % Lowpass filter image
[M,N] = size(I);
%
I = I(1:dwn:M,1:dwn:N);          % Downsample unfiltered image
subplot (1,2,1); imshow(I);      %  and display
  title('No Filtering');
% Downsample filtered image and display
I_lowass = I_lowpass(1:dwn: M,1:dwn:N);
subplot(1,2,2); imshow(I_lowpass);
  title ('Lowpass Filtered');
```

The lowpass cutoff frequency used in Example 11.5 was determined empirically. Although the cutoff frequency was fairly high ($f_S/4$), this filter still produced substantial reduction in aliasing in the downsampled image.

SPATIAL TRANSFORMATIONS

Several useful transformations take place entirely in the spatial domain. Such transformations include image resizing, rotation, cropping, stretching, shearing, and image projections. Spatial transformations perform a remapping of pixels and often require some form of interpolation in addition to possible anti-aliasing. The primary approach to anti-aliasing is lowpass filtering, as demonstrated above. For interpolation, there are three methods popularly used in image processing, and MATLAB supports all three. All three interpolation strategies use the same basic approach: the interpolated pixel in the output image is the weighted sum of pixels in the vicinity of the original pixel after transformation. The methods differ primarily in how many neighbors are considered.

As mentioned above, spatial transforms involve a remapping of one set of pixels (i.e., image) to another. In this regard, the original image can be considered as the input to the remapping process and the transformed image is the output of this process. If images were continuous, then remapping would not require interpolation, but the discrete nature of pixels usually necessitates remapping.* The simplest interpolation method is the *nearest neighbor* method in which the output pixel is assigned the value of the closest pixel in the transformed image, Figure 11.7. If the transformed image is larger than the original and involves more pixels, then a remapped input pixel may fall into two or

---

*A few transformations may not require interpolation such as rotation by 90 or 180 degrees.

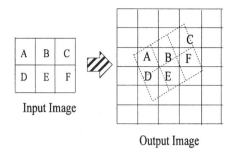

FIGURE 11.7 A rotation transform using the nearest neighbor interpolation method. Pixel values in the output image (solid grid) are assigned values from the nearest pixel in the transformed input image (dashed grid).

more output pixels. In the bilinear interpolation method, the output pixel is the weighted average of transformed pixels in the nearest 2 by 2 neighborhood, and in bicubic interpolation the weighted average is taken over a 4 by 4 neighborhood.

Computational complexity and accuracy increase with the number of pixels that are considered in the interpolation, so there is a trade-off between quality and computational time. In MATLAB, the functions that require interpolation have an optional argument that specifies the method. For most functions, the default method is nearest neighbor. This method produces acceptable results on all image classes and is the only method appropriate for indexed images. The method is also the most appropriate for binary images. For RGB and intensity image classes, the bilinear or bicubic interpolation method is recommended since they lead to better results.

MATLAB provides several routines that can be used to generate a variety of complex spatial transformations such as image projections or specialized distortions. These transformations can be particularly useful when trying to overlay (register) images of the same structure taken at different times or with different modalities (e.g., PET scans and MRI images). While MATLAB's spatial transformations routines allow for any imaginable transformation, only two types of transformation will be discussed here: *affine* transformations and *projective* transformations. Affine transformations are defined as transformations in which straight lines remain straight and parallel lines remain parallel, but rectangles may become parallelograms. These transformations include rotation, scaling, stretching, and shearing. In projective translations, straight lines still remain straight, but parallel lines often converge toward *vanishing points*. These transformations are discussed in the following MATLAB implementation section.

MATLAB Implementation

Affine Transformations

MATLAB provides a procedure described below for implementing any affine transformation; however, some of these transformations are so popular they are supported by separate routines. These include image resizing, cropping, and rotation. Image resizing and cropping are both techniques to change the dimensions of an image: the latter is interactive using the mouse and display while the former is under program control. To change the size of an image, MATLAB provides the 'imresize' command given below.

```
I_resize = imresize(I, arg or [M N], method);
```

where I is the original image and I_resize is the resized image. If the second argument is a scalar arg, then it gives a magnification factor, and if it is a vector, [M N], it indicates the desired new dimensions in vertical and horizontal pixels, *M*, *N*. If arg > 1, then the image is increased (magnified) in size proportionally and if arg < 1, it is reduced in size (minified). This will change image size proportionally. If the vector [M N] is used to specify the output size, image proportions can be modified: the image can be stretched or compressed along a given dimension. The argument method specifies the type of interpolation to be used and can be either 'nearest', 'bilinear', or 'bicubic', referring to the three interpolation methods described above. The nearest neighbor (nearest) is the default. If image size is reduced, then imresize automatically applies an anti- aliasing, lowpass filter unless the interpolation method is nearest; i.e., the default. The logic of this is that the nearest neighbor interpolation method would usually only be used with indexed images, and lowpass filtering is not really appropriate for these images.

Image cropping is an interactive command:

```
I_resize = imcrop;
```

The imcrop routine waits for the operator to draw an on-screen cropping rectangle using the mouse. The current image is resized to include only the image within the rectangle.

Image rotation is straightforward using the imrotate command:

```
I_rotate = imrotate(I, deg, method, bbox);
```

where I is the input image, I_rotate is the rotated image, deg is the degrees of rotation (counterclockwise if positive, and clockwise if negative), and method describes the interpolation method as in imresize. Again, the nearest neighbor method is the default even though the other methods are preferred except for indexed images. After rotation, the image will not, in general, fit into the same rectangular boundary as the original image. In this situation, the rotated image can be cropped to fit within the original boundaries or the image size can be increased to fit the rotated image. Specifying the bbox argument as 'crop' will produce a cropped image having the dimensions of the original image, while setting bbox to 'loose' will produce a larger image that contains the entire original, unrotated, image. The loose option is the default. In either case, additional pixels will be required to fit the rotated image into a rectangular space (except for orthogonal rotations), and imrotate pads these with zeros producing a black background to the rotated image (see Figure 11.8).

Application of the imresize and imrotate routines is shown in Example 11.5 below. Application of imcrop is presented in one of the problems at the end of this chapter.

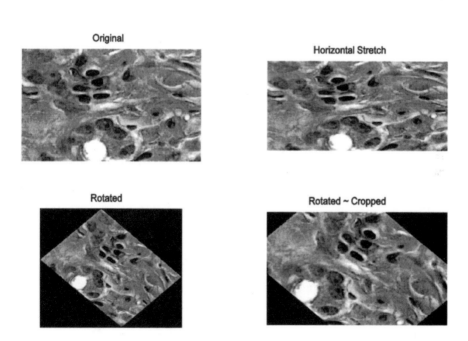

FIGURE 11.8 Two spatial transformations (horizontal stretching and rotation) applied to an image of bone marrow. The rotated images are cropped either to include the full image (lower left), or to have the same dimensions are the original image (lower right). Stained image courtesy of Alan W. Partin, M.D., Ph.D., Johns Hopkins University School of Medicine.

Example 11.5   Demonstrate resizing and rotation spatial transformations. Load the image of stained tissue (`hestain.png`) and transform it so that the horizontal dimension is 25% longer than in the original, keeping the vertical dimension unchanged. Rotate the original image 45 degrees clockwise, with and without cropping. Display the original and transformed images in a single figure.

```
% Example 11.5 and Figure 11.8
% Example of various Spatial Transformations
% Input the image of bone marrow (bonemarr.tif) and perform
%   two spatial transformations:
%   1) Stretch the object by 25% in the horizontal direction;
%   2) Rotate the image clockwise by 30 deg. with and without
%   cropping.
% Display the original and transformed images.
%
.......read image and convert if necessary .......
%
% Rotate image with and without cropping
I_rotate = imrotate(I,-45,'bilinear');
I_rotate_crop = imrotate (I, -45, 'bilinear', 'crop');
%
[M N] = size(I);
% Stretch by 25% horin.
I_stretch = imresize (I,[M N*1.25], 'bilinear');
%
.......display the images .........
```

The images produced by this code are shown in Figure 11.8.

General Affine Transformations

In the MATLAB Image Processing Toolbox, both affine and projective spatial transformations are defined by a `Tform` structure which is constructed using one of two routines: the routine `maketform` uses parameters supplied by the user to construct the transformation while `cp2tform` uses control points, or *landmarks*, placed on different images to generate the transformation. Both routines are very flexible and powerful, but that also means they are quite involved. This section describes aspects of the `maketform` routine, while the `cp2tfrom` routine will be presented in context with image registration.

Irrespective of the way in which the desired transformation is specified, it is implemented using the routine `imtransform`. This routine is only slightly less complicated than the transformation specification routines, and only some of its features will be discussed here. (The associated help file should be consulted for more detail.) The basic calling structure used to implement the spatial transformation is:

```
B = imtransform(A, Tform, 'Param1', value1, 'Param2',
   value2,....);
```

where A and B are the input and output arrays, respectively, and Tform provides the transformation specifications as generated by maketform or cp2tform. The additional arguments are optional. The optional parameters are specified as pairs of arguments: a string containing the name of the optional parameter (i.e., 'Param1') followed by the value.* These parameters can (1) specify the pixels to be used from the input image (the default is the entire image), (2) permit a change in pixel size, (3) specify how to fill any extra background pixels generated by the transformation, and (4) specify the size and range of the output array. Only the parameters that specify output range will be discussed here, as they can be used to override the automatic rescaling of image size performed by imtransform. To specify output image range and size, parameters 'XData' and 'YData' are followed by a two-variable vector that gives the x or y coordinates of the first and last elements of the output array, B. To keep the size and range in the output image the same as the input image, simply specify the horizontal and vertical size of the input array, i.e.:

```
[M N] = size(A);
...
B = imtransform(A, Tform, 'Xdata', [1 N], 'Ydata', [1 M]);
```

As with the transform specification routines, imtransform uses the *spatial coordinate system* described at the beginning of the Chapter 10. In this system, the first dimension is the x coordinate while the second is the y, the reverse of the matrix subscripting convention used by MATLAB. (However the y coordinate still increases in the downward direction.) In addition, non-integer values for x and y indexes are allowed.

The routine maketform can be used to generate the spatial transformation descriptor, Tform. There are two alternative approaches to specifying the transformation, but the most straightforward uses simple geometrical objects to define the transformation. The calling structure under this approach is:

```
Tform = maketform('type', U, X);
```

where 'type' defines the type of transformation and U and X are vectors that define the specific transformation by defining the input (U) and output (X) geometries. While maketform supports a variety of transformation types, including

---

*This is a common approach used in many MATLAB routines when a large number of arguments are possible, especially when many of these arguments are optional. It allows the arguments to be specified in any order.

custom, user-defined types, only the affine and projective transformations will be discussed here. These are specified by the `type` parameters `'affine'` and `'projective'`.

Only three points are required to define an affine transformation, so, for this transformation type, U and X define corresponding vertices of input and output triangles. Specifically, U and X are 3 by 2 matrices where each 2-column row defines a corresponding vertex that maps input to output geometry. For example, to stretch an image vertically, define an output triangle that is taller than the input triangle. Assuming an input image of size M by N, to increase the vertical dimension by 50% define input (`U`) and output (`X`) triangles as:

```
U = [1, 1; 1, M; N, M]'    X = [1, 1-.5M; 1, M; N, M];
```

In this example, the input triangle, `U`, is simply the upper left, lower left, and lower right corners of the image. The output triangle, `X`, has its top, left vertex increased by 50%. (Recall the coordinate pairs are given as x,y and y increases negatively. Note that negative coordinates are acceptable). To increase the vertical dimension symmetrically, change `X` to:

```
X = [1, 1-.25M; 1, 1.25*M; N, 1.25*M];
```

In this case, the upper vertex is increased by only 25%, and the two lower vertexes are lowered in the y direction by increasing the y coordinate value by 25%. This transformation could be done with `imresize`, but this would also change the dimension of the output image. When this transform is implemented with `imtransform`, it is possible to control output size as described below. Hence this approach, although more complicated, allows greater control of the transformation. Of course, if output image size is kept the same, the contents of the original image, when stretched, may exceed the boundaries of the image and will be lost. An example of the use of this approach to change image proportions is given in Problem 6.

The `maketform` routine can be used to implement other affine transformations such as *shearing*. For example, to shear an image to the left, define an output triangle that is skewed by the desired amount with respect to the input triangle, Figure 11.9. In Figure 11.9, the input triangle is specified as: `U = [N/2 1; 1 M; N M]`, (solid line) and the output triangle as `X = [1 1; 1 M; N M]` (solid line). This shearing transform is implemented in Example 11.6.

Projective Transformations

In *projective* transformations, straight lines remain straight but parallel lines may converge. Projective transformations can be used to give objects perspective. Projective transformations require *four points* for definition; hence, the

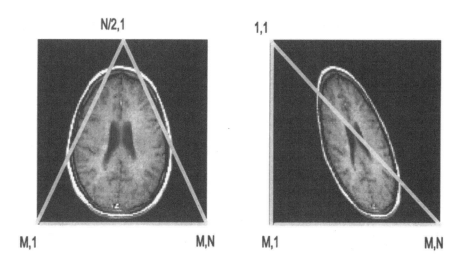

FIGURE 11.9 An affine transformation can be defined by three points. The transformation shown here is defined by an input (left) and output (right) triangle and produces a sheared image. *M,N* are indicated in this figure as row, column, but are actually specified in the algorithm in reverse order, as *x,y*. (Original image from the MATLAB Image Processing Toolbox. Copyright 1993–2003, The Math Work, Inc. Reprinted with permission.)

defining geometrical objects are quadrilaterals. Figure 11.10 shows a projective transformation in which the original image would appear to be tilted back. In this transformation, vertical lines in the original image would converge in the transformed image. In addition to adding perspective, these transformations are of value in correcting for relative tilts between image planes during image registration. In fact, most of these spatial transformations will be revisited in the section on image registration. Example 11.6 illustrates the use of these general image transformations for affine and projective transformations.

Example 11.6 General spatial transformations. Apply the affine and projective spatial transformation to one frame of the MRI image in `mri.tif`. The affine transformation should skew the top of the image to the left, just as shown in Figure 11.9. The projective transformation should tilt the image back as shown in Figure 11.10. This example will also use projective transformation to tilt the image forward, or opposite to that shown in Figure 11.10.

After the image is loaded, the affine input triangle is defined as an equilateral triangle inscribed within the full image. The output triangle is defined by shifting the top point to the left side, so the output triangle is now a right triangle (see Figure 11.9). In the projective transformation, the input quadrilateral is a

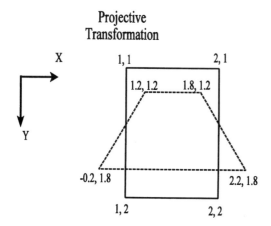

FIGURE 11.10 Specification of a projective transformation by defining two quadrilaterals. The solid lines define the input quadrilateral and the dashed line defines the desired output quadrilateral.

rectangle the same size as the input image. The output quadrilateral is generated by moving the upper points inward and down by an equal amount while the lower points are moved outward and up, also by a fixed amount. The second projective transformation is achieved by reversing the operations performed on the corners.

```
% Example 11.6 General Spatial Transformations
% Load a frame of the MRI image (mri.tif)
%   and perform two spatial transformations
%   1) An affine transformation that shears the image to the left
%   2) A projective transformation that tilts the image backward
%   3) A projective transformation that tilts the image forward
clear all; close all;
%
%   .......load frame 18 .......
%
% Define affine transformation
U1 = [N/2 1; 1 M; N M];         % Input triangle
X1 = [1 1; 1 M; N M];           % Output triangle
% Generate transform
Tform1 = maketform('affine', U1, X1);
% Apply transform
I_affine = imtransform(I, Tform1, 'Size', [M N]);
%
% Define projective transformation vectors
offset = .25*N;
U = [1 1; 1 M; N M; N 1];       % Input quadrilateral
```

```
X = [1-offset 1+offset; 1+offset M-offset; ...
  N-offset M-offset; N+offset 1+offset];
%
% Define transformation based on vectors U and X
Tform2 = maketform('projective', U, X);
I_proj1 = imtransform(I,Tform2,'Xdata',[1 N],'Ydata', ...
  [1 M]);
%
% Second transformation. Define new output quadrilateral
X = [1+offset 1+offset; 1-offset M-offset; ...
  N+offset M-offset; N-offset 1+offset];
% Generate transform
Tform3 = maketform('projective', U, X);
% Apply transform
I_proj2 = imtransform(I,Tform3, 'Xdata',[1 N],
  'Ydata',[1 M]);
%
.......display images .......
```

The images produced by this code are shown in Figure 11.11.

Of course, a great many other transforms can be constructed by redefining the output (or input) triangles or quadrilaterals. Some of these alternative transformations are explored in the problems.

All of these transforms can be applied to produce a series of images having slightly different projections. When these multiple images are shown as a movie, they will give an object the appearance of moving through space, perhaps in three dimensions. The last three problems at the end of this chapter explore these features. The following example demonstrates the construction of such a movie.

Example 11.7 Construct a series of projective transformations, that when shown as a movie, give the appearance of the image tilting backward in space. Use one of the frames of the MRI image.

Solution The code below uses the projective transformation to generate a series of images that appear to tilt back because of the geometry used. The approach is based on the second projective transformation in Example 11.7, but adjusts the transformation to produce a slightly larger apparent tilt in each frame. The program fills 24 frames in such a way that the first 12 have increasing angles of tilt and the last 12 frames have decreasing tilt. When shown as a movie, the image will appear to rock backward and forward. This same approach will also be used in Problem 7. Note that as the images are being generated by imtransform, they are converted to indexed images using gray2ind since this is the format required by immovie. The grayscale map generated by gray2ind is used (at the default level of 64), but any other map could be substituted in immovie to produce a pseudocolor image.

Original

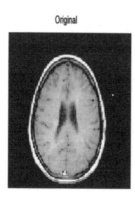

Affine Transformation

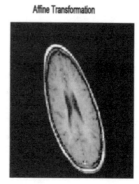

Projective Transformation 1

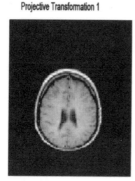

Projective Transformation 2

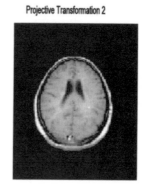

FIGURE 11.11 Original MR image and three spatial transformations. Upper right: An affine transformation that shears the image to the left. Lower left: A projective transform in which the image is made to appear tilted forward. Lower right: A projective transformation in which the image is made to appear tilted backward. (Original image from the MATLAB Image Processing Toolbox, Copyright 1993–2003, The Math Works, Inc. Reprinted with permission.)

```
% Example 11.7 Spatial Transformation movie
% Load a frame of the MRI image (mri.tif). Use the projective
%  transformation to make a movie of the image as it tilts
%  horizontally.
%
clear all; close all;
Nu_frame = 12;              % Number of frames in each direction
Max_tilt = .5;              % Maximum tilt achieved
    ........load MRI frame 12 as in previous examples .......
```

```
%
U = [1 1; 1 M; N M; N 1];      % Input quadrilateral
for i = 1:Nu_frame              % Construct Nu_frame * 2 movie frames
% Define projective transformation Vary offset up to Max_tilt
  offset = Max_tilt*N*i/Nu_frame;
  X = [1+offset 1+offset; 1-offset M-offset; N+offset ...
    M-offset; N-offset...1+offset];
  Tform2 = maketform('projective', U, X);
  [I_proj(:,:,1,i), map] = gray2ind(imtransform(I,Tform2,...
    'Xdata',[1 N],'Ydata',[1 M]));
  % Make image tilt back and forth
  I_proj(:,:,1,2*Nu_frame+1-i) = I_proj(:,:,1,i);
end
%
% Display first 12 images as a montage
montage(I_proj(:,:,:,1:12),map);
mov = immovie(I_proj,map);     % Display as movie
movie(mov,5);
```

While it is not possible to show the movie that is produced by this code, the various frames are shown as a montage in Figure 11.12. The last three problems in the problem set explore the use of spatial transformations used in combination to make movies.

IMAGE REGISTRATION

Image registration is the alignment of two or more images so they best superimpose. This task has become increasingly important in medical imaging as it is used for merging images acquired using different modalities (for example, MRI and PET). Registration is also useful for comparing images taken of the same structure at different points in time. In functional magnetic resonance imaging (fMRI), image alignment is needed for images taken sequentially in time as well as between images that have different resolutions. To achieve the best alignment, it may be necessary to transform the images using any or all of the transformations described previously. Image registration can be quite challenging even when the images are identical or very similar (as will be the case in the examples and problems given here). Frequently the images to be aligned are not that similar, perhaps because they have been acquired using different modalities. The difficulty in accurately aligning images that are only moderately similar presents a significant challenge to image registration algorithms, so the task is often aided by a human intervention or the use of embedded markers for reference.

Approaches to image registration can be divided into two broad categories: unassisted image registration where the algorithm generates the alignment without human intervention, and interactive registration where a human operator

Tilting Brain Movie

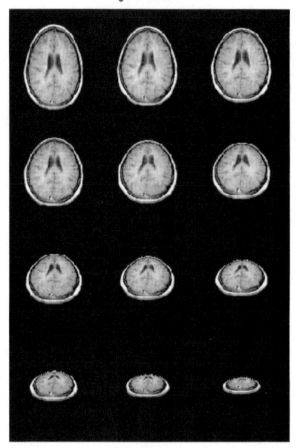

FIGURE 11.12 Montage display of the movie produced by the code in Example 11.7. The various projections give the appearance of the brain slice tilting and moving back in space. Only half the 24 frames are shown here as the rest are the same, just presented in reverse order to give the appearance of the brain rocking back and forth. (Original image from the MATLAB Image Processing Toolbox. Copyright 1993–2003, The Math Works, Inc. Reprinted with permission.)

guides or aids the registration process. The former approach usually relies on some optimization technique to maximize the correlation between the images. In the latter approach, a human operator may aid the alignment process by selecting corresponding reference points in the images to be aligned: corresponding features are identified by the operator and tagged using some interactive graphics procedure. This approach is well supported in MATLAB's Image Processing Toolbox. Both of these approaches are demonstrated in the examples and problems.

Unaided Image Registration

Unaided image registration usually involves the application of an optimization algorithm to maximize the correlation, or other measure of similarity, between the images. In this strategy, the appropriate transformation is applied to one of the images, the *input image*, and a comparison is made between this transformed image and the *reference image* (also termed the *base image*). The optimization routine seeks to vary the transformation in some manner until the comparison is best possible. The problem with this approach is the same as with all optimization techniques: the optimization process may converge on a sub-optimal solution (a so-called *local maximum*), not the optimal solution (the *global maximum*). Often the solution achieved depends on the starting values of the transformation variables. An example of convergence to a sub-optimal solution and dependency on initial variables is found in Problem 8.

Example 11.8 below uses the optimization routine that is part of the basic MATLAB package, `fminsearch` (formerly `fmins`). This routine is based on the simplex (direct search) method, and will adjust any number of parameters to minimize a function specified though a user routine. To *maximize* the correspondence between the reference image and the input image, the *negative* of the correlation between the two images is *minimized*. The routine `fminsearch` will automatically adjust the transformation variables to achieve this minimum (remember that this may not be the absolute minimum).

To implement an optimization search, a routine is required that applies the transformation variables supplied by `fminsearch`, performs an appropriate trial transformation on the input image, then compares the trial image with the reference image. Following convergence, the optimization routine returns the values of the transformation variables that produce the best comparison. These can then be applied to produce the final aligned image. Note that the programmer must specify the actual structure of the transformation since the optimization routine works blindly and simply seeks a set of variables that produces a minimum output. The transformation selected should be based on the possible mechanisms for misalignment: translations, size changes, rotations, skewness, projective misalignment, or other more complex distortions. For efficiency, the transformation should be one that requires the least number of defining variables. Reducing the number of variables increases the likelihood of optimal convergence and substantially reduces computation time. To minimize the number of transformation variables, the simplest transformation that will compensate for the possible mechanisms of distortions should be used.*

Example 11.8   This is an example of unaided image registration requiring an affine transformation. The input image, the image to be aligned, is a distorted version of the reference image. Specifically, it has been stretched horizontally, compressed vertically, and tilted, all using a single affine transformation. The problem is to find a transformation that will realign this image with the reference image.

Solution   MATLAB's optimization routine `fminsearch` will be used to determine an optimized transformation that will make the two images as similar as possible. MATLAB's `fminsearch` routine calls the user routine `rescale` to perform the transformation and make the comparison between the two images. The `rescale` routine assumes that an affine transformation is required and that only the horizontal, vertical, and tilt dimensions need to be adjusted. (It does not, for example, take into account possible translations between the two images, although this would not be too difficult to incorporate.) The `fminsearch` routine requires as input arguments, the name of the routine whose output is to be minimized (in this example, `rescale`), and the initial values of the transformation variables (in this example, all 1's). The routine uses the size of the initial value vector to determine how many variables it needs to adjust (in this case, three variables). Any additional input arguments following an optional vector specifying operational features are passed to `rescale` immediately following the transformation variables. The optimization routine will continue to call `rescale` automatically until it has found an acceptable minimum for the error (or until some maximum number of iterations is reached, see the associated help file).

```
% Example 11.8 and Figure 11.13
% Image registration after spatial transformation
% Load a frame of the MRI image (mri.tif). Transform the original
%   image by increasing it horizontally, decreasing it vertically,
%   and tilting it to the right. Also decrease image contrast
%   slightly
% Use MATLAB's basic optimization routine, 'fminsearch' to find
%   the transformation that restores the original image shape.
%
```

---

*The number of defining variables depends on the transformation. For example rotation alone only requires one variable, linear transformations require two variables, affine transformations require 3 variables while projective transformations require 4 variables. Two additional variables are required for translations.

Reference Image   Input Image   Aligned Image

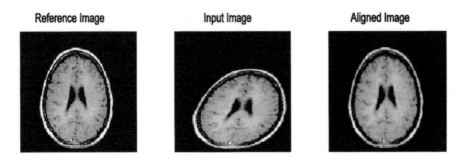

FIGURE 11.13 Unaided image registration requiring several affine transformations. The left image is the original (reference) image and the distorted center image is to be aligned with that image. After a transformation determined by optimization, the right image is quite similar to the reference image. (Original image from the same as fig 11.12.)

```
clear all; close all;
H_scale = .25;            % Define distorting parameters
V_scale = .2;             % Horizontal, vertical, and tilt
tilt = .2;                %  in percent

.......load mri.tif, frame 18.......

[M N]= size(I);
H_scale = H_scale * N/2; % Convert percent scale to pixels
V_scale = V_scale * M;
tilt = tilt * N
%
% Construct distorted image.
U = [1 1; 1 M; N M];       % Input triangle
X = [1-H_scale+tilt 1+V_scale; 1-H_scale M; N+H_scale M];
Tform = maketform('affine', U, X);
I_transform = (imtransform(I,Tform,'Xdata',[1 N], ...
   'Ydata', [1 M]))*.8;
%
% Now find transformation to realign image
initial_scale = [1 1 1]; % Set initial values
[scale,Fval] = fminsearch('rescale',initial_scale,[ ], ...
   I, I_transform);
disp(Fval)                 % Display final correlation
%
% Realign image using optimized transform
```

```
X = [1+scale(1)+scale(3) 1 + scale(2); 1+scale(1) M; ...
  N-scale(1) M];
Tform = maketform('affine', U, X);
I_aligned = imtransform(I_transform,Tform,'Xdata',[1 N],
  'Ydata',[1 M]);
%
subplot(1,3,1); imshow(I);   %Display the images
  title('Original Image');
subplot(1,3,2); imshow(I_transform);
  title('Transformed Image');
subplot(1,3,3); imshow(I_aligned);
  title('Aligned Image');
```

The rescale routine is used by fminsearch. This routine takes in the transformation variables supplied by fminsearch, performs a trial transformation, and compares the trial image with the reference image. The routine then returns the error to be minimized calculated as the negative of the correlation between the two images.

```
function err = rescale(scale, I, I_transform);
% Function used by 'fminsearch' to rescale an image
%  horizontally, vertically, and with tilt.
% Performs transformation and computes correlation between
%  original and newly transformed image.
% Inputs:
%  scale              Current scale factor (from 'fminsearch')
%  I                  original image
%  I_transform        image to be realigned
% Outputs:
%  Negative correlation between original and transformed image.
%
[M N]= size(I);
U = [1 1; 1 M; N M];      % Input triangle
%
% Perform trial transformation
X = [1+scale(1)+scale(3) 1 + scale(2); 1+scale(1) M; ...
  N-scale(1) M];
Tform = maketform('affine', U, X);
I_aligned = imtransform(I_transform,Tform,'Xdata', ...
  [1 N], 'Ydata',[1 M]);
%
% Calculate negative correlation
err = -abs(corr2(I_aligned,I));
```

The results achieved by this registration routine are shown in Figure 11.13. The original reference image is shown on the left, and the input image is in the center. As noted above, this image is the same as the reference except that it has been distorted by several affine transformations (horizontal scratching, vertical compression, and a tilt). The aligned image achieved by the optimization is shown on the right. This image is very similar to the reference image. This optimization was fairly robust: it converged to a correlation of 0.99 from both positive and negative initial values. However, in many cases, convergence can depend on the initial values as demonstrated in Problem 8. This program took about 1 minute to run on a 1 GHz PC.

Interactive Image Registration

Several strategies may be used to guide the registration process. In the example used here, registration will depend on reference marks provided by a human operator. Interactive image registration is well supported by the MATLAB Image Processing Toolbox and includes a graphically based program, `cpselect`, that automates the process of establishing corresponding reference marks. Under this procedure, the user interactively identifies a number of corresponding features in the reference and input image, and a transform is constructed from these pairs of reference points. The program must specify the type of transformation to be performed (*linear, affine, projective*, etc.), and the minimum number of reference pairs required will depend on the type of transformation. The number of reference pairs required is the same as the number of variables needed to define a transformation: an affine transformation will require a minimum of three reference points while a projective transformation requires four variables. Linear transformations require only two pairs, while other more complex transformations may require six or more point pairs. In most cases, the alignment is improved if more than the minimal number of point pairs is given.

In Example 11.9, an alignment requiring a projective transformation is presented. This Example uses the routine `cp2tform` to produce a transformation in `Tform` format, based on point pairs obtained interactively. The `cp2tform` routine has a large number of options, but the basic calling structure is:

```
Tform = cp2tform(input_points, base_points, 'type');
```

where `input_points` is a *m* by 2 matrix consisting of *x,y* coordinates of the reference points in the input image; `base_points` is a matrix containing the same information for the reference image. This routine assumes that the points are entered in the same order, i.e., that corresponding rows in the two vectors describe corresponding points. The `type` variable is the same as in `maketform` and specifies the type of transform (`'affine'`, `'projective'`, etc.). The use of this routine is demonstrated in Example 11.9.

Example 11.9 An example of interactive image registration. In this example, an input image is generated by transforming the reference image with a projective transformation including vertical and horizontal translations. The program then opens two windows displaying the reference and input image, and takes in eight reference points for each image from the operator using the MATLAB ginput routine. As each point is taken it, it is displayed as an '*' overlaid on the image. Once all 16 points have been acquired (eight from each image), a transformation is constructed using cp2tform. This transformation is then applied to the input image using imtransform. The reference, input, and realigned images are displayed.

```
% Example 11.9 Interactive Image Registration
% Load a frame of the MRI image (mri.tif) and perform a spatial
%  transformation that tilts the image backward and displaces
%  it horizontally and vertically.
% Uses interactive registration and the MATLAB function
%  'cp2tform' to realign the image
%
clear all; close all;
nu_points = 8;                  % Number of reference points

    .......Load mri.tif, frame 18 .......

[M N] = size(I);
%
% Construct input image. Perform projective transformation
U = [1 1; 1 M; N M; N 1];
offset = .15*N;                 % Projection offset
H = .2 * N;                     % Horizontal translation
V = .15 * M;                    % Vertical translation
X = [1-offset+H 1+offset-V; 1+offset+H M-offset-V; ...
   N-offset+H M-offset-V; ...N+offset+H 1+offset-V];
 Tform1 = maketform('projective', U, X);
I_transform = imtransform(I,Tform1,'Xdata',[1 N], ...
   'Ydata', [1 M]);
%
% Acquire reference points
% First open two display windows
fig(1) = figure;
  imshow(I);
fig(2) = figure;
  imshow(I_transform);
%
%
for i = 1:2                              % Get reference points: both
                                         %  images

   figure(fig(i));                       % Open window i
   hold on;
```

```
title('Enter four reference points');
for j = 1:nu_points
  [x(j,i), y(j,i)] = ginput(1); % Get reference point
  plot(x(j,i), y(j,i),'*');      % Mark reference point
                                 %  with *
  end
end
%
% Construct transformation with cp2tform and implement with
%  imtransform
%
[Tform2, inpts, base_pts] = cp2tform([x(:,2) y(:,2)], ...
  [x(:,1) y(:,1)],'projective');
I_aligned = imtransform(I_transform,Tform2,'Xdata', ...
  [1 N],'Ydata',[1 M]);
%
figure;
subplot(1,3,1); imshow(I);        % Display the images
  title('Original');
subplot(1,3,2); imshow(I_transform);
  title('Transformation');
subplot(1,3,3); imshow(I_aligned);
  title('Realigned');
```

The reference and input windows are shown along with the reference points selected in Figure 11.14A and B. Eight points were used rather than the minimal four, because this was found to produce a better result. The influence of the number of reference point used is explored in Problem 9. The result of the transformation is presented in Figure 11.15. This figure shows that the realignment was less that perfect, and, in fact, the correlation after alignment was only 0.78. Nonetheless, the primary advantage of this method is that it couples into the extraordinary abilities of human visual identification and, hence, can be applied to images that are only vaguely similar when correlation-based methods would surely fail.

PROBLEMS

1. Load the MATLAB test pattern image `testpat1.png` used in Example 11.5. Generate and plot the Fourier transform of this image. First plot only the 25 points on either side of the center of this transform, then plot the entire function, but first take the log for better display.

2. Load the horizontal chirp pattern shown in Figure 11.1 (found on the disk as `imchirp.tif`) and take the Fourier transform as in the above problem. Then multiply the Fourier transform (in complex form) in the horizontal direction by

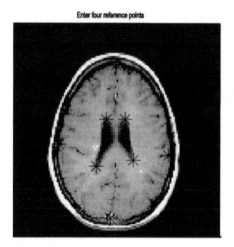

FIGURE 11.14A   A reference image used in Example 11.9 showing the reference points as black. (Original image from the MATLAB Image Processing Toolbox. Copyright 1993–2003, The Math Works, Inc. Reprinted with permission.)

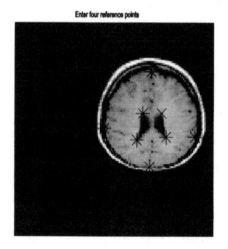

FIGURE 11.14B   Input image showing reference points corresponding to those shown in Figure 11.14A.

Reference Image   Input Image   Realigned

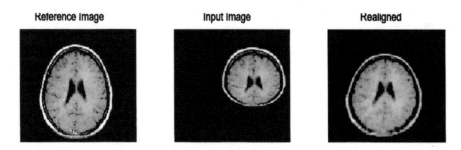

FIGURE 11.15 Image registration using a transformation developed interactively. The original (reference) image is seen on the left, and the input image in the center. The image after transformation is similar, but not identical to the reference image. The correlation between the two is 0.79. (Original image from the MATLAB Image Processing Toolbox. Copyright 1993–2003, The Math Works, Inc. Reprinted with permission.)

a half-wave sine function of same length. Now take the inverse Fourier transform of this windowed function and plot alongside the original image. Also apply the window in the vertical direction, take the inverse Fourier transform, and plot the resulting image. Do not apply `fftshift` to the Fourier transform as the inverse Fourier transform routine, `ifft2` expects the DC component to be in the upper left corner as `fft2` presents it. Also you should take the absolute value at the inverse Fourier transform before display, to eliminate any imaginary components. (The chirp image is square, so you do not have to recompute the half-wave sine function; however, you may want to plot the sine wave to verify that you have a correct half-wave sine function). You should be able to explain the resulting images. (*Hint*: Recall the frequency characteristics of the *two-point central difference* algorithm used for taking the derivative.)

3.   Load the blood cell image (`blood1.tif`). Design and implement your own 3 by 3 filter that enhances vertical edges that go from dark to light. Repeat for a filter that enhances horizontal edges that go from light to dark. Plot the two images along with the original. Convert the first image (vertical edge enhancement) to a binary image and adjust the threshold to emphasize the edges. Plot this image with the others in the same figure. Plot the three-dimensional frequency representations of the two filters together in another figure.

4.   Load the chirp image (`imchirp.tif`) used in Problem 2. Design a one-dimensional 64th-order narrowband bandpass filter with cutoff frequencies of 0.1 and 0.125 Hz and apply it the chirp image. Plot the modified image with the original. Repeat for a 128th-order filter and plot the result with the others. (This may take a while to run.) In another figure, plot the three-dimensional frequency representation of a 64th-order filter.

5. Produce a movie of the rotating brain. Load frame 16 of the MRI image (`mri.tif`). Make a multiframe image of the basic image by rotating that image through 360 degrees. Use 36 frames (10 degrees per rotation) to cover the complete 360 degrees. (If your resources permit, you could use 64 frames with 5 degrees per rotation.) Submit a montage plot of those frames that cover the first 90 degrees of rotation; i.e., the first eight images (or 16, if you use 64 frames).

6. Back in the 1960's, people were into "expanding their minds" through meditation, drugs, rock and roll, or other "mind-expanding" experiences. In this problem, you will expand the brain in a movie using an affine transformation. (Note: `imresize` will not work because it changes the number of pixels in the image and `immovie` requires that all images have the same dimensions.) Load frame 18 of the MRI image (`mri.tif`). Make a movie where the brain stretches in and out horizontally from 75% to 150% of normal size. The image will probably exceed the frame size during its larger excursions, but this is acceptable. The image should grow symmetrically about the center (i.e., in both directions.) Use around 24 frames with the latter half of the frames being the reverse of the first as in Example 11.7, so the brain appears to grow then shrink. Submit a montage of the first 12 frames. Note: use some care in getting the range of image sizes to be between 75% and 150%. (*Hint*: to simplify the computation of the output triangle, it is best to define the input triangle at three of the image corners. Note that all three triangle vertices will have to be modified to stretch the image in both directions, symmetrically about the center.)

7. Produce a spatial transformation movie using a projective transformation. Load a frame of the MRI image (`mri.tif`, your choice of frame). Use the projective transformation to make a movie of the image as it tilts vertically. Use 24 frames as in Example 11.7: the first 12 will tilt the image back while the rest tilt the image back to its original position. You can use any reasonable transformation that gives a vertical tilt or rotation. Submit a montage of the first 12 images.

8. Load frame 12 of `mri.tif` and use `imrotate` to rotate the image by 15 degrees clockwise. Also reduce image contrast of the rotated image by 25%. Use MATLAB's basic optimization program `fminsearch` to align the image that has been rotated. (You will need to write a function similar to `rescale` in Example 11.8 that rotates the image based on the first input parameter, then computes the negative correlation between the rotated image and the original image.)

9. Load a frame of the MRI image (`mri.tif`) and perform a spatial transformation that first expands the image horizontally by 20% then rotates the image by 20 degrees. Use interactive registration and the MATLAB function `cp2tform` to transform the image. Use (A) the minimum number of points and (B) twice the minimum number of points. Compare the correlation between the original and the realigned image using the two different number of reference points.

12

Image Segmentation

Image segmentation is the identification and isolation of an image into regions that—one hopes—correspond to structural units. It is an especially important operation in biomedical image processing since it is used to isolate physiological and biological structures of interest. The problems associated with segmentation have been well studied and a large number of approaches have been developed, many specific to a particular image. General approaches to segmentation can be grouped into three classes: pixel-based methods, regional methods, and edge-based methods. Pixel-based methods are the easiest to understand and to implement, but are also the least powerful and, since they operate on one element at time, are particularly susceptible to noise. Continuity-based and edge-based methods approach the segmentation problem from opposing sides: edge-based methods search for differences while continuity-based methods search for similarities.

PIXEL-BASED METHODS

The most straightforward and common of the pixel-based methods is *thresholding* in which all pixels having intensity values above, or below, some level are classified as part of the segment. Thresholding is an integral part of converting an intensity image to a binary image as described in Chapter 10. Thresholding is usually quite fast and can be done in real time allowing for interactive setting of the threshold. The basic concept of thresholding can be extended to include both upper and lower boundaries, an operation termed *slicing* since it isolates a specific range of pixels. Slicing can be generalized to include a number of different upper and lower boundaries, each encoded into a different number. An example of multiple slicing was presented in Chapter 10 using the MATLAB `gray2slice` routine. Finally, when RGB color or pseudocolor images are involved, thresholding can be applied to each color plane separately. The resulting image could be either a thresholded RGB image, or a single image composed of a logical combination (AND or OR) of the three image planes after thresholding. An example of this approach is seen in the problems.

A technique that can aid in all image analysis, but is particularly useful in pixel-based methods, is intensity remapping. In this global procedure, the pixel values are rescaled so as to extend over different maximum and minimum values. Usually the rescaling is linear, so each point is adjusted proportionally with a possible offset. MATLAB supports rescaling with the routine `imadjust` described below, which also provides a few common nonlinear rescaling options. Of course, any rescaling operation is possible using MATLAB code if the intensity images are of *class double*, or the image arithmetic routines described in Chapter 10 are used.

Threshold Level Adjustment

A major concern in these pixel-based methods is setting the threshold or slicing level(s) appropriately. Usually these levels are set by the program, although in some situations they can be set interactively by the user.

Finding an appropriate threshold level can be aided by a plot of pixel intensity distribution over the whole image, regardless of whether you adjust the pixel level interactively or automatically. Such a plot is termed the *intensity histogram* and is supported by the MATLAB routine `imhist` detailed below. Figure 12.1 shows an x-ray image of the spine image with its associated density histogram. Figure 12.1 also shows the binary image obtained by applying a threshold at a specific point on the histogram. When RGB color images are being analyzed, intensity histograms can be obtained from all three color planes and different thresholds established for each color plane with the aid of the corresponding histogram.

Intensity histograms can be very helpful in selecting threshold levels, not only for the original image, but for images produced by various segmentation algorithms described later. Intensity histograms can also be useful in evaluating the efficacy of different processing schemes: as the separation between structures improves, histogram peaks should become more distinctive. This relationship between separation and histogram shape is demonstrated in Figures 12.2 and, more dramatically, in Figures 12.3 and 12.4.

Original Figure

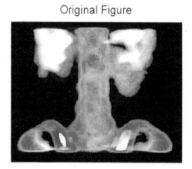

Threshold: 0.34047

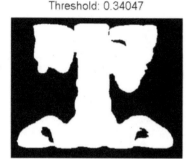

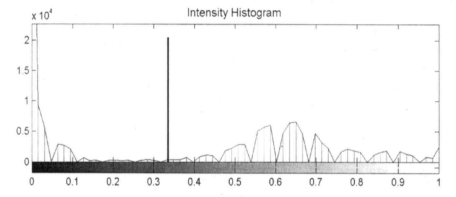

FIGURE 12.1 An image of bone marrow, upper left, and its associated intensity histogram, lower plot. The upper right image is obtained by thresholding the original image at a value corresponding to the vertical line on the histogram plot. (Original image from the MATLAB Image Processing Toolbox. Copyright 1993–2003, The Math Works, Inc. Reprinted with permission.)

Intensity histograms contain no information on position, yet it is spatial information that is of prime importance in problems of segmentation, so some strategies have been developed for determining threshold(s) from the histogram (Sonka et al. 1993). If the intensity histogram is, or can be assumed as, bimodal (or multi-modal), a common strategy is to search for low points, or minima, in the histogram. This is the strategy used in Figure 12.1, where the threshold was set at 0.34, the intensity value at which the histogram shows an approximate minimum. Such points represent the fewest number of pixels and should produce minimal classification errors; however, the histogram minima are often difficult to determine due to variability.

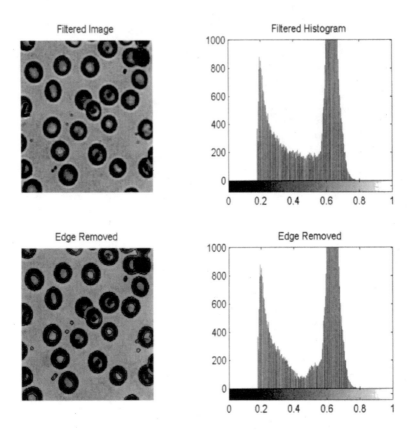

FIGURE 12.2 Image of bloods cells with (upper) and without (lower) intermediate boundaries removed. The associated histograms (right side) show improved separability when the boundaries are eliminated. The code that generated these images is given in Example 12.1. (Original image reprinted with permission from the Image Processing Handbook 2nd edition. Copyright CRC Press, Boca Raton, Florida.)

An approach to improve the determination of histogram minima is based on the observation that many boundary points carry values intermediate to the values on either side of the boundary. These intermediate values will be associated with the region between the actual boundary values and may mask the optimal threshold value. However, these intermediate points also have the highest gradient, and it should be possible to identify them using a gradient-sensitive filter, such as the Sobel or Canny filter. After these boundary points are identified, they can be eliminated from the image, and a new histogram is computed with a distribution that is possibly more definitive. This strategy is used in

Threshold Original Image   Threshold Masked Image

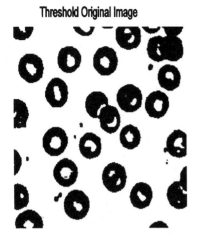
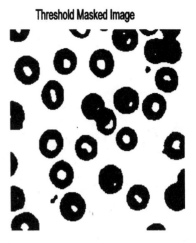

FIGURE 12.3   Thresholded blood cell images. *Optimal* thresholds were applied to the blood cell images in Figure 12.2 with (left) and without (right) boundaries pixel masked. Fewer inappropriate pixels are seen in the right image.

Example 12.1, and Figure 12.2 shows images and associated histograms before and after removal of boundary points as identified using Canny filtering. The reduction in the number of intermediate points can be seen in the middle of the histogram (around 0.45). As shown in Figure 12.3, this leads to slightly better segmentation of the blood cells.

Another histogram-based strategy that can be used if the distribution is bimodal is to assume that each mode is the result of a unimodal, Gaussian distribution. An estimate is then made of the underlying distributions, and the point at which the two estimated distributions intersect should provide the optimal threshold. The principal problem with this approach is that the distributions are unlikely to be truly Gaussian.

A threshold strategy that does not use the histogram is based on the concept of minimizing the variance between presumed foreground and background elements. Although the method assumes two different gray levels, it works well even when the distribution is not bimodal (Sonka et al., 1993). The approach uses an iterative process to find a threshold that minimizes the variance between the intensity values on either side of the threshold level (Outso's method). This approach is implemented using the MATLAB routine `grayslice` (see Example 12.1).

A pixel-based technique that provides a segment boundary directly is *contour mapping*. Contours are lines of equal intensity, and in a continuous image they are necessarily continuous: they cannot end within the image, although

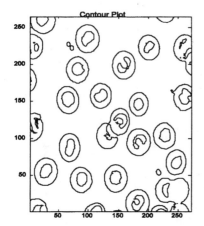 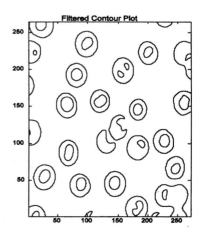

FIGURE 12.4 Contour maps drawn from the blood cell image of Figures 12.2 and 12.3. The right image was pre-filtered with a Gaussian lowpass filter (alpha = 3) before the contour lines were drawn. The contour values were set manually to provide good images.

they can branch or loop back on themselves. In digital images, these same properties exist but the value of any given contour line will not generally equal the values of the pixels it traverses. Rather, it usually reflects values intermediate between adjacent pixels. To use contour mapping to identify image structures requires accurate setting of the contour levels, and this carries the same burdens as thresholding. Nonetheless, contour maps do provide boundaries directly, and, if subpixel interpolation is used in establishing the contour position, they may be spatially more accurate. Contour maps are easy to implement in MATLAB, as shown in the next section on MATLAB Implementation. Figure 12.4 shows contours maps for the blood cell images shown in Figure 12.2. The right image was pre-filtered with a Gaussian lowpass filter which reduces noise slightly and improves the resultant contour image.

Pixel-based approaches can lead to serious errors, even when the average intensities of the various segments are clearly different, due to noise-induced intensity variation within the structure. Such variation could be acquired during image acquisition, but could also be inherent in the structure itself. Figure 12.5 shows two regions with quite different average intensities. Even with optimal threshold selection, many inappropriate pixels are found in both segments due to intensity variations within the segments Fig 12.3 (right). Techniques for improving separation in such images are explored in the sections on continuity-based approaches.

Original Image

Thresholded

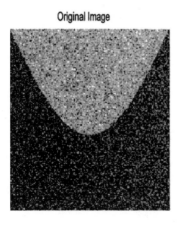
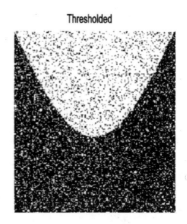

FIGURE 12.5 An image with two regions having different average gray levels. The two regions are clearly distinguishable; however, using thresholding alone, it is not possible to completely separate the two regions because of noise.

MATLAB Implementation

Some of the routines for implementing pixel-based operations such as im2bw and grayslice have been described in preceding chapters. The image intensity histogram routine is produced by imhist without the output arguments:

```
[counts, x] = imhist(I, N);
```

where counts is the histogram value at a given x, I is the image, and N is an optional argument specifying the number of histogram bins (the default is 255). As mentioned above, imhist is usually invoked without the output arguments, count and x, to produce a plot directly.

The rescale routine is:

```
I_rescale = imscale(I, [low high], [bottom top], gamma);
```

where I_rescale is the rescaled output image, I is the input image. The range between low and high in the input image is rescaled to be between bottom and top in the output image.

Several pixel-based techniques are presented in Example 12.1.

Example 12.1 An example of segmentation using pixel-based methods. Load the image of blood cells, and display along with the intensity histogram. Remove the edge pixels from the image and display the histogram of this modi-

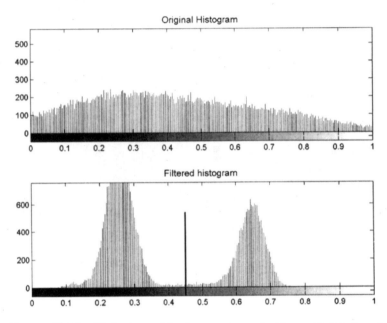

FIGURE 12.6A Histogram of the image shown in Figure 12.3 before (upper) and after (lower) lowpass filtering. Before filtering the two regions overlap to such an extend that they cannot be identified. After lowpass filtering, the two regions are evident, and the boundary found by minimum variance is shown. The application of this boundary to the filtered image results in perfect separation as shown in Figure 12.4B.

fied image. Determine thresholds using the minimal variance iterative technique described above, and apply this approach to threshold both images. Display the resultant thresholded images.

    Solution   To remove the edge boundaries, first identify these boundaries using an edge detection scheme. While any of the edge detection filters described previously can be used, this application will use the Canny filter as it is most robust to noise. This filter is implemented as an option of MATLAB's `edge` routine, which produces a binary image of the boundaries. This binary image will be converted to a boundary *mask* by inverting the image using `imcomplement`. After inversion, the edge pixels will be zero while all other pixels will be one. Multiplying the original image by the boundary mask will produce an image in which the boundary points are removed (i.e., set to zero, or black). All the images involved in this process, including the original image, will then be plotted.

Filtered Figure   Tresholded and Filtered

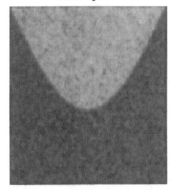 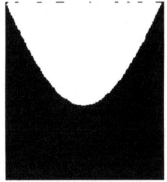

FIGURE 12.6B Left side: The same image shown in Figure 12.5 after lowpass filtering. Right side: This filtered image can now be perfectly separated by thresholding.

```
% Example 12.1 and Figure 12.2 and Figure 12.3
% Lowpass filter blood cell image, then display histograms
%   before and after edge point removal.
% Applies "optimal" threshold routine to both original and
%   "masked" images and display the results
%
........input image and convert to double.......
h = fspecial('gaussian',12,2);        % Construct gaussian
                                      %   filter
I_f = imfilter(I,h,'replicate');      % Filter image
%
I_edge = edge.(I_f,'canny',.3);       % To remove edge
I_rem = I_f .* imcomplement(I_edge);  %   points, find edge,
                                      %   complement and use
                                      %   as mask
%
subplot(2,2,1); imshow(I_f);          % Display images and
                                      %   histograms
    title('Original Figure');
subplot(2,2,2); imhist(I_f); axis([0 1 0 1000]);
    title('Filtered histogram');
subplot(2,2,3); imshow(I_rem);
    title('Edge Removed');
subplot(2,2,4); imhist(I_rem); axis([0 1 0 1000]);
    title('Edge Removed histogram');
```

```
%
figure;                                    % Threshold and
                                           %   display images
t1 = graythresh(I);                        % Use minimum variance
                                           %   thresholds
t2 = graythresh(I_f);
subplot(1,2,1); imshow(im2bw(I,t1));
  title('Threshold Original Image');
subplot(1,2,2); imshow(im2bw(I_f,t2));
  title('Threshold Masked Image');
```

The results have been shown previously in Figures 12.2 and 12.3, and the improvement in the histogram and threshold separation has been mentioned. While the change in the histogram is fairly small (Figure 12.2), it does lead to a reduction in artifacts in the thresholded image, as shown in Figure 12.3. This small improvement could be quite significant in some applications. Methods for removing the small remaining artifacts will be described in the section on morphological operations.

CONTINUITY-BASED METHODS

These approaches look for similarities or consistency in the search for structural units. As demonstrated in the examples below, these approaches can be very effective in segmentation tasks, but they all suffer from a lack of edge definition. This is because they are based on neighborhood operations and these tend to blur edge regions, as edge pixels are combined with structural segment pixels. The larger the neighborhood used, the more poorly edges will be defined. Unfortunately, increasing neighborhood size usually improves the power of any given continuity-based operation, setting up a compromise between identification ability and edge definition. One easy technique that is based on continuity is lowpass filtering. Since a lowpass filter is a sliding neighborhood operation that takes a weighted average over a region, it enhances consistent characteristics. Figure 12.6A shows histograms of the image in Figure 12.5 before and after filtering with a Gaussian lowpass filter (alpha = 1.5). Note the substantial improvement in separability suggested by the associated histograms. Applying a threshold to the filtered image results in perfectly isolated segments as shown in Figure 12.6B. The thresholded images in both Figures 12.5 and 12.4B used the same minimum variance technique to set the threshold, yet the improvement brought about by simple lowpass filtering is remarkable.

Image features related to *texture* can be particularly useful in segmentation. Figure 12.7 shows three regions that have approximately the same average intensity values, but are readily distinguished visually because of differences in texture. Several neighborhood-based operations can be used to distinguish textures: the small segment Fourier transform, local variance (or standard deviation), the *Laplacian* operator, the *range* operator (the difference between maximum and minimum pixel values in the neighborhood), the *Hurst* operator (maximum difference as a function of pixel separation), and the *Haralick* operator (a measure of distance moment). Many of these approaches are either directly supported in MATLAB, or can be implement using the `nlfilter` routine described in Chapter 10.

MATLAB Implementation

Example 12.2 attempts to separate the three regions shown in Figure 12.7 by applying one of these operators to convert the texture pattern to a difference in intensity that can then be separated using thresholding.

Example 12.2   Separate out the three segments in Figure 12.7 that differ only in texture. Use one of the texture operators described above and demonstrate the improvement in separability through histogram plots. Determine appropriate threshold levels for the three segments from the histogram plot.

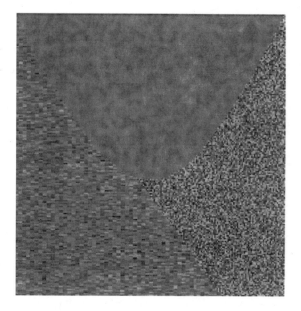

FIGURE 12.7   An image containing three regions having approximately the same intensity, but different textures. While these areas can be distinguished visually, separation based on intensity or edges will surely fail. (Note the single peak in the intensity histogram in Figure 12.9–upper plot.)

Solution   Use the nonlinear *range* filter to convert the textural patterns into differences in intensity. The range operator is a sliding neighborhood procedure that takes the difference between the maximum and minimum pixel value with a neighborhood. Implement this operation using MATLAB's `nlfilter` routine with a 7-by-7 neighborhood.

```
% Example 12.2 Figures 12.8, 12.9, and 12.10
% Load image 'texture3.tif' which contains three regions having
%  the same average intensities, but different textural patterns.
%  Apply the "range" nonlinear operator using 'nlfilter'
%  Plot original and range histograms and filtered image
%
clear all; close all;
[I] = imread('texture3.tif');  % Load image and
I = im2double(I);              % Convert to double
%
range = inline('max(max(x))-  % Define Range function
   min(min(x))');
I_f = nlfilter(I,[7 7], range); % Compute local range
I_f = mat2gray(I_f);           % Rescale intensities
```

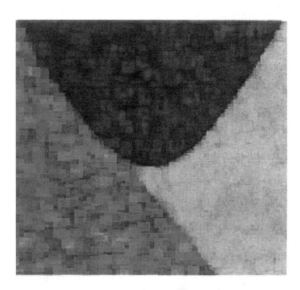

FIGURE 12.8 The texture pattern shown in Figure 12.7 after application of the nonlinear range operation. This operator converts the textural properties in the original figure into a difference in intensities. The three regions are now clearly visible as intensity differences and can be isolated using thresholding.

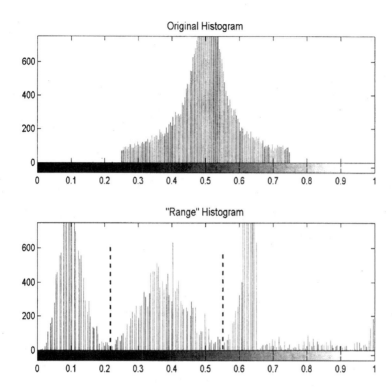

FIGURE 12.9 Histogram of original texture pattern before (upper) and after non-linear filtering using the *range* operator (lower). After filtering, the three intensity regions are clearly seen. The thresholds used to isolate the three segments are indicated.

```
%
imshow(I_f);                          % Display results
  title('"Range" Image');
figure;
subplot(2,1,1); imhist(I);            % Display both histograms
  title('Original Histogram')
subplot(2,1,2); imhist(I_f);
  title('"Range" Histogram');
figure;
subplot(1,3,1); imshow(im2bw         % Display three segments
  (I_f,.22));
subplot(1,3,2); imshow(islice        % Uses 'islice' (see below)
  (I_f,.22,.54));
subplot(1,3,3); imshow(im2bw(I_f,.54));
```

The image produced by the range filter is shown in Figure 12.8, and a clear distinction in intensity level can now be seen between the three regions. This is also demonstrated in the histogram plots of Figure 12.9. The histogram of the original figure (upper plot) shows a single Gaussian-like distribution with no evidence of the three patterns.* After filtering, the three patterns emerge as three distinct distributions. Using this distribution, two thresholds were chosen at minima between the distributions (at 0.22 and 0.54: the solid vertical lines in Figure 12.9) and the three segments isolated based on these thresholds. The two end patterns could be isolated using im2bw, but the center pattern used a special routine, islice. This routine sets pixels to one whose values fall between an upper and lower boundary; if the pixel has values above or below these boundaries, it is set to zero. (This routine is on the disk.) The three fairly well separated regions are shown in Figure 12.10. A few artifacts remain in the isolated images, and subsequent methods can be used to eliminate or reduce these erroneous pixels.

Occasionally, segments will have similar intensities and textural properties, except that the texture differs in orientation. Such patterns can be distinguished using a variety of filters that have orientation-specific properties. The local Fourier transform can also be used to distinguish orientation. Figure 12.11 shows a pattern with texture regions that are different only in terms of their orientation. In this figure, also given in Example 12.3, orientation was identified

Isolated Images

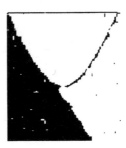 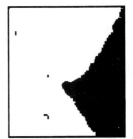

FIGURE 12.10 Isolated regions of the texture pattern in Figure 12.7. Although there are some artifact, the segmentation is quite good considering the original image. Methods for reducing the small artifacts will be given in the section on edge detection.

---

*In fact, the distribution is Gaussian since the image patterns were generated by filtering an array filled with Gaussianly distributed numbers generated by **randn**.

FIGURE 12.11 Textural pattern used in Example 12.3. The horizontal and vertical patterns have the same textural characteristics except for their orientation. As in Figure 12.7, the three patterns have the same average intensity.

by application of a direction operator that operates only in the horizontal direction. This is followed by a lowpass filter to improve separability. The intensity histograms in Figure 12.12 shown at the end of the example demonstrate the intensity separations achieved by the directional range operator and the improvement provided by the lowpass filter. The different regions are then isolated using threshold techniques.

Example 12.3 Isolate segments from a texture pattern that includes two patterns with the same textural characteristics except for orientation. Note that the approach used in Example 12.2 will fail: the similarity in the statistical properties of the vertical and horizontal patterns will give rise to similar intensities following a range operation.

Solution Apply a filter that has directional sensitivity. A Sobel or Prewitt filter could be used, followed by the range or similar operator, or the operations could be done in a single step by using a directional range operator. The choice made in this example is to use a horizontal range operator implemented with `nlfilter`. This is followed by a lowpass filter (Gaussian, alpha = 4) to improve separation by removing intensity variation. Two segments are then isolated using standard thresholding. In this example, the third segment was constructed

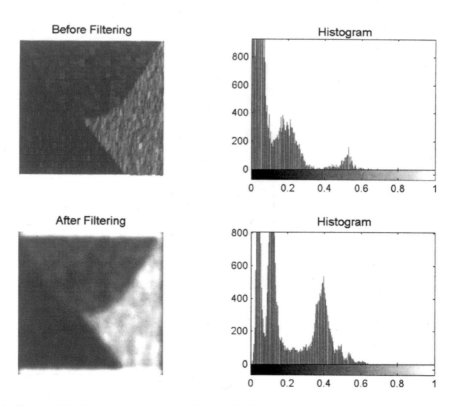

FIGURE 12.12 Images produced by application of a direction range operator applied to the image in Figure 12.11 before (upper) and after (lower) lowpass filtering. The histograms demonstrate the improved separability of the filter image showing deeper minima in the filtered histogram.

by applying a logical operation to the other two segments. Alternatively, the islice routine could have been used as in Example 12.2.

```
% Example 12.3 and Figures 12.11, 12.12, and 12.13
% Analysis of texture pattern having similar textural
%   characteristics but with different orientations. Use a
%   direction-specific filter.
%
clear all; close all;
I = imread('texture4.tif');       % Load "orientation" texture
I = im2double(I);                 % Convert to double
```

Isolated Segments

 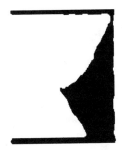 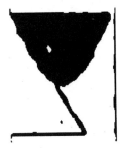

FIGURE 12.13 Isolated segments produced by thresholding the lowpass filtered image in Figure 12.12. The rightmost segment was found by applying logical operations to the other two images.

```
%
% Define filters and functions: I-D range function
range = inline ('max(x)—min(x)');
h_lp = fspecial ('gaussian', 20, 4);
%
% Directional nonlinear filter
I_nl = nlfilter(I, [9 1], range);
I_h = imfilter(I_nl*2, h_lp);     % Average (lowpass filter)
%
subplot(2,2,1); imshow              % Display image and histogram
   (I_nl*2);                        %   before lowpass filtering
   title('Modified Image');         %   and after lowpass filtering
subplot(2,2,2); imhist(I_nl);
   title('Histogram');
subplot(2,2,3); imshow(I_h*2);      % Display modified image
   title('Modified Image');
subplot(2,2,4); imhist(I_h);
   title('Histogram');
%
figure;
BW1 = im2bw(I_h,.08);               % Threshold to isolate segments
BW2 = ~im2bw(I_h,.29);
BW3 = ~(BW1 & BW2);                 % Find third image from other
                                    %   two

subplot(1,3,1); imshow(BW1);        % Display segments
subplot(1,3,2); imshow(BW2);
subplot(1,3,3); imshow(BW3);
```

The image produced by the horizontal range operator with, and without, lowpass filtering is shown in Figure 12.12. Note the improvement in separation produced by the lowpass filtering as indicated by a better defined histogram. The thresholded images are shown in Figure 12.13. As in Example 12.2, the separation is not perfect, but is quite good considering the challenges posed by the original image.

Multi-Thresholding

The results of several different segmentation approaches can be combined either by adding the images together or, more commonly, by first thresholding the images into separate binary images and then combining them using logical operations. Either the AND or OR operator would be used depending on the characteristics of each segmentation procedure. If each procedure identified all of the segments, but also included non-desired areas, the AND operator could be used to reduce artifacts. An example of the use of the AND operation was found in Example 12.3 where one segment was found using the inverse of a logical AND of the other two segments. Alternatively, if each procedure identified some portion of the segment(s), then the OR operator could be used to combine the various portions. This approach is illustrated in Example 12.4 where first two, then three, thresholded images are combined to improve segment identification. The structure of interest is a cell which is shown on a gray background. Threshold levels above and below the gray background are combined (after one is inverted) to provide improved isolation. Including a third binary image obtained by thresholding a texture image further improves the identification.

Example 12.4   Isolate the cell structures from the image of a cell shown in Figure 12.14.

Solution   Since the cell is projected against a gray background it is possible to isolate some portions of the cell by thresholding above and below the background level. After inversion of the lower threshold image (the one that is below the background level), the images are combined using a logical OR. Since the cell also shows some textural features, a texture image is constructed by taking the regional standard deviation (Figure 12.14). After thresholding, this texture-based image is also combined with the other two images.

```
% Example 12.4 and Figures 12.14 and 12.15
% Analysis of the image of a cell using texture and intensity
%  information then combining the resultant binary images
%  with a logical OR operation.
clear all; close all;
I = imread('cell.tif');              % Load "orientation" texture
```

Original Image

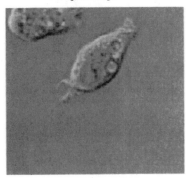

Filtered Texture Image

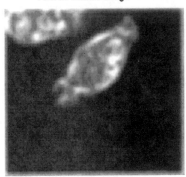

FIGURE 12.14 Image of cells (left) on a gray background. The textural image (right) was created based on local variance (standard deviation) and shows somewhat more definition. (Cancer cell from rat prostate, courtesy of Alan W. Partin, M.D., Ph.D., Johns Hopkins University School of Medicine.)

```
I = im2double(I);                  % Convert to double
%
h = fspecial('gaussian', 20, 2);   % Gaussian lowpass filter
%
subplot(1,2,1); imshow(I);         % Display original image
   title('Original Image');
I_std = (nlfilter(I,[3 3],         % Texture operation
   'std2'))*6;
I_lp = imfilter(I_std, h);         % Average (lowpass filter)
%
subplot(1,2,2); imshow(I_lp*2);    % Display texture image
   title('Filtered image');
%
figure;
BW_th = im2bw(I,.5);               % Threshold image
BW_thc = ~im2bw(I,.42);            %   and its complement
BW_std = im2bw(I_std,.2);          % Threshold texture image
BW1 = BW_th | BW_thc;              % Combine two thresholded
                                   %   images
BW2 = BW_std | BW_th | BW_thc;     % Combine all three images
subplot(2,2,1); imshow(BW_th);     % Display thresholded and
subplot(2,2,2); imshow(BW_thc);    %   combined images
subplot(2,2,3); imshow(BW1);
```

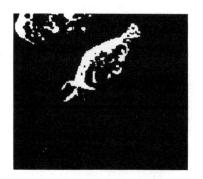

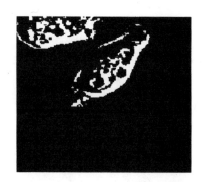

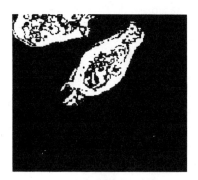

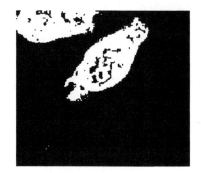

FIGURE 12.15 Isolated portions of the cells shown in Figure 12.14. The upper images were created by thresholding the intensity. The lower left image is a combination (logical OR) of the upper images and the lower right image adds a thresholded texture-based image.

The original and texture images are shown in Figure 12.14. Note that the texture image has been scaled up, first by a factor of six, then by an additional factor of two, to bring it within a nominal image range. The intensity thresholded images are shown in Figure 12.15 (upper images; the upper right image has been inverted). These images are combined in the lower left image. The lower right image shows the combination of both intensity-based images with the thresholded texture image. This method of combining images can be extended to any number of different segmentation approaches.

MORPHOLOGICAL OPERATIONS

Morphological operations have to do with processing shapes. In this sense they are continuity-based techniques, but in some applications they also operate on edges, making them useful in edge-based approaches as well. In fact, morphological operations have many image processing applications in addition to segmentation, and they are well represented and supported in the MATLAB Image Processing Toolbox.

The two most common morphological operations are *dilation* and *erosion*. In dilation the rich get richer and in erosion the poor get poorer. Specifically, in dilation, the center or active pixel is set to the maximum of its neighbors, and in erosion it is set to the minimum of its neighbors. Since these operations are often performed on binary images, dilation tends to expand edges, borders, or regions, while erosion tends to decrease or even eliminate small regions. Obviously, the size and shape of the neighborhood used will have a very strong influence on the effect produced by either operation.

The two processes can be done in tandem, over the same area. Since both erosion and dilation are nonlinear operations, they are not *invertible* transformations; that is, one followed by the other will not generally result in the original image. If erosion is followed by dilation, the operation is termed *opening*. If the image is binary, this combined operation will tend to remove small objects without changing the shape and size of larger objects. Basically, the initial erosion tends to reduce all objects, but some of the smaller objects will disappear altogether. The subsequent dilation will restore those objects that were not eliminated by erosion. If the order is reversed and dilation is performed first followed by erosion, the combined process is called *closing*. Closing connects objects that are close to each other, tends to fill up small holes, and smooths an object's outline by filling small gaps. As with the more fundamental operations of dilation and erosion, the size of objects removed by opening or filled by closing depends on the size and shape of the neighborhood that is selected.

An example of the opening operation is shown in Figure 12.16 including the erosion and dilation steps. This is applied to the blood cell image after thresholding, the same image shown in Figure 12.3 (left side). Since we wish to eliminate black artifacts in the background, we first invert the image as shown in Figure 12.16. As can be seen in the final, opened image, there is a reduction in the number of artifacts seen in the background, but there is also now a gap created in one of the cell walls. The opening operation would be more effective on the image in which intermediate values were masked out (Figure 12.3, right side), and this is given as a problem at the end of the chapter.

Figure 12.17 shows an example of closing applied to the same blood cell image. Again the operation was performed on the inverted image. This operation tends to fill the gaps in the center of the cells; but it also has filled in gaps between the cells. A much more effective approach to filling holes is to use the `imfill` routine described in the section on MATLAB implementation.

Other MATLAB morphological routines provide local maxima and minima, and allows for manipulating the image's maxima and minima, which implement various fill-in effects.

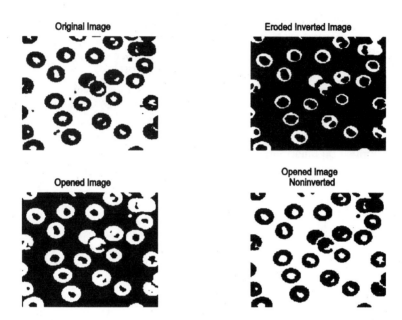

FIGURE 12.16 Example of the *opening* operation to remove small artifacts. Note that the final image has fewer background spots, but now one of the cells has a gap in the wall.

MATLAB Implementation

The erosion and dilation could be implemented using the nonlinear filter routine `nlfilter`, although this routine limits the shape of the neighborhood to a rectangle. The MATLAB routines `imdilate` and `imerode` provide for a variety of neighborhood shapes and are much faster than `nlfilter`. As mentioned above, opening consists of erosion followed by dilation and closing is the reverse. MATLAB also provide routines for implementing these two operations in one statement.

To specify the neighborhood used by all of these routines, MATLAB uses a *structuring element*.* A structuring element can be defined by a binary array, where the ones represent the neighborhood and the zeros are irrelevant. This allows for easy specification of neighborhoods that are nonrectangular, indeed that can have any arbitrary shape. In addition, MATLAB makes a number of popular shapes directly available, just as the `fspecial` routine makes a number

---

*Not to be confused with a similar term, *structural unit*, used in the beginning of this chapter. A *structural unit* is the object of interest in the image.

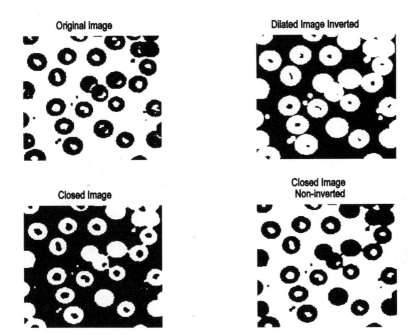

FIGURE 12.17 Example of *closing* to fill gaps. In the closed image, some of the cells are now filled, but some of the gaps between cells have been erroneously filled in.

of popular two-dimensional filter functions available. The routine to specify the structuring element is `strel` and is called as:

```
structure = strel(shape, NH, arg);
```

where `shape` is the type of shape desired, `NH` usually specifies the size of the neighborhood, and `arg` and an argument, frequently optional, that depends on `shape`. If `shape` is `'arbitrary'`, or simply omitted, then `NH` is an array that specifies the neighborhood in terms of ones as described above. Prepackaged shapes include:

`'disk'`	a circle of radius `NH` (in pixels)
`'line'`	a line of length `NH` and angle `arg` in degrees
`'rectangle'`	a rectangle where `NH` is a two element vector specifying rows and columns
`'diamond'`	a diamond where `NH` is the distance from the center to each corner
`'square'`	a square with linear dimensions `NH`

For many of these shapes, the routine strel produces a *decomposed* structure that runs significantly faster.

Based on the structure, the statements for dilation, erosion, opening, and closing are:

```
I1 = imdilate(I, structure);
I1 = imerode(I, structure);
I1 = imopen(I, structuure);
I1 = imclose(I, structure);
```

where I1 is the output image, I is the input image and structure is the neighborhood specification given by strel, as described above. In all cases, structure can be replaced by an array specifying the neighborhood as ones, bypassing the strel routine. In addition, imdilate and imerode have optional arguments that provide packing and unpacking of the binary input or output images.

Example 12.5 Apply opening and closing to the thresholded blood cell images of Figure 12–3 in an effort to remove small background artifacts and to fill holes. Use a circular structure with a diameter of four pixels.

```
% Example 12.5 and Figures 12.16 and 12.17
% Demonstration of morphological opening to eliminate small
%   artifacts and of morphological closing to fill gaps
% These operations will be applied to the thresholded blood cell
%   images of Figure 12.3 (left image).
% Uses a circular or disk shaped structure 4 pixels in diameter
%
clear all; close all;
I = imread('blood1.tif');   % Get image and threshold
I = im2double(I);
BW = ~im2bw(I,thresh(I));
%
SE = strel('disk',4);        % Define structure: disk of radius
                             %   4 pixels
BW1= imerode(BW,SE);         % Opening operation: erode
BW2 = imdilate(BW1,SE);      %   image first, then dilate
%
   .......display images.....
%
BW3= imdilate(BW,SE);        % Closing operation, dilate image
BW4 = imerode(BW3,SE);       %   first then erode
%
   .......display images.....
```

This example produced the images in Figures 12.15 and 12.16.

Example 12.6   Apply an opening operation to remove the dark patches seen in the thresholded cell image of Figure 12.15.

```
% Figures 12.6 and 12.18
% Use opening to remove the dark patches in the thresholded cell
%   image of Figure 12.15
%
close all; clear all;
%
SE = strel('square',5);      % Define closing structure:
                             %  square 5 pixels on a side
load fig12_15;               % Get data of Figure 12.15 (BW2)
BW1= ~imopen(~BW2,SE);       % Opening operation
   .......Display images.....
```

The result of this operation is shown in Figure 12.18. In this case, the closing operation is able to remove completely the dark patches in the center of the cell image. A 5-by-5 pixel square structural element was used. The size (and shape) of the structural element controlled the size of artifact removed, and no attempt was made to optimize its shape. The size was set here as the minimum that would still remove all of the dark patches. The opening operation in this example used the single statement `imopen`. Again, the opening operation operates on activated (i.e., white pixels), so to remove dark artifacts it is necessary to invert the image (using the logical NOT operator, ~) before performing the opening operation. The *opened* image is then inverted again before display.

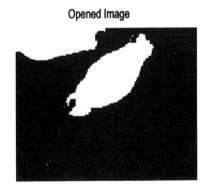

Original Thresholded Image	Opened Image

FIGURE 12.18 Application of the open operation to remove the dark patches in the binary cell image in Figure 12.15 (lower right). Using a 5 by 5 square structural element resulted in eliminating all of the dark patches.

MATLAB morphology routines also allow for manipulation of maxima and minima in an image. This is useful for identifying objects, and for filling. Of the many other morphological operations supported by MATLAB, only the imfill operation will be described here. This operation begins at a designated pixel and changes connected background pixels (0's) to foreground pixels (1's), stopping only when a boundary is reached. For grayscale images, imfill brings the intensity levels of the dark areas that are surrounded by lighter areas up to the same intensity level as surrounding pixels. (In effect, imfill removes regional minima that are not connected to the image border.) The initial pixel can be supplied to the routine or obtained interactively. Connectivity can be defined as either *four connected* or *eight connected*. In four connectivity, only the four pixels bordering the four edges of the pixel are considered, while in eight connectivity all pixel that touch, including those that touch only at the corners, are considered connected.

The basic imfill statement is:

```
I_out = imfill(I, [r c], con);
```

where I is the input image, I_out is the output image, [r c] is a two-element vector specifying the beginning point, and con is an optional argument that is set to 8 for eight connectivity (four connectivity is the default). (See the help file to use imfill interactively.) A special option of imfill is available specifically for filling holes. If the image is binary, a hole is a set of background pixels that cannot be reached by filling in the background from the edge of the image. If the image is an intensity image, a hole is an area of dark pixels surrounded by lighter pixels. To invoke this option, the argument following the input image should be holes. Figure 12.19 shows the operation performed on the blood cell image by the statement:

```
I_out = imfill(I, 'holes');
```

EDGE-BASED SEGMENTATION

Historically, edge-based methods were the first set of tools developed for segmentation. To move from edges to segments, it is necessary to group edges into chains that correspond to the sides of structural units, i.e., the structural boundaries. Approaches vary in how much prior information they use, that is, how much is used of what is known about the possible shape. False edges and missed edges are two of the more obvious, and more common, problems associated with this approach.

The first step in edge-based methods is to identify edges which then become candidates for boundaries. Some of the filters presented in Chapter 11

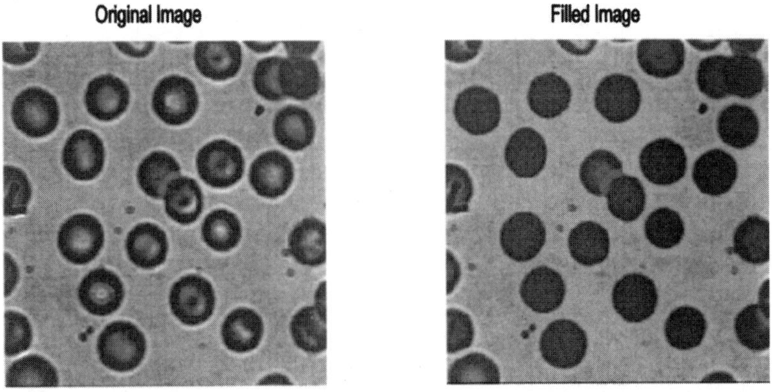

Original Image   Filled Image

FIGURE 12.19 Hole filling operation produced by `imfill`. Note that neither the edge cell (at the upper image boundary) or the overlapped cell in the center are filled since they are not actually holes. (Original image reprinted with permission from the Image Processing Handbook 2nd edition. Copyright CRC Press, Boca Raton, Florida.)

perform edge enhancement, including the Sobel, Prewitt, and Log filters. In addition, the Laplacian, which takes the spatial second derivative, can be used to find edge candidates. The Canny filter is the most advanced edge detector supported by MATLAB, but it necessarily produces a binary output while many of the secondary operations require a graded edge image.

Edge relaxation is one approach used to build chains from individual edge candidate pixels. This approach takes into account the local neighborhood: weak edges positioned between strong edges are probably part of the edge, while strong edges in isolation are likely spurious. The Canny filter incorporates a type of edge relaxation. Various formal schemes have been devised under this category. A useful method is described in Sonka (1995) that establishes edges between pixels (so-called *crack edges*) based on the pixels located at the end points of the edge.

Another method for extending edges into chains is termed *graph searching*. In this approach, the endpoints (which could both be the same point in a closed boundary) are specified, and the edge is determined based on minimizing some *cost function*. Possible pathways between the endpoints are selected from candidate pixels, those that exceed some threshold. The actual path is selected based on a minimization of the cost function. The cost function could include features such as the strength of an edge pixel and total length, curvature, and proximity of the edge to other candidate borders. This approach allows for a great deal of flexibility. Finally, dynamic programming can be used which is also based on minimizing a cost function.

The methods briefly described above use local information to build up the boundaries of the structural elements. Details of these methods can be found in Sonka et al. (1995). Model-based edge detection methods can be used to exploit prior knowledge of the structural unit. For example, if the shape and size of the image is known, then a simple matching approach based on correlation can be used (matched filtering). When the general shape is known, but not the size, the *Hough transform* can be used. This approach was originally designed for identifying straight lines and curves, but can be expanded to other shapes provided the shape can be described analytically.

The basic idea behind the Hough transform is to transform the image into a parameter space that is constructed specifically to describe the desired shape analytically. Maxima in this parameter space then correspond to the presence of the desired image in image space. For example, if the desired object is a straight line (the original application of the Hough transform), one analytic representation for this shape is $y = mx + b$,* and such shapes can be completely defined by a two-dimensional parameter space of m and b parameters. All straight lines in image space map to points in parameter space (also known as the *accumulator array* for reasons that will become obvious). Operating on a binary image of edge pixels, all possible lines through a given pixel are transformed into m,b combinations, which then increment the accumulator array. Hence, the accumulator array accumulates the number of *potential* lines that could exist in the image. Any active pixel will give rise to a large number of possible line slopes, m, but only a limited number of m,b combinations. If the image actually contains a line, then the accumulator element that corresponds to that particular line's m,b parameters will have accumulated a large number. The accumulator array is searched for maxima, or supra threshold locations, and these locations identify a line or lines in the image.

This concept can be generalized to any shape that can be described analytically, although the parameter space (i.e., the accumulator) may have to include several dimensions. For example, to search for circles note that a circle can be defined in terms of three parameters, a, s, and r for the equation given below.

$$(y = a)^2 + (x - b)^2 = r^2 \tag{1}$$

where a and b define the center point of the circle and r is the radius. Hence the accumulator space must be three-dimensional to represent a, b, and r.

---

*This representation of a line will not be able to represent vertical lines since $m \to \infty$ for a vertical line. However, lines can also be represented in two dimensions using cylindrical coordinates, r and θ: $y = r \cos \theta + r \sin \theta$.

MATLAB Implementation

Of the techniques described above, only the Hough transform is supported by MATLAB image processing routines, and then only for straight lines. It is supported as the *Radon transform* which computes projections of the image along a straight line, but this projection can be done at any angle.* This results in a projection matrix that is the same as the accumulator array for a straight line Hough transform when expressed in cylindrical coordinates.

The Radon transform is implemented by the statement:

```
[R, xp] = radon(BW, theta);
```

where BW is a binary input image and theta is the projection angle in degrees, usually a vector of angles. If not specified, theta defaults to (1:179). R is the projection array where each column is the projection at a specific angle. (R is a column vector if theta is a constant). Hence, maxima in R correspond to the positions (encoded as an angle and distance) in the image. An example of the use of radon to perform the Hough transformation is given in Example 12.7.

Example 12.7   Find the strongest line in the image of Saturn in image file `saturn.tif`. Plot that line superimposed on the image.

Solution   First convert the image to an edge array using MATLAB's edge routine. Use the Hough transform (implemented for straight lines using radon) to build an accumulator array. Find the maximum point in that array (using max) which will give theta, the angle perpendicular to the line, and the distance along that perpendicular line of the intersection. Convert that line to rectangular coordinates, then plot the line superimposed on the image.

```
% Example 12.7 Example of the Hough transform
%  (implemented using 'radon') to identify lines in an image.
% Use the image of Saturn in 'saturn.tif'
%
clear all; close all;
radians = 2*pi/360;          % Convert from degrees to radians
I = imread('saturn.tif');    % Get image of Saturn
theta = 0:179;               % Define projection angles
BW = edge(I,.02);            % Threshold image, threshold set
[R,xp] = radon(BW,theta);    % Hough (Radon) transform
% Convert to indexed image
[X, map] = gray2ind (mat2gray(R));
```

---

*The Radon transform is an important concept in computed tomography (CT) as described in a following section.

```
%
subplot(1,2,1); imshow(BW)    % Display results
  title('Saturn ~ Thresholded');
subplot(1,2,2); imshow(X, hot);
                              % The hot colormap gives better
                              %  reproduction
%
[M, c] = max(max(R));         % Find maximum element
[M, r] = max(R(:,c));
% Convert to rectangular coordinates
[ri ci] = size(BW);           % Size of image array
[ra ca] = size(R);            % Size of accumulator array
m = tan((c-90)*radians);      % Slope from theta
b = -r/cos((c-90)*radians);   % Intercept from basic
                              %  trigonometry
x = (0:ci);
y = m*x + b;                  % Construct line
subplot(1,2,1); hold on;
  plot(x,-y,'r');             % Plot line on graph
subplot(1,2,1); hold on;
  plot(c, ra-r,'*k');         % Plot maximum point in
                              %  accumulator
```

This example produces the images shown in Figure 12.20. The broad white line superimposed is the line found as the most dominant using the Hough transform. The location of this in the accumulator or parameter space array is shown in the right-hand image. Other points nearly as strong (i.e., bright) can be seen in the parameter array which represent other lines in the image. Of course, it is possible to identify these lines as well by searching for maxima other than the global maximum. This is done in a problem below.

PROBLEMS

1. Load the blood cell image (`blood1.tif`) Filter the image with two lowpass filters, one having a weak cutoff (for example, Gaussian with an `alpha` of 0.5) and the other having a strong cutoff (`alpha` > 4). Threshold the two filtered images using the maximum variance routine (`graythresh`). Display the original and filtered images along with their histograms. Also display the thresholded images.

2. The Laplacian filter which calculates the second derivative can also be used to find edges. In this case edges will be located where the second derivative is near zero. Load the image of the spine (`'spine.tif'`) and filter using the Laplacian filter (use the default constant). Then threshold this image using

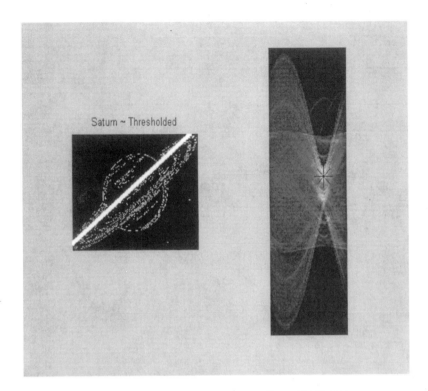

FIGURE 12.20 Thresholded image of Saturn (from MATLAB's `saturn.tif`) with the dominant line found by the Hough transform. The right image is the accumulator array with the maximum point indicated by an '*'. (Original image is a public domain image courtesy of NASA, Voyger 2 image, 1981-08-24.)

`islice`. The threshold values should be on either side of zero and should be quite small (< 0.02) since you are interested in values quite close to zero.

3.   Load image `'texture3.tif'` which contains three regions having the same average intensities but different textural patterns. Before applying the nonlinear range operator used in Example 12.2, preprocess with a Laplacian filter (alpha = 0.5). Apply the range operator as in Example 12.2 using `nlfilter`. Plot original and *range* images along with their histograms. Threshold the range image to isolate the segments and compare with the figures in the book. (*Hint*: You may have to adjust the thresholds slightly, but you do not have to rerun the time-consuming range operator to adjust these thresholds.) You should observe a modest improvement: one of the segments can now be perfectly separated.

4. Load the texture orientation image `texture4.tif`. Separate the segments as well as possible by using a Sobel operator followed by a standard deviation operator implemented using `nlfilter`. (Note you will have to multiply the standard deviation image by around 4 to get it into an appropriate range.) Plot the histogram and use it to determine the best boundaries for separating the three segments. Display the three segments as white objects.

5. Load the thresholded image of Figure 12.5 (found as `Fig12_5.tif` on the disk) and use *opening* to eliminate as many points as possible in the upper field without affecting the lower field. Then use *closing* to try to blacken as many points as possible in the lower field without affecting the upper field. (You should be able to blacken the lower field completely except for edge effects.)

13

Image Reconstruction

Medical imaging utilizes several different physical principals or imaging *modalities*. Common modalities used clinically include x-ray, computed tomography (CT), positron emission tomography (PET), single photon emission computed tomography (SPECT), and ultrasound. Other approaches under development include optical imaging* and impedence tomography. Except for simple x-ray images which provide a shadow of intervening structures, some form of image processing is required to produce a useful image. The algorithms used for image reconstruction depend on the modality. In magnetic resonance imaging (MRI), reconstruction techniques are fairly straightforward, requiring only a two-dimensional inverse Fourier transform (described later in this chapter). Positron emission tomography (PET) and computed tomography use *projections* from collimated beams and the reconstruction algorithm is critical. The quality of the image is strongly dependent on the image reconstruction algorithm.†

---

*Of course, optical imaging is used in microscopy, but because of scattering it presents serious problems when deep tissues are imaged. A number of advanced image processing methods are under development to overcome problems due to scattering and provide useful images using either coherent or noncoherent light.

†CT may be the first instance where the analysis software is an essential component of medical diagnosis and comes between the physician and patient: the physician has no recourse but to trust the software.

375

CT, PET, AND SPECT

Reconstructed images from PET, SPECT, and CT all use collimated beams directed through the target, but they vary in the mechanism used to produce these collimated beams. CT is based on x-ray beams produced by an external source that are collimated by the detector: the detector includes a *collimator*, usually a long tube that absorbs diagonal or off-axis photons. A similar approach is used for SPECT, but here the photons are produced by the decay of a radioactive isotope within the patient. Because of the nature of the source, the beams are not as well collimated in SPECT, and this leads to an unavoidable reduction in image resolution. Although PET is also based on photons emitted from a radioactive isotope, the underlying physics provide an opportunity to improve beam collimation through so-called *electronic collimation*. In PET, the radioactive isotope emits a positron. Positrons are short lived, and after traveling only a short distance, they interact with an electron. During this interaction, their masses are annihilated and two photons are generated traveling in opposite directions, 180 deg. from one another. If two separate detectors are activated at essentially the same time, then it is likely a positron annihilation occurred somewhere along a line connecting these two detectors. This *coincident detection* provides an electronic mechanism for establishing a collimated path that traverses the original positron emission. Note that since the positron does not decay immediately, but may travel several cm in any direction before annihilation, there is an inherent limitation on resolution.

In all three modalities, the basic data consists of measurements of the absorption of x-rays (CT) or concentrations of radioactive material (PET and SPECT), along a known beam path. From this basic information, the reconstruction algorithm must generate an image of either the tissue absorption characteristics or isotope concentrations. The mathematics are fairly similar for both absorption and emission processes and will be described here in terms of absorption processes; i.e., CT. (See Kak and Slaney (1988) for a mathematical description of emission processes.)

In CT, the intensity of an x-ray beam is dependent on the intensity of the source, I_o, the absorption coefficient, μ, and length, ℓ, of the intervening tissue:

$$I(x,y) = I_o e^{-\mu \ell} \tag{1}$$

where $I(x,y)$ is the beam intensity (proportional to number of photons) at position x,y. If the beam passes through tissue components having different absorption coefficients then, assuming the tissue is divided into equal sections $\Delta \ell$, Eq. (1) becomes:

$$I(x,y) = I_o exp\left(-\sum_i \mu(x,y)\Delta \ell\right) \tag{2}$$

The *projection p(x,y)*, is the log of the intensity ratio, and is obtained by dividing out I_o and taking the natural log:

$$p(x,y) = \ln\left(\frac{I_o}{I(x,y)}\right) = \sum_i \mu_i(x,y)\Delta\ell \tag{3}$$

Eq. (3) is also expressed as a continuous equation where it becomes the line integral of the attenuation coefficients from the source to the detector:

$$p(x,y) = \int_{\text{Source}}^{\text{Detector}} \mu(x,y)d\ell \tag{4}$$

Figure 13.1A shows a series of collimated parallel beams traveling through tissue.* All of these beams are at the same angle, θ, with respect to the reference axis. The output of each beam is just the projection of absorption characteristics of the intervening tissue as defined in Eq. (4). The projections of all the individual parallel beams constitute a *projection profile* of the intervening

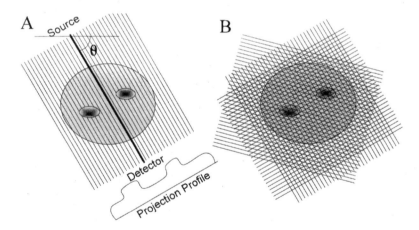

FIGURE 13.1 (A) A series of parallel beam paths at a given angle, θ, is projected through biological tissue. The net absorption of each beam can be plotted as a projection profile. (B) A large number of such parallel paths, each at a different angle, is required to obtain enough information to reconstruct the image.

---

*In modern CT scanners, the beams are not parallel, but dispersed in a spreading pattern from a single source to an array of detectors, a so-called fan beam pattern. To simplify the analysis presented here, we will assume a parallel beam geometry. Kak and Slaney (1988) also cover the derivation of reconstruction algorithms for fan beam geometry.

tissue absorption coefficients. With only one projection profile, it is not possible to determine how the tissue absorptions are distributed along the paths. However, if a large number of projections are taken at different angles through the tissue, Figure 13.1B, it ought to be possible, at least in principle, to estimate the distribution of absorption coefficients from some combined analysis applied to all of the projections. This analysis is the challenge given to the CT reconstruction algorithm.

If the problem were reversed, that is, if the distribution of tissue absorption coefficients was known, determining the projection profile produced by a set of parallel beams would be straightforward. As stated in Eq. (13-4), the output of each beam is the line integral over the beam path through the tissue. If the beam is at an angle, θ (Figure 13-2), then the equation for a line passing through the origin at angle θ is:

$$x \cos \theta + y \sin \theta = 0 \tag{5}$$

and the projection for that single line at a fixed angle, p_θ, becomes:

$$p_\theta = \int_{-\infty}^{\infty} \int_{-\infty}^{\infty} I(x,y)(x \cos\theta + y \sin\theta) \, dxdy \tag{6}$$

where $I(x,y)$ is the distribution of absorption coefficients as Eq. (2). If the beam is displaced a distance, r, from the axis in a direction perpendicular to θ, Figure 13.2, the equation for that path is:

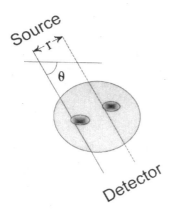

FIGURE 13.2 A single beam path is defined mathematically by the equation given in Eq. (5).

$$x \cos \theta + y \sin \theta - r = 0 \qquad (7)$$

The whole family of parallel paths can be mathematically defined using Eqs. (6) and (7) combined with the Dirac delta distribution, δ, to represent the discrete parallel beams. The equation describing the entire projection profile, $p_\theta(r)$, becomes:

$$p_\theta(r) = \int_{-\infty}^{\infty} \int_{-\infty}^{\infty} I(x,y) \, \delta(x \cos\theta + y \sin\theta - r) \, dxdy \qquad (8)$$

This equation is known as the *Radon transform*, $\mathcal{R}$. It is the same as the Hough transform (Chapter 12) for the case of straight lines. The expression for $p_\theta(r)$ can also be written succinctly as:

$$p_\theta(r) = \mathcal{R}[I(x,y)] \qquad (9)$$

The forward Radon transform can be used to generate raw CT data from image data, useful in problems, examples, and simulations. This is the approach that is used in some of the examples given in the MATLAB Implementation section, and also to generate the CT data used in the problems.

The Radon transform is helpful in understanding the problem, but does not help in the actual reconstruction. Reconstructing the image from the projection profiles is a classic *inverse problem*. You know what comes out—the projection profiles—but want to know the image (or, in the more general case, the system), that produced that output. From the definition of the Radon transform in Eq. (9), the image should result from the application of an inverse Radon transform $\mathcal{R}^{-1}$, to the projection profiles, $p_\theta(r)$:

$$I(x,y) = \mathcal{R}^{-1}[p_\theta(r)] \qquad (10)$$

While the Radon transform (Eqs. (8) and (9)) and inverse Radon transform (Eq. (10)) are expressed in terms of continuous variables, in imaging systems the absorption coefficients are given in terms of discrete pixels, $I(n,m)$, and the integrals in the above equations become summations. In the discrete situation, the absorption of each pixel is an unknown, and each beam path provides a single projection ratio that is the solution to a multi-variable equation. If the image contains N by M pixels, and there are $N \times M$ different projections (beam paths) available, then the system is adequately determined, and the reconstruction problem is simply a matter of solving a large number of simultaneous equations. Unfortunately, the number of simultaneous equations that must be solved is generally so large that a direct solution becomes unworkable. The early attempts at CT reconstruction used an iterative approach called the *algebraic reconstruction algorithm* or *ART*. In this algorithm, each pixel was updated based on errors between projections that would be obtained from the current pixel values and the actual projections. When many pixels are involved, convergence was slow and the algorithm was computationally intensive and time-consuming. Current approaches can be classified as either transform methods or series expansion methods. The *filtered back-projection* method described below falls into the first category and is one of the most popular of CT reconstruction approaches.

Filtered back-projection can be described in either the spatial or spatial frequency domain. While often implemented in the latter, the former is more intuitive. In back-projection, each pixel absorption coefficient is set to the sum (or average) of the values of all projections that traverse the pixel. In other words, each projection that traverses a pixel contributes its full value to the pixel, and the contributions from all of the beam paths that traverse that pixel are simply added or averaged. Figure 13.3 shows a simple 3-by-3 pixel grid with a highly absorbing center pixel (absorption coefficient of 8) against a background of lessor absorbing pixels. Three projection profiles are shown traversing the grid horizontally, vertically, and diagonally. The lower grid shows the image that would be reconstructed using back-projection alone. Each grid contains the average of the projections though that pixel. This reconstructed image resembles the original with a large central value surrounded by smaller values, but the background is no longer constant. This background variation is the result of blurring or smearing the central image over the background.

To correct the blurring or smoothing associated with the back-projection method, a spatial filter can be used. Since the distortion is in the form of a blurring or smoothing, spatial differentiation is appropriate. The most common filter is a pure derivative up to some maximum spatial frequency. In the frequency domain, this filter, termed the *Ram-Lak* filter, is a ramp up to some maximum cutoff frequency. As with all derivative filters, high-frequency noise will be increased, so this filter is often modified by the addition of a lowpass filter. Lowpass filters that can be used include the Hamming window, the Hanning window, a cosine window, or a sinc function window (the *Shepp-Logan* filter). (The frequency characteristics of these filters are shown in Figure 13.4). Figure 13.5 shows a simple image of a light square on a dark background. The projection profiles produced by the image are also shown (calculated using the Radon transform).

The back-projection reconstruction of this image shows a blurred version of the basic square form with indistinct borders. Application of a highpass filter sharpens the image (Figure 13.4). The MATLAB implementation of the inverse Radon transform, `iradon` described in the next section, uses the filtered back-projection method and also provides for all of the filter options.

Filtered back-projection is easiest to implement in the frequency domain. The *Fourier slice theorem* states that the one-dimensional Fourier transform of a projection profile forms a single, radial line in the two-dimensional Fourier transform of the image. This radial line will have the same angle in the spatial

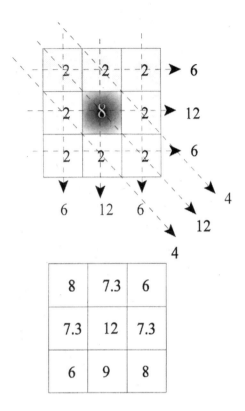

FIGURE 13.3 Example of back-projection on a simple 3-by-3 pixel grid. The upper grid represents the original image which contains a dark (absorption 8) center pixel surrounded by lighter (absorption 2) pixels. The projections are taken as the linear addition of all intervening pixels. In the lower reconstructed image, each pixel is set to the average of all beams that cross that pixel. (Normally the sum would be taken over a much larger set of pixels.) The center pixel is still higher in absorption, but the background is no longer the same. This represents a smearing of the original image.

frequency domain as the projection angle (Figure 13.6). Once the two-dimensional Fourier transform space is filled from the individual one-dimensional Fourier transforms of the projection profiles, the image can be constructed by applying the inverse two-dimensional Fourier transform to this space. Before the inverse transform is done, the appropriate filter can be applied directly in the frequency domain using multiplication.

As with other images, reconstructed CT images can suffer from alaising if they are undersampled. Undersampling can be the result of an insufficient

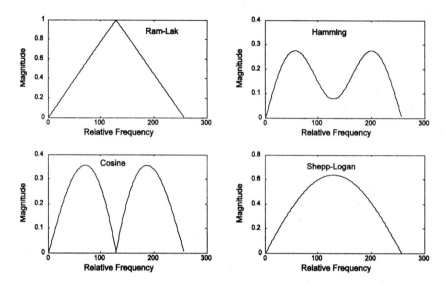

FIGURE 13.4 Magnitude frequency characteristics of four common filters used in filtered back-projection. They all show highpass characteristics at lower frequencies. The *cosine* filter has the same frequency characteristics as the two-point central difference algorithm.

number of parallel beams in the projection profile or too few rotation angles. The former is explored in Figure 13.7 which shows the square pattern of Figure 13.5 sampled with one-half (left-hand image) and one-quarter (right-hand image) the number of parallel beams used in Figure 13.5. The images have been multiplied by a factor of 10 to enhance the faint aliasing artifacts. One of the problems at the end of this chapter explores the influence of undersampling by reducing the number of angular rotations an well as reducing the number of parallel beams.

Fan Beam Geometry

For practical reasons, modern CT scanners use fan beam geometry. This geometry usually involves a single source and a ring of detectors. The source rotates around the patient while those detectors in the beam path acquire the data. This allows very high speed image acquisition, as short as half a second. The source fan beam is shaped so that the beam hits a number of detections simultaneously, Figure 13.8. MATLAB provides several routines that provide the Radon and inverse Radon transform for fan beam geometry.

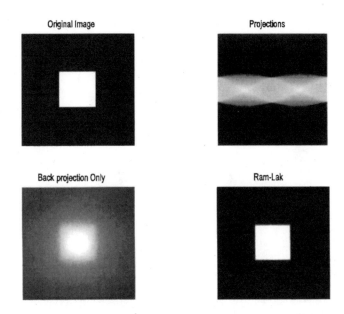

Original Image

Projections

Back projection Only

Ram-Lak

FIGURE 13.5 Image reconstruction of a simple white square against a black background. Back-projection alone produces a smeared image which can be corrected with a spatial derivative filter. These images were generated using the code given in Example 13.1.

MATLAB Implementation

Radon Transform

The MATLAB Image Processing Toolbox contains routines that perform both the Radon and inverse Radon transforms. The Radon transform routine has already been introduced as an implementation of the Hough transform for straight line objects. The procedure here is essentially the same, except that an intensity image is used as the input instead of the binary image used in the Hough transform.

```
[p, xp] = radon(I, theta);
```

where I is the image of interest and theta is the production angle in degs.s, usually a vector of angles. If not specified, theta defaults to (1:179). The output parameter p is the projection array, where each column is the projection profile at a specific angle. The optional output parameter, xp gives the radial coordinates for each row of p and can be used in displaying the projection data.

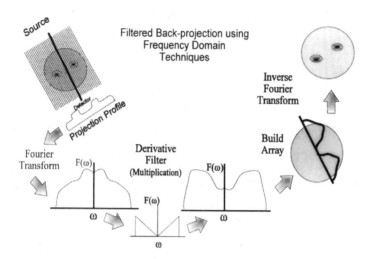

FIGURE 13.6 Schematic representation of the steps in filtered back-projection using frequency domain techniques. The steps shown are for a single projection profile and would be repeated for each projection angle.

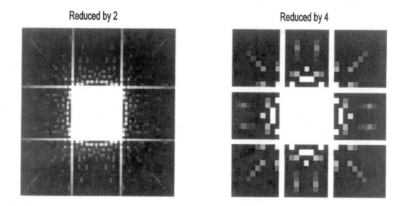

FIGURE 13.7 Image reconstructions of the same simple pattern shown in Figure 13.4, but undersampled by a factor of two (left image) or four (right image). The contrast has been increased by a factor of ten to enhance the relatively low-intensity aliasing patterns.

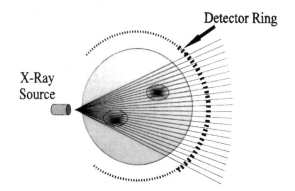

FIGURE 13.8 A series of beams is projected from a single source in a fan-like pattern. The beams fall upon a number of detectors arranged in a ring around the patient. Fan beams typically range between 30 to 60 deg. In the most recent CT scanners (so-called *fourth-generation* machines) the detectors completely encircle the patient, and the source can rotate continuously.

Inverse Radon Transform: Parallel Beam Geometry

MATLAB's inverse Radon transform is based on filtered back-projection and uses the frequency domain approach illustrated in Figure 13.6. A variety of filtering options are available and are implemented directly in the frequency domain.

The calling structure of the inverse Radon transform is:

```
[I,f] = iradon(p,theta,interp,filter,d,n);
```

where **p** is the only required input argument and is a matrix where each column contains one projection profile. The angle of the projection profiles is specified by **theta** in one of two ways: if **theta** is a scalar, it specifies the angular spacing (in degs.) between projection profiles (with an assumed range of zero to number of columns − 1); if **theta** is a vector, it specifies the angles themselves, which must be evenly spaced. The default **theta** is 180 deg. divided by the number of columns. During reconstruction, **iradon** assumes that the center of rotation is half the number of rows (i.e., the midpoint of the projection profile: **ceil(size (p,1)/2)**).

The optional argument **interp** is a string specifying the back-projection interpolation method: `'nearest'`, `'linear'` (the default), and `'spline'`. The filter option is also specified as a string. The 'Ram-Lak' option is the default and consists of a ramp in frequency (i.e., an ideal derivative) up to some maximum frequency (Figure 13.4 (on p. 382)). Since this filter is prone to high-frequency noise, other options multiply the ramp function by a lowpass function. These lowpass functions are the same as described above: Hamming window ('Hamming'), Hanning window ('Hann'), cosine ('cosine'), and sinc ('Shepp-Logan') function. Frequency plots of several of these filters are shown in Figure 13.4. The filter's frequency characteristics can be modified by the optional parameter, d, which scales the frequency axis: if d is less than one (the default value is one) then filter transfer function values above d, in normalized frequency, are set to 0. Hence, decreasing d increases the lowpass filter effect. The optional input argument, n, can be reused to rescale the image. These filter options are explored in several of the problems.

The image is contained in the output matrix I (class double), and the optional output vector, h, contains the filter's frequency response. (This output vector was used to generate the filter frequency curves of Figure 13.4.) An application of the inverse Radon transform is given in Example 13.1.

Example 13.1 Example of the use of back-projection and filtered back-projection. After a simple image of a white square against a dark background is generated, the CT projections are constructed using the forward Radon transform. The original image is reconstructed from these projections using both the filtered and unfiltered back-projection algorithm. The original image, the projections, and the two reconstructed images are displayed in Figure 13.5 on page 385.

```
% Example 13.1 and Figure 13.4.
% Image Reconstruction using back-projection and filtered
%   back-projection.
% Uses MATLAB's 'iradon' for filtered back-projection and
%   'i_back' for unfiltered back-projection.
%   (This routine is a version of 'iradon' modified to eliminate
%   the filter.)
% Construct a simple image consisting of a white square against
%   a black background. Then apply back-projection without
%   filtering and with the derivative (Ram-Lak) filters.
% Display the original and reconstructed images along with the
%   projections.
%
clear all; close all;
%
I = zeros(128,128);          % Construct image: black
I(44:84,44:84) = 1;          %   background with a central
                             %   white square
```

```
%
% Generate the projections using 'radon'
theta = (1:180);              % Angle between projections
                              %  is 1 deg.

[p,xp] = radon(I, theta);
%
% Now reconstruct the image
I_back = i_back(p,delta_theta);  % Back-projection alone
I_back = mat2gray(I_back);       % Convert to grayscale
I_filter_back = iradon           % Filtered back-projection
  (p,delta_theta);
%
.......Display images.......
```

The display generated by this code is given in Figure 13.4. Example 13.2 explores the effect of filtering on the reconstructed images.

Example 13.2 The inverse Radon transform filters. Generate CT data by applying the Radon transform to an MRI image of the brain (an unusual example of mixed modalities!). Reconstruct the image using the inverse Radon transform with the Ram-Lak (derivative) filter and the cosine filter with a maximum relative frequency of 0.4. Display the original and reconstructed images.

```
% Example 13.2 and Figure 13.9 Image Reconstruction using
%  filtered back-projection
% Uses MATLAB's 'iradon' for filtered backprojection
% Load a frame of the MRI image (mri.tif) and construct the CT
%  projections using 'radon'. Then apply backprojection with
%  two different filters: Ram-Lak and cosine (with 0.4 as
%  highest frequency
%
clear all; close all;
frame = 18;                   % Use MR image slice 18
[I(:,:,:,1), map ] = imread('mri.tif',frame);
if isempty(map) == 0          % Check to see if Indexed data
    I = ind2gray(I,map);      % If so, convert to Intensity
                              %  image
end
I = im2double(I);             % Convert to double and scale
%
% Construct projections of MR image
delta_theta = (1:180);

[p,xp] = radon(I,delta_theta);  % Angle between projections
                                %  is 1 deg.
```

```
%
% Reconstruct image using Ram-Lak filter
I_RamLak = iradon(p,delta_theta,'Ram-Lak');
%
.......Display images.......
```

Radon and Inverse Radon Transform: Fan Beam Geometry

The MATLAB routines for performing the Radon and inverse Radon transform using fan beam geometry are termed `fanbeam` and `ifanbeam`, respectively, and have the form:

```
fan = fanbeam(I,D)
```

where `I` is the input image and `D` is a scalar that specifies the distance between the beam vertex and the center of rotation of the beams. The output, `fan`, is a matrix containing the fan bean projection profiles, where each column contains the sensor samples at one rotation angle. It is assumed that the sensors have a one-deg. spacing and the rotation angles are spaced equally over 0 to 359 deg. A number of optional input variables specify different geometries, sensor spacing, and rotation increments.

The inverse Radon transform for fan beam projections is specified as:

```
I = ifanbeam(fan,D)
```

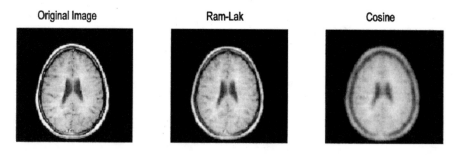

FIGURE 13.9 Original MR image and reconstructed images using the inverse Radon transform with the Ram-Lak derivative and the cosine filter. The cosine filter's lowpass cutoff has been modified by setting its maximum relative frequency to 0.4. The Ram-Lak reconstruction is not as sharp as the original image and sharpness is reduced further by the cosine filter with its lowered bandwidth. (Original image from the MATLAB Image Processing Toolbox. Copyright 1993–2003, The Math Works, Inc. Reprinted with permission.)

where `fan` is the matrix of projections and `D` is the distance between beam vertex and the center of rotation. The output, `I`, is the reconstructed image. Again there are a number of optional input arguments specifying the same type of information as in `fanbeam`. This routine first converts the fan beam geometry into a parallel geometry, then applies filtered back-projection as in `iradon`. During the filtered back-projection stage, it is possible to specify filter options as in `iradon`. To specify, the string `'Filter'` should precede the filter name (`'Hamming'`, `'Hann'`, `'cosine'`, etc.).

Example 13.3   Fan beam geometry. Apply the fan beam and parallel beam Radon transform to the simple square shown in Figure 13.4. Reconstruct the image using the inverse Radon transform for both geometries.

```
% Example 13.3 and Figure 13.10
% Example of reconstruction using the Fan Beam Geometry
% Reconstructs a pattern of 4 square of different intensities
%   using parallel beam and fan beam approaches.
%
clear all; close all;
D = 150;                        % Distance between fan beam vertex
                                %   and center of rotation
theta = (1:180);                % Angle between parallel
                                %   projections is 1 deg.
%
I = zeros(128,128);             % Generate image
I(22:54,22:52) = .25;           % Four squares of different shades
I(76;106,22:52) = .5;           %   against a black background
I(22:52,76:106) = .75;
I(76:106,76:106) = 1;
%
% Construct projections: Fan and parallel beam
[F,Floc,Fangles] = fanbeam (I,D,'FanSensorSpacing',.5);
[R,xp] = radon(I,theta);
%
% Reconstruct images. Use Shepp-Logan filter
I_rfb = ifanbeam(F,D,'FanSensorSpacing',.5,'Filter', ...
  'Shepp-Logan');
I_filter_back = iradon(R,theta,'Shepp-Logan');
%
% Display images
subplot(1,2,1);
  imshow(I_rfb); title('Fan Beam')
subplot(1,2,2);
  imshow(I_filter_back); title('Parallel Beam')
```

The images generated by this example are shown in Figure 13.10. There are small artifacts due to the distance between the beam source and the center of rotation. The affect of this distance is explored in one of the problems.

MAGNETIC RESONANCE IMAGING

Basic Principles

MRI images can be acquired in a number of ways using different image acquisition protocols. One of the more common protocols, the *spin echo pulse sequence*, will be described with the understanding that a fair number of alternatives are commonly used. In this sequence, the image is constructed on a slice-by-slice basis, although the data are obtained on a line-by-line basis. For each slice, the raw MRI data encode the image as a variation in signal frequency in one dimension, and in signal phase in the other. To reconstruct the image only requires the application of a two-dimensional inverse Fourier transform to this frequency/phase encoded data. If desired, spatial filtering can be implemented in the frequency domain before applying the inverse Fourier transform.

The physics underlying MRI is involved and requires quantum mechanics for a complete description. However, most descriptions are approximations that use classical mechanics. The description provided here will be even more abbreviated than most. (For a detailed classical description of the MRI physics see Wright's chapter in Enderle et al., 2000.). Nuclear magnetism occurs in nuclei with an odd number of nucleons (protons and/or neutrons). In the presence of a magnetic field such nuclei possess a magnetic dipole due to a quantum mechani-

Fan Beam   Parallel Beam

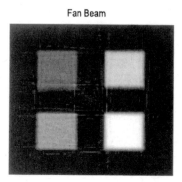 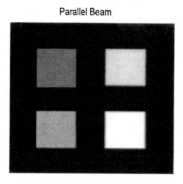

FIGURE 13.10 Reconstruction of an image of four squares at different intensities using parallel beam and fan beam geometry. Some artifact is seen in the fan beam geometry due to the distance between the beam source and object (see Problem 3).

cal property known as spin.* In MRI lingo, the nucleus and/or the associated magnetic dipole is termed a *spin*. For clinical imaging, the hydrogen proton is used because it occurs in large numbers in biological tissue. Although there are a large number of hydrogen protons, or spins, in biological tissue (1 mm^3 of water contains 6.7×10^{19} protons), the net magnetic moment that can be produced, even if they were all aligned, is small due to the near balance between spin-up (½) and spin-down (−½) states. When they are placed in a magnetic field, the magnetic dipoles are not static, but rotate around the axis of the applied magnetic field like spinning tops, Figure 13.11A (hence, the spins themselves spin). A group of these spins produces a net moment in the direction of the magnetic field, z, but since they are not in phase, any horizontal moment in the x and y direction tends to cancel (Figure 13.11B).

While the various spins do not have the same relative phase, they do all rotate at the same frequency, a frequency given by the *Larmor equation*:

$$\omega_o = \gamma H \tag{11}$$

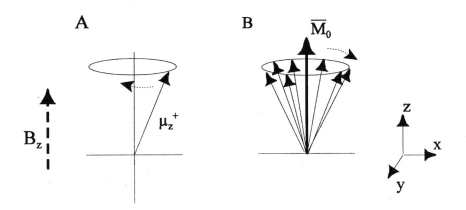

FIGURE 13.11 (A) A single proton has a magnetic moment which rotates in the presence of an applied magnet field, B_z. This dipole moment could be up or down with a slight favoritism towards up, as shown. (B) A group of upward dipoles create a net moment in the same direction as the magnetic field, but any horizontal moments (x or y) tend to cancel. Note that all of these dipole vectors should be rotating, but for obvious reasons they are shown as stationary with the assumption that they rotate, or more rigorously, that the coordinate system is rotating.

---

*Nuclear spin is not really a spin, but another one of those mysterious quantum mechanical properties. Nuclear spin can take on values of ±1/2, with +1/2 slightly favored in a magnetic field.

where ω_0 is the frequency in radians, H is the magnitude of the magnitude field, and γ is a constant termed the *gyromagnetic constant*. Although γ is primarily a function of the type of nucleus it also depends slightly on the local chemical environment. As shown below, this equation contains the key to spatial localization in MRI: variations in local magnetic field will encode as variations in rotational frequency of the protons.

If these rotating spins are exposed to electromagnetic energy at the rotational or *Larmor frequency* specified in Eq. (11), they will absorb this energy and rotate further and further from their equilibrium position near the z axis: they are *tipped* away from the z axis (Figure 13.12A). They will also be synchronized by this energy, so that they now have a net horizontal moment. For protons, the Larmor frequency is in the radio frequency (rf) range, so an rf pulse of the appropriate frequency in the xy-plane will tip the spins away from the z-axis an amount that depends on the length of the pulse:

$$\theta = \gamma H T_p \tag{12}$$

where θ is the *tip angle* and T_p pulse time. Usually T_p is adjusted to tip the angle either 90 or 180 deg. As described subsequently, a 90 deg. tip is used to generate the strongest possible signal and an 180 deg tip, which changes the sign of the

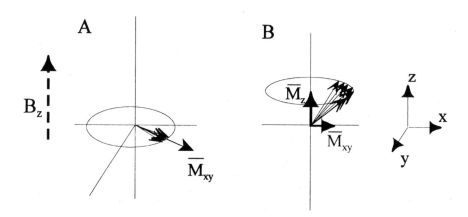

FIGURE 13.12 (A) After an rf pulse that tips the spins 90 deg., the net magnetic moment looks like a vector, M_{xy}, rotating in the xy-plane. The net vector in the z direction is zero. (B) After the rf energy is removed, all of the spins begin to relax back to their equilibrium position, increasing the z component, M_z, and decreasing the xy component, M_{xy}. The xy component also decreases as the spins desynchronize.

moment, is used to generate an *echo* signal. Note that a given 90 or 180 deg. T_p will only flip those spins that are exposed to the appropriate local magnetic field, H.

When all of the spins in a region are tipped 90 deg. and synchronized, there will be a net magnetic moment rotating in the xy-plane, but the component of the moment in the z direction will be zero (Figure 13.12A). When the rf pulse ends, the rotating magnetic field will generate its own rf signal, also at the Larmor frequency. This signal is known as the *free induction decay* (FID) signal. It is this signal that induces a small voltage in the receiver coil, and it is this signal that is used to construct the MR image. Immediately after the pulse ends, the signal generated is given by:

$$S(t) = \rho \sin(\theta) \cos(\omega_o t) \tag{13}$$

where ω_o is the Larmor frequency, θ is the tip angle, and ρ is the density of spins. Note that a tip angle of 90 deg. produces the strongest signal.

Over time the spins will tend to relax towards the equilibrium position (Figure 13.12B). This relaxation is known as the *longitudinal* or *spin-lattice* relaxation time and is approximately exponential with a time constant denoted as "T_1." As seen in Figure 13.12B, it has the effect of increasing the horizontal moment, M_z, and decreasing the xy moment, M_{xy}. The xy moment is decreased even further, and much faster, by a loss of synchronization of the collective spins, since they are all exposed to a slightly different magnetic environment from neighboring atoms (Figure 13.12B). This so-called *transverse* or *spin-spin* relaxation time is also exponential and decays with a time constant termed "T_2." The spin-spin relaxation time is always less than the spin lattice relaxation time, so that by the time the net moment returns to equilibrium position along the z axis the individual spins are completely de-phased. Local inhomogeneities in the applied magnetic field cause an even faster de-phasing of the spins. When the de-phasing time constant is modified to include this effect, it is termed T_2^* (pronounced *tee two star*). This time constant also includes the T_2 influences. When these relaxation processes are included, the equation for the FID signals becomes:

$$S(t) = \rho \cos(\omega_o t) \, e^{-t/T_2^*} \, e^{-t/T_1} \tag{14}$$

While frequency dependence (i.e., the Larmor equation) is used to achieve localization, the various relation times as well as proton density are used to achieve image contrast. Proton density, ρ, for any given collection of spins is a relatively straightforward measurement: it is proportional to FID signal amplitude as shown in Eq. (14). Measuring the local T_1 and T_2 (or T_2^*) relaxation times is more complicated and is done through clever manipulations of the rf pulse and local magnetic field gradients, as briefly described in the next section.

Data Acquisition: Pulse Sequences

A combination of rf pulses, magnetic gradient pulses, delays, and data acquisition periods is termed a *pulse sequence*. One of the clever manipulations used in many pulse sequences is the *spin echo* technique, a trick for eliminating the de-phasing caused by local magnetic field inhomogeneities and related artifacts (the T_2^* decay). One possibility might be to sample immediately after the rf pulse ends, but this is not practical. The alternative is to sample a realigned echo. After the spins have begun to spread out, if their direction is suddenly reversed they will come together again after a known delay. The classic example is that of a group of runners who are told to reverse direction at the same time, say one minute after the start. In principal, they all should get back to the start line at the same time (one minute after reversing) since the fastest runners will have the farthest to go at the time of reversal. In MRI, the reversal is accomplished by a phase-reversing 180 rf pulse. The realignment will occur with the same time constant, T_2^*, as the misalignment. This echo approach will only cancel the de-phasing due to magnetic inhomogeneities, not the variations due to the sample itself: i.e., those that produce the T_2 relaxation. That is actually desirable because the sample variations that cause T_2 relaxation are often of interest.

As mentioned above, the Larmor equation (Eq. (11)) is the key to localization. If each position in the sample is subjected to a different magnetic field strength, then the locations are tagged by their resonant frequencies. Two approaches could be used to identify the signal from a particular region. Use an rf pulse with only one frequency component, and if each location has a unique magnetic field strength then only the spins in one region will be excited, those whose magnetic field correlates with the rf frequency (by the Larmor equation). Alternatively excite a broader region, then vary the magnetic field strength so that different regions are given different resonant frequencies. In clinical MRI, both approaches are used.

Magnetic field strength is varied by the application of gradient fields applied by electromagnets, so-called *gradient coils*, in the three dimensions. The gradient fields provide a linear change in magnetic field strength over a limited area within the MR imager. The gradient field in the z direction, G_z, can be used to isolate a specific xy slice in the object, a process known as *slice selection*.* In the absence of any other gradients, the application of a linear gradient in the z direction will mean that only the spins in one xy-plane will have a resonant frequency that matches a specific rf pulse frequency. Hence, by adjusting the

---

*Selected slices can be in any plane, x, y, z, or any combination, by appropriate activation of the gradients during the rf pulse. For simplicity, this discussion assumes the slice is selected by the z-gradient so spins in an xy-plane are excited.

gradient, different *xy*-slices will be associated with (by the Larmor equation), and excited by, a specific rf frequency. Since the rf pulse is of finite duration it cannot consist of a single frequency, but rather has a range of frequencies, i.e., a finite bandwidth. The thickness of the slice, that is, the region in the *z*-direction over which the spins are excited, will depend on the steepness of the gradient field and the bandwidth of the rf pulse:

$$\Delta z \propto \gamma G_z z(\Delta \omega) \tag{15}$$

Very thin slices, Δz, would require a very narrowband pulse, $\Delta \omega$, in combination with a steep gradient field, G_z.

If all three gradients, G_x, G_y, and G_z, were activated prior to the rf pulse then only the spins in one unique volume would be excited. However, only one data point would be acquired for each pulse repetition, and to acquire a large volume would be quite time-consuming. Other strategies allow the acquisition of entire lines, planes, or even volumes with one pulse excitation. One popular pulse sequence, the spin-echo pulse sequence, acquires one line of data in the spatial frequency domain. The sequence begins with a shaped rf pulse in conjunction with a G_z pulse that provides slice selection (Figure 13.13). The G_z includes a reversal at the end to cancel a *z*-dependent phase shift. Next, a *y*-gradient pulse of a given amplitude is used to phase encode the data. This is followed by a second rf/G_z combination to produce the echo. As the echo regroups the spins, an *x*-gradient pulse frequency encodes the signal. The reformed signal constitutes one line in the ferquency domain (termed *k-space* in MRI), and is sampled over this period. Since the echo signal duration is several hundred microseconds, high-speed data acquisition is necessary to sample up to 256 points during this signal period.

As with slice thickness, the ultimate pixel size will depend on the strength of the magnetic gradients. Pixel size is directly related to the number of pixels in the reconstructed image and the actual size of the imaged area, the so-called *field-of-view* (FOV). Most modern imagers are capable of a 2 cm FOV with samples up to 256 by 256 pixels, giving a pixel size of 0.078 mm. In practice, image resolution is usually limited by signal-to-noise considerations since, as pixel area decreases, the number of spins available to generate a signal diminishes proportionately. In some circumstances special receiver coils can be used to increase the signal-to-noise ratio and improve image quality and/or resolution. Figure 13.14A shows an image of the *Shepp-Logan phantom* and the same image acquired with different levels of detector noise.* As with other forms of signal processing, MR image noise can be improved by averaging. Figure

---

*The Shepp-Logan phantom was developed to demonstrate the difficulty of identifying a tumor in a medical image.

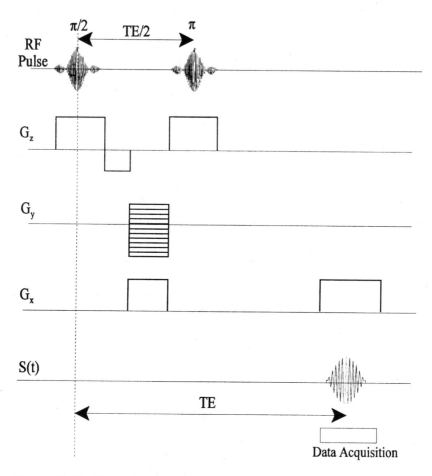

FIGURE 13.13 The spin-echo pulse sequence. Events are timed with respect to the initial rf pulse. See text for explanation.

13.14D shows the noise reduction resulting from averaging four of the images taken under the same noise conditions as Figure 13.14C. Unfortunately, this strategy increases scan time in direct proportion to the number of images averaged.

Functional Magnetic Resonance Imaging

Image processing for MR images is generally the same as that used on other images. In fact, MR images have been used in a number of examples and problems in previous chapters. One application of MRI does have some unique im-

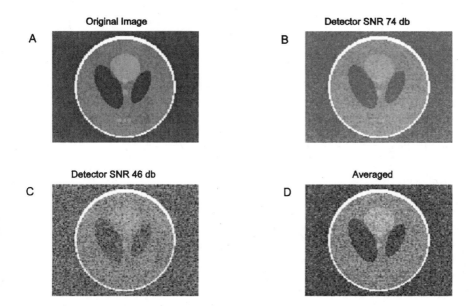

FIGURE 13.14 (A) MRI reconstruction of a Shepp-Logan phantom. (B) and (C) Reconstruction of the phantom with detector noise added to the frequency domain signal. (D) Frequency domain average of four images taken with noise similar to C. Improvement in the image is apparent. (Original image from the MATLAB Image Processing Toolbox. Copyright 1993–2003, The Math Works, Inc. Reprinted with permission.)

age processing requirements: the area of functional magnetic resonance imaging (fMRI). In this approach, neural areas that are active in specific tasks are identified by increases in local blood flow. MRI can detect cerebral blood changes using an approach known as *BOLD*: blood oxygenation level dependent. Special pulse sequences have been developed that can acquire images very quickly, and these images are sensitive to the BOLD phenomenon. However, the effect is very small: changes in signal level are only a few percent.

During a typical fMRI experiment, the subject is given a task which is either physical (such a finger tapping), purely sensory (such as a flashing visual stimulus), purely mental (such as performing mathematical calculations), or involves sensorimotor activity (such as pushing a button whenever a given image appears). In single-task protocols, the task alternates with non-task or baseline activity period. Task periods are usually 20–30 seconds long, but can be shorter and can even be single events under certain protocols. Multiple task protocols are possible and increasingly popular. During each task a number of MR images are acquired. The primary role of the analysis software is to identify pixels that have some relationship to the task/non-task activity.

There are a number of software packages available that perform fMRI analysis, some written in MATLAB such as *SPM*, (statistical parametric mapping), others in c-language such as *AFNI* (analysis of neural images). Some packages can be obtained at no charge off the Web. In addition to identifying the active pixels, these packages perform various preprocessing functions such as aligning the sequential images and reshaping the images to conform to standard models of the brain.

Following preprocessing, there are a number of different approaches to identifying regions where local blood flow correlates with the task/non-task timing. One approach is simply to use correlation, that is correlate the change in signal level, on a pixel-by-pixel basis, with a task-related function. This function could represent the task by a one and the non-task by a zero, producing a square wave-like function. More complicated task functions account for the dynamics of the BOLD process which has a 4 to 6 second time constant. Finally, some new approaches based on independent component analysis (ICA, Chapter 9) can be used to extract the task function from the data itself. The use of correlation and ICA analysis is explored in the MATLAB Implementation section and in the problems. Other univariate statistical techniques are common such as *t*-tests and *f*-tests, particularly in the multi-task protocols (Friston, 2002).

MATLAB Implementation

Techniques for fMRI analysis can be implemented using standard MATLAB routines. The identification of active pixels using correlation with a task protocol function will be presented in Example 13.4. Several files have been created on the disk that simulate regions of activity in the brain. The variations in pixel intensity are small, and noise and other artifacts have been added to the image data, as would be the case with real data. The analysis presented here is done on each pixel independently. In most fMRI analyses, the identification procedure might require activity in a number of adjoining pixels for identification. Lowpass filtering can also be used to smooth the image.

Example 13.4 Use correlation to identify potentially active areas from MRI images of the brain. In this experiment, 24 frames were taken (typical fMRI experiments would contain at least twice that number): the first 6 frames were acquired during baseline activity and the next 6 during the task. This off-on cycle was then repeated for the next 12 frames. Load the image in MATLAB file `fmri1`, which contains all 24 frames. Generate a function that represents the off-on task protocol and correlate this function with each pixel's variation over the 24 frames. Identify pixels that have correlation above a given threshold and mark the image where these pixels occur. (Usually this would be done in color with higher correlations given brighter color.) Finally display the time sequence of one of the active pixels. (Most fMRI analysis packages can display the time variation of pixels or regions, usually selected interactively.)

```
% Example 13.4 Example of identification of active area
%   using correlation.
% Load the 24 frames of the image stored in fmri1.mat.
% Construct a stimulus profile.
% In this fMRI experiment the first 6 frames were taken during
%   no-task conditions, the next six frames during the task
%   condition, and this cycle was repeated.
% Correlate each pixel's variation over the 24 frames with the
%   task profile. Pixels that correlate above a certain threshold
%   (use 0.5) should be identified in the image by a pixel
%   whose intensity is the same as the correlation values
%
clear all; close all
thresh = .5;                    % Correlation threshold
load fmri1;                     % Get data
i_stim2 = ones(24,1);           % Construct task profile
i_stim2(1:6) = 0;               % First 6 frames are no-task
i_stim2(13:18) = 0;             % Frames 13 through 18
                                %   are also no-task
%
% Do correlation: pixel by pixel over the 24 frames
I_fmri_marked = I_fmri;
active = [0 0];
for i = 1:128
  for j = 1:128
    for k = 1:24
      temp(k) = I_fmri(i,j,1,k);
    end
    cor_temp = corrcoef([temp'i_stim2]);
    corr(i,j) = cor_temp(2,1); % Get correlation value
    if corr(i,j) > thresh
      I_fmri_marked(i,j,:,1) = I_fmri(i,j,:,1) + corr(i,j);
      active = [active; i,j];    % Save supra-threshold
                                 %   locations
    end
  end
end
%
% Display marked image
imshow(I_fmri_marked(:,:,:,1)); title('fMRI Image');
figure;
% Display one of the active areas
for i = 1:24       % Plot one of the active areas
```

```
active_neuron(i)  =  I_fmri(active(2,1),active(2,2),:,i);
end
plot(active_neuron); title('Active neuron');
```

The marked image produced by this program is shown in Figure 13.15. The actual active area is the rectangular area on the right side of the image slightly above the centerline. However, a number of other error pixels are present due to noise that happens to have a sufficiently high correlation with the task profile (a correlation of 0.5 in this case). In Figure 13.16, the correlation threshold has been increased to 0.7 and most of the error pixels have been

Correlation 0.5

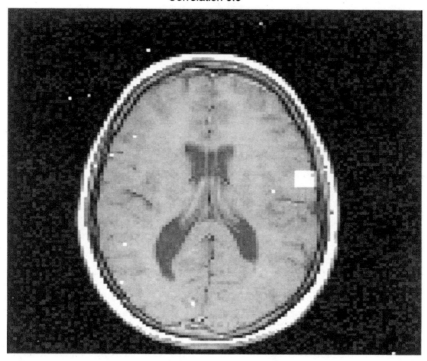

FIGURE 13.15 White pixels were identified as active based on correlation with the task profile. The actual active area is the rectangle on the right side slightly above the center line. Due to inherent noise, false pixels are also identified, some even outside of the brain. The correlation threshold was set a 0.5 for this image. (Original image from the MATLAB Image Processing Toolbox. Copyright 1993–2003, The Math Works, Inc. Reprinted with permission.)

Correlation 0.7

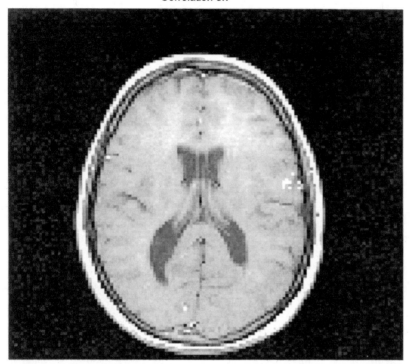

FIGURE 13.16 The same image as in Figure 13.15 with a higher correlation threshold (0.7). Fewer errors are seen, but the active area is only partially identified.

eliminated, but now the active region is only partially identified. An intermediate threshold might result in a better compromise, and this is explored in one of the problems.

Functional MRI software packages allow isolation of specific *regions of interest* (ROI), usually though interactive graphics. Pixel values in these regions of interest can be plotted over time and subsequent processing can be done on the isolated region. Figure 13.17 shows the variation over time (actually, over the number of frames) of one of the active pixels. Note the very approximate correlation with the square wave-like task profile also shown. The poor correlation is due to noise and other artifacts, and is fairly typical of fMRI data. Identifying the very small signal within the background noise is the one of the major challenges for fMRI image processing algorithms.

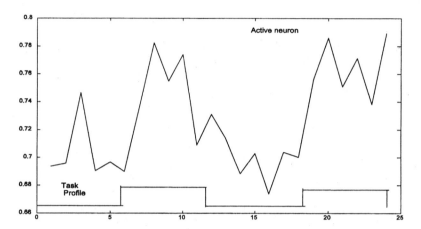

FIGURE 13.17 Variation in intensity of a single pixel within the active area of Figures 13.15 and 13.16. A correlation with the task profile is seen, but considerable noise is also present.

Principal Component and Independent Component Analysis

In the above analysis, active pixels were identified by correlation with the task profile. However, the neuronal response would not be expected to follow the task temporal pattern exactly because of the dynamics of the blood flow response (i.e., blood *hemodynamics*) which requires around 4 to 6 seconds to reach its peak. In addition, there may be other processes at work that systematically affect either neural activity or pixel intensity. For example, respiration can alter pixel intensity in a consistent manner. Identifying the actual dynamics of the fMRI process and any consistent artifacts might be possible by a direct analysis of the data. One approach would be to search for components related to blood flow dynamics or artifacts using either principal component analysis (PCA) or independent component analysis (ICA).

Regions of interest are first identified using either standard correlation or other statistical methods so that the new tools need not be applied to the entire image. Then the isolated data from each frame is re-formatted so that it is one-dimensional by stringing the image rows, or columns, together. The data from each frame are now arranged as a single vector. ICA or PCA is applied to the transposed ensemble of frame vectors so that each pixel is treated as a different source and each frame is an observation of that source. If there are pixels whose intensity varies in a non-random manner, this should produce one or more components in the analyses. The component that is most like the task profile can then be used as a more accurate estimate of blood flow hemodynamics in the correlation analysis: the isolated component is used for the comparison instead of the task profile. An example of this approach is given in Example 13.5.

Example 13.5 Select a region of interest from the data of Figure 13.16, specifically an area that surrounds and includes the potentially active pixels. Normally this area would be selected interactively by an operator. Reformat the images so that each frame is a single row vector and constitutes one row of an ensemble composed of the different frames. Perform both an ICA and PCA analysis and plot the resulting components.

```
% Example 13.5 and Figure 13.18 and 13.19
% Example of the use of PCA and ICA to identify signal
%   and artifact components in a region of interest
%   containing some active neurons.
% Load the region of interest then re-format to a images so that
%   each of the 24 frames is a row then transpose this ensemble
%   so that the rows are pixels and the columns are frames.
% Apply PCA and ICA analysis. Plot the first four principal
%   components and the first two independent components.
%
close all; clear all;
nu_comp = 2;
% Number of independent components
load roi2;                    % Get ROI data
% Find number of frames %
[r c dummy frames] = size(ROI);
% Convert each image frame to a column and construct an
%   ensemble were each column is a different frame
%
for i = 1:frames
  for j = 1:r
    row = ROI(j,:,:,i);    % Convert frame to a row
    if j == 1
      temp = row;
    else
      temp = [temp row];
    end
  end
  if i == 1
    data = temp;                % Concatenate rows
  else
    data = [data;temp];
  end
end
%
% Now apply PCA analysis
[U,S,pc]= svd(data',0);  % Use singular value decomposition
eigen = diag(S).^2;
for i = 1:length(eigen)
```

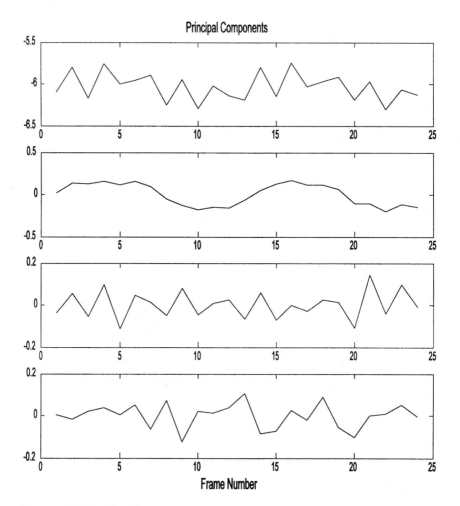

FIGURE 13.18 First four components from a principal component analysis applied to a region of interest in Figure 13.15 that includes the active area. A function similar to the task is seen in the second component. The third component also has a possible repetitive structure that could be related to respiration.

```
    pc(:,i) = pc(:,i) * sqrt(eigen(i));
end
%
% Determine the independent components
w = jadeR(data',nu_comp);
ica = (w* data');
```

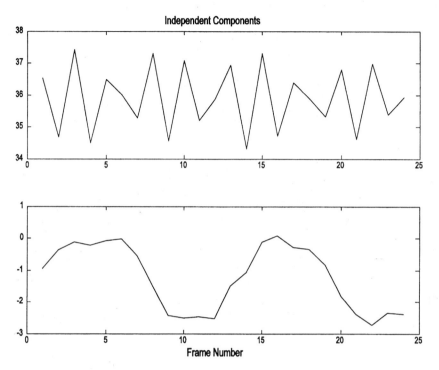

FIGURE 13.19 Two components found by independent component analysis. The task-related function and the respiration artifact are now clearly identified.

```
%
.......Display components.......
```

The principal components produced by this analysis are shown in Figure 13.18. A waveform similar to the task profile is seen in the second plot down. Since this waveform derived from the data, it should more closely represent the actual blood flow hemodynamics. The third waveform shows a regular pattern, possibly due to respiration artifact. The other two components may also contain some of that artifact, but do not show any other obvious pattern.

The two patterns in the data are better separated by ICA. Figure 13.19 shows the first two independent components and both the blood flow hemodynamics and the artifact are clearly shown. The former can be used instead of the task profile in the correlation analysis. The results of using the profile obtained through ICA are shown in Figure 13.20A and B. Both activity maps were obtained from the same data using the same correlation threshold. In Figure 13.20A, the task profile function was used, while in Figure 13.20B the hemody-

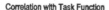

Correlation with Task Function

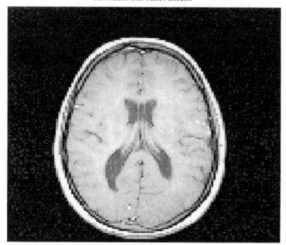

FIGURE 13.20A   Activity map obtained by correlating pixels with the square-wave task function. The correlation threshold was 0.55. (Original image from the MATLAB Image Processing Toolbox. Copyright 1993–2003, The Math Works, Inc. Reprinted with permission.)

Correlation with Profile from Example 13-5

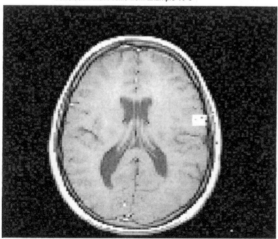

FIGURE 13.20B   Activity map obtained by correlating pixels with the estimated hemodynamic profile obtained from ICA. The correlation threshold was 0.55.

namic profile (the function in the lower plot of Figure 13.19) was used in the correlation. The improvement in identification is apparent. When the task function is used, very few of the areas actually active are identified and a number of error pixels are identified. Figure 13.20B contains about the same number of errors, but all of the active areas are identified. Of course, the number of active areas identified using the task profile could be improved by lowering the threshold of correlation, but this would also increase the errors.

PROBLEMS

1.   Load slice 13 of the MR image used in Example 13.3 (`mri.tif`). Construct parallel beam projections of this image using the Radon transform with two different angular spacings between rotations: 5 deg. and 10 deg. In addition, reduce spacing of the 5 deg. data by a factor of two. Reconstruct the three images (5 deg. unreduced, 5 deg. reduced, and 10 deg.) and display along with the original image. Multiply the images by a factor of 10 to enhance any variations in the background.

2.   The data file `data_prob_13_2` contains projections of the test pattern image, `testpat1.png` with noise added. Reconstruct the image using the inverse Radon transform with two filter options: the `Ram-Lak` filter (the default), and the `Hamming` filter with a maximum frequency of 0.5.

3.   Load the image `squares.tif`. Use `fanbeam` to construct fan beam projections and `ifanbeam` to produce the reconstructed image. Repeat for two different beam distances: 100 and 300 (pixels). Plot the reconstructed images. Use a `FanSensorSpacing` of 1.

4.   The rf-pulse used in MRI is a *shaped pulse* consisting of a sinusoid at the base frequency that is amplitude modulated by some pulse shaping waveform. The sinc waveform $(\sin(x)/x)$ is commonly used. Construct a shaped pulse consisting of $\cos(\omega_2)$ modulated by $\mathrm{sinc}(\omega_2)$. Pulse duration should be such that ω_2 ranges between $\pm\pi$: $-2\pi \le \omega_2 \le 2\pi$. The sinusoidal frequency, ω_1, should be 10 ω_2. Use the inverse Fourier transform to plot the magnitude frequency spectrum of this slice selection pulse. (*Note*: the MATLAB `sinc` function is normalized to π, so the range of the vector input to this function should be ± 2. In this case, the `cos` function will need to multiplied by 2π, as well as by 10.)

5.   Load the 24 frames of image `fmri3.mat`. This contains the 4-D variable, `I_fmri`, which has 24 frames. Construct a stimulus profile. Assume the same task profile as in Example 13.4: the first 6 frames were taken during no-task conditions, the next six frames during the task condition, then the cycle was repeated. Rearrange Example 13.4 so that the correlations coefficients are computed first, then the thresholds are applied (so each new threshold value does not

require another calculation of correlation coefficients). Search for the optimal threshold. Note these images contain more noise than those used in Example 13.4, so even the best thresholded will contain error pixels.

6.   Example of identification of active area using correlation. Repeat Problem 6 except filter the matrix containing the pixel correlations before applying the threshold. Use a 4 by 4 averaging filter. (**fspecial** can be helpful here.)

7.   Example of using principal component analysis and independent component analysis to identify signal and artifact. Load the region of interest file **roi4.mat** which contains variable ROI. This variable contains 24 frames of a small region around the active area of **fmri3.mat**. Reformat to a matrix as in Example 13.5 and apply PCA and ICA analysis. Plot the first four principal components and the first two independent components. Note the very slow time constant of the blood flow hemodynamics.

Annotated Bibliography

The following is a very selective list of books or articles that will be of value of in providing greater depth and mathematical rigor to the material presented in this text. Comments regarding the particular strengths of the reference are included.

Akansu, A. N. and Haddad, R. A., *Multiresolution Signal Decomposition: Transforms, subbands, wavelets*. Academic Press, San Diego CA, 1992. A modern classic that presents, among other things, some of the underlying theoretical aspects of wavelet analysis.

Aldroubi A and Unser, M. (eds) *Wavelets in Medicine and Biology*, CRC Press, Boca Raton, FL, 1996. Presents a variety of applications of wavelet analysis to biomedical engineering.

Boashash, B. *Time-Frequency Signal Analysis*, Longman Cheshire Pty Ltd., 1992. Early chapters provide a very useful introduction to time–frequency analysis followed by a number of medical applications.

Boashash, B. and Black, P.J. An efficient real-time implementation of the Wigner-Ville Distribution, *IEEE Trans. Acoust. Speech Sig. Proc.* ASSP-35:1611–1618, 1987. Practical information on calculating the Wigner-Ville distribution.

Boudreaux-Bartels, G. F. and Murry, R. Time-frequency signal representations for biomedical signals. In: *The Biomedical Engineering Handbook*. J. Bronzino (ed.) CRC Press, Boca Raton, Florida and IEEE Press, Piscataway, N.J., 1995. This article presents an exhaustive, or very nearly so, compilation of Cohen's class of time-frequency distributions.

Bruce, E. N. *Biomedical Signal Processing and Signal Modeling*, John Wiley and Sons,

New York, 2001. Rigorous treatment with more of an emphasis on linear systems than signal processing. Introduces nonlinear concepts such as chaos.

Cichicki, A and Amari S. *Adaptive Bilnd Signal and Image Processing*: *Learning Algorithms and Applications*, John Wiley and Sons, Inc. New York, 2002. Rigorous, somewhat dense, treatment of a wide range of principal component and independent component approaches. Includes disk.

Cohen, L. Time-frequency distributions—A review. *Proc. IEEE* 77:941–981, 1989. Classic review article on the various time-frequency methods in Cohen's class of time–frequency distributions.

Ferrara, E. and Widrow, B. Fetal Electrocardiogram enhancement by time-sequenced adaptive filtering. *IEEE Trans. Biomed. Engr.* BME-29:458–459, 1982. Early application of adaptive noise cancellation to a biomedical engineering problem by one of the founders of the field. See also Widrow below.

Friston, K. Statistical Parametric Mapping On-line at: *http://www.fil.ion.ucl.ac.uk/spm/course/note02/* Through discussion of practical aspects of fMRI analysis including pre-processing, statistical methods, and experimental design. Based around SPM analysis software capabilities.

Haykin, S. *Adaptive Filter Theory* (2nd ed.), Prentice-Hall, Inc., Englewood Cliffs, N.J., 1991. The definitive text on adaptive filters including Weiner filters and gradient-based algorithms.

Hyvärinen, A. Karhunen, J. and Oja, E. *Independent Component Analysis*, John Wiley and Sons, Inc. New York, 2001. Fundamental, comprehensive, yet readable book on independent component analysis. Also provides a good review of principal component analysis.

Hubbard B.B. *The World According to Wavelets* (2nd ed.) A.K. Peters, Ltd. Natick, MA, 1998. Very readable introductory book on wavelengths including an excellent section on the foyer transformed. Can be read by a non-signal processing friend.

Ingle, V.K. and Proakis, J. G. *Digital Signal Processing with MATLAB*, Brooks/Cole, Inc. Pacific Grove, CA, 2000. Excellent treatment of classical signal processing methods including the Fourier transform and both FIR and IIR digital filters. Brief, but informative section on adaptive filtering.

Jackson, J. E. A User's Guide to Principal Components, John Wiley and Sons, New York, 1991. Classic book providing everything you ever want to know about principal component analysis. Also covers linear modeling and introduces factor analysis.

Johnson, D.D. Applied Multivariate Methods for Data Analysis, Brooks/Cole, Pacific Grove, CA, 1988. Careful, detailed coverage of multivariate methods including principal components analysis. Good coverage of discriminant analysis techniques.

Kak, A.C and Slaney M. *Principles of Computerized Tomographic Imaging*. IEEE Press, New York, 1988. Thorough, understandable treatment of algorithms for reconstruction of tomographic images including both parallel and fan-beam geometry. Also includes techniques used in reflection tomography as occurs in ultrasound imaging.

Marple, S.L. *Digital Spectral Analysis with Applications*, Prentice-Hall, Englewood Cliffs, NJ, 1987. Classic text on modern spectral analysis methods. In-depth, rigorous treatment of Fourier transform, parametric modeling methods (including AR and ARMA), and eigenanalysis-based techniques.

Rao, R.M. and Bopardikar, *A.S. Wavelet Transforms*: *Introduction to Theory and Appli-*

cations, Addison-Wesley, Inc., Reading, MA, 1998. Good development of wavelet analysis including both the continuous and discreet wavelet transforms.

Shiavi, R *Introduction to Applied Statistical Signal Analysis*, (2nd ed), Academic Press, San Diego, CA, 1999. Emphasizes spectral analysis of signals buried in noise. Excellent coverage of Fourier analysis, and autoregressive methods. Good introduction to statistical signal processing concepts.

Sonka, M., Hlavac V., and Boyle R. Image processing, analysis, and machine vision. Chapman and Hall Computing, London, 1993. A good description of edge-based and other segmentation methods.

Strang, G and Nguyen, T. *Wavelets and Filter Banks*, Wellesley-Cambridge Press, Wellesley, MA, 1997. Thorough coverage of wavelet filter banks including extensive mathematical background.

Stearns, S.D. and David, R.A *Signal Processing Algorithms in MATLAB*, Prentice Hall, Upper Saddle River, NJ, 1996. Good treatment of the classical Fourier transform and digital filters. Also covers the LMS adaptive filter algorithm. Disk enclosed.

Wickerhauser, M.V. *Adapted Wavelet Analysis from Theory to Software*, A.K. Peters, Ltd. and IEEE Press, Wellesley, MA, 1994. Rigorous, extensive treatment of wavelet analysis.

Widrow, B. Adaptive noise cancelling: Principles and applications. *Proc IEEE* 63:1692–1716, 1975. Classic original article on adaptive noise cancellation.

Wright S. Nuclear Magnetic Resonance and Magnetic Resonance Imaging. In: *Introduction to Biomedical Engineering* (Enderle, Blanchard and Bronzino, Eds.) Academic Press, San Diego, CA, 2000. Good mathematical development of the physics of MRI using classical concepts.

Index